AF789285

DRAINAGE DESIGN

Edited by

P. SMART

and

J.G. HERBERTSON

Department of Civil Engineering
University of Glasgow

Springer Science+Business Media, LLC

Originally published by Blackie and Son Ltd in 1992
First published 1992

16 15 14 13 12 10 9 8 7 6 5 4 3 2 1

British Library Cataloguing in Publication Data

Drainage design.
I. Smart, P. II. Herbertson, J.G.
627

ISBN 978-1-4757-5029-4 ISBN 978-1-4757-5027-0 (eBook)
DOI 10.1007/978-1-4757-5027-0

Library of Congress CIP data available

Preface

This book provides a review of the principles and methods of drainage with an emphasis on design. The whole field of drainage is covered, and although the book concentrates mainly on the practice in North America, Europe and Britain, the practice in developing countries is also included. The book is directed primarily at the graduate engineer entering professional practice, but will also provide a useful reference for more senior engineers and for those in adjunct professions.

Chapter 1 outlines the necessity for drainage on a large or small scale, for rural and urban areas. As the drainage engineer must decide how much unwanted water there will be and when it will occur, the chapter discusses climatic types, prediction of rainfall, evapotranspiration effects, return periods (of design storms and runoff events), river flow and flood prediction, and various sensing systems for providing short term predictions of rainfall, runoff, streamflow and flood warning. Chapter 2 gives a thorough review of the properties of soil in the context of drainage design. The extensive mathematical theories which relate to the crucial area of soil water movement are outlined and due attention is paid to the growing importance of predicting soil water movement in partially saturated soils. Chapter 3 tries to bridge the gap between agricultural and civil drainage engineers by outlining the types of schemes which the civil engineer may expect to encounter, as in many countries civil engineers are not responsible for, and therefore are ignorant of, agricultural field drainage practice: an area for which agricultural engineers and farmers are generally responsible. In addition, as the world's population rises so the pressure on the natural environment increases dramatically, and therefore a discussion of the purpose and design of small scale drainage schemes is provided. Chapter 4 concentrates on giving an informed account of the various practices which are being used to minimise and control soil erosion in tropical countries. Commonly engineers designing field drainage schemes are also responsible for providing irrigation water, but as this water contains dissolved salts the consequences of salt precipitation and accumulation need to be considered. Removal is often by flushing excess irrigation water through the soil, and examples of typical design calculations are given. Modern views of urban drainage are reviewed in chapter 5, and after examining the physical nature of the urban environment and the interactions between the various elements of the system, the chapter then discusses design methods. A special feature of this chapter is the thorough discussion of the modern computer models for prediction and forecasting which are used to design and evaluate urban drainage schemes.

Closely associated with urban drainage, but extending also to the rural and industrial environments, is pollution control. In industrial countries increasingly stringent regulations are being introduced to reduce the problem. Chapter 6 starts by discussing the various types of polluting agents and their effects on water, and follows with a brief review of current water quality standards and legislation. Practical methods for the control of discharge quality are outlined before discussing the powerful new mathematical techniques currently being used to predict pollutant behaviour in existing systems and in new systems. Chapter 7 discusses how drainage waters find their way into river systems, and how increasingly these systems are coming under pressure due to changes in climate, land use, and expanding populations. There is extensive discussion of how computer models predict the effects of such changes, and calculations extend from those for a single reach of river to the numerical representation of a complete river network. The chapter also discusses flow regimes affecting flood plains and ends with practical advice on flood alleviation and control.

Chapter 8 gives an overview of the various improvements which are constantly being made to river systems. The various types of watercourse are outlined, and this is followed by a discussion of modern examples of river control structures. As several recent bridge failures have been attributed to scour, a brief review covers both the phenomenon and control methods. Finally an exposition is provided of the various steps for designing river engineering works. Chapter 9 discusses pumped drainage, which is required when very low-lying rural and urban land has to be drained. This is an expensive method, and for these reasons pumped drainage schemes must be designed with great care. This chapter provides a step-by-step guide to the design of pumped drainage schemes, and explains the engineering decisions which need to be taken. The final two chapters—on deep drainage and dewatering—were written as a complementary pair. The chapter on deep drainage starts with a discussion of aquifer geology, the engineering properties of aquifers and a reminder of the modelling methods used, followed by an overview of the full spectrum of ground water flow regimes and ends with a discussion on the engineering aspects of deep drainage. The dewatering chapter firstly reviews methods for dewatering excavations by pumping and then discusses how to exclude ground water from excavations. Finally, control of ground water during embankment construction, and methods for permanent dewatering are outlined.

The compilation of this multi-authored book would not have been possible without the willing co-operation of many individuals and organisations, and this we gratefully acknowledge. In addition we wish to thank Dr D.A. Ervine, who wrote the section on two-stage channels.

P.S.
J.G.H

Contributors

Mr Paul Carter Babtie Geotechnical, 95 Bothwell Street, Glasgow G2 7HX

Mr Peter Cook Ministry of Agriculture, Fisheries and Food, Lincoln (now of 24 Shaftesbury Avenue, Lincoln LN6 0QN)

Dr John Ellis Consultant Engineer, 12 Craigfern Drive, Blanefield, Glasgow G63 9DP

Dr Eric Farr Scottish Agricultural College, School of Agriculture, 581 King Street, Aberdeen AB9 1UD

Ir G.D. Geldof Tauw Infra Consult BV, PO Box 479, 7400 AL Deventer, The Netherlands

Mr William C. Henderson Department of Agriculture and Fisheries for Scotland, New St Andrews House, Edinburgh EH14 1TW

Dr J. Graham Herbertson Civil Engineering Department, Glasgow University, Glasgow G12 8QQ

Dr Peter B. Leeds-Harrison Silsoe College, Cranfield Institute of Technology, Silsoe, Bedfordshire MK45 4DT

Ir A.J.M. Nelen Delft University of Technology, Faculty of Civil Engineering, Department of Water Management, PO Box 5048, 2600 GA Delft, The Netherlands

Mr Martin Osborne Hydraulics Research Ltd, Wallingford, Oxfordshire OX10 8BA

Dr Judy A. Payne Hydraulics Research Ltd, Wallingford, Oxfordshire OX10 8BA

Miss R.J. Rickson Silsoe College,Cranfield Institute of Technology, Silsoe, Bedfordshire MK45 4DT

Mr Nicholas S. Robins British Geological Survey, Maclean Building, Crowmarsh Gifford, Wallingford, Oxfordshire OX10 8BB

Miss Elizabeth M. Shaw 9 Phillimore Place, London W8 7BY

Dr Peter Smart Civil Engineering Department, Glasgow University, Glasgow G12 8QQ

Dr Ir F.H.M. Van de Ven Delft University of Technology, Faculty of Civil Engineering, Department of Water Management, PO Box 5048, 2600 GA Delft, The Netherlands

Mr M.J. Wakelin Lewin, Fryer and Partners, Grove House, 100 High Street, Hampton, Middlesex TW12 2ST

Professor Edward G. Youngs Silsoe College, Cranfield Institute of Technology, Silsoe, Bedfordshire MK45 4DT

Contents

1 Surface hydrology

E.M. SHAW

1.1 Introduction

Hydrological studies are a vital prerequisite for the design of drainage systems. Civil engineering problems range from providing adequate drainage for small developing areas in urban centres and for larger areas of agricultural land to the successful containment of major rivers in flood. Consequently, the hydrological events producing superfluous water may be an intensive local storm, the accumulation of excess rainfall over a wet spell of a few days or, on a longer time scale, the seasonal flood from warm rain falling on a melting winter snow pack lying on frozen ground. A whole range of events lies between these extremes.

Catchment topography, channel gradients and the nature of the ground surface play a large part in determining drainage needs. Impervious surfaces of city buildings and the concrete expanses of car parks and airport runways provide a rapid response to heavy rainfall. Sandy soils and porous geological strata may readily absorb the rainfall according to their initial state, and the overall catchment response is thereby delayed. Ground cover in the form of vegetation, either natural or agricultural crops, also has an important role in the determination of catchment response. Deciduous and coniferous forests with their seasonal differences nevertheless are efficient rainfall interceptors, and all vegetation causes a reduction in runoff by active transpiration of moisture back to the atmosphere. In assessing the drainage needs of irrigated land, the crop water use is a vital component of the water balance.

The variation in hydrological causes of excessive water requiring assisted drainage from problem sites is a direct result of geographical location. The differing climatic regimes around the world are a major factor to be considered. While the regions of high average precipitation are well-known and mapped, the temporal variability is often less well appreciated owing to the shortage of reliable long-term records, particularly of short-duration falls. More significantly, serious rainfall excesses can be experienced in semiarid regions from rare intensive thunderstorms. Reductions in surplus rainfall by evaporation are more effective in warm climates, but high relative humidity of the air may inhibit the evaporation process.

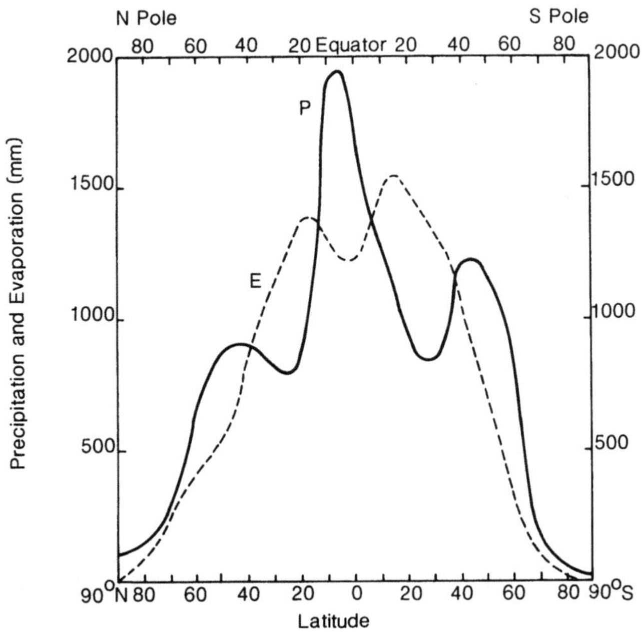

Figure 1.1 Average latitudinal values of annual precipitation (P) and evaporation (E) (after Sellars, 1965).

The average values for annual precipitation and evaporation from the equator to the poles are shown in Figure 1.1. The differences between the two hemispheres result from the greater landmasses in the north and the much larger areal proportion of oceans in the south. In general, on an annual basis, rainfall excess occurs in the zones within 10° of the equator and polewards of the 40° latitude. Between 10 and 40° north and south of the equator, the average curves are influenced by the hot desert regions of the world.

As already indicated, the structure and composition of an area to be drained has a most important bearing on the catchment response to extreme climatological conditions and consequently on the possible quantities of excess water. The design of a drainage system requires knowledge of the chance of occurrence and timing of peak flows and maximum volumes. This chapter will deal with the hydrological processes operating above the ground surface which contribute to the production of drainage design criteria.

1.2 Rainfall

The main component of the hydrological cycle forming the principal source of water on the global land areas is precipitation, which can be in liquid or solid forms. Except for melting snow already lying on the ground, it is the liquid form, rainfall, which gives the larger quantities in the shorter durations and thereby gives the drainage engineer the greater cause for concern.

1.2.1 *Formation*

The formation of rainfall comes within the province of the meteorologist or cloud physicist (McIlveen, 1986). Before the atmospheric water vapour, evaporated mainly from the oceans, can condense, the air must be nearly saturated. Even then, condensation is scarcely possible without the presence of aerosols, small airborne particles. These condensation nuclei may be hygroscopic particles having affinity for water vapour before the air is saturated or non-hygroscopic particles needing some degree of super-saturation before causing condensation. The character and particle size of the aerosols are the chief criteria in the formation of cloud droplets. At temperatures below 0°C in the atmosphere, ice nuclei attract water vapour to form ice crystals. Thus with increasing height above ground, there is a succession of large cloud droplets from hygroscopic nuclei, often particles from evaporated seaspray, diminishing to small droplets from fine dust particles then followed at greater heights in the drier, freezing zones by tiny ice crystals. Then the cloud droplets and ice crystals must grow before they become potential raindrops. The conventional borderline between cloud droplets and raindrops is a radius of 100 μm. Cloud droplets do not reach raindrop size through continuous condensation since the competition for the water vapour is too great (1 million droplets radius 10 μm = 1 raindrop radius 1 mm).

There are several theories of rainfall formation, and the effectiveness of the various mechanisms is dependent on the air temperature and humidity, the mixture of cloud droplet sizes and/or the mixture of cloud droplets and ice crystals. The growth of a large droplet by collision and coalescence with smaller droplets is the mechanism most probably found in deep cumulus and cumulonimbus clouds with large liquid water content and moderate updraughts. These are the conditions favourable to intense rainfalls.

The occurrence of rainfall depends therefore on the existence of favourable atmospheric conditions, and these are found in distinctive weather patterns which give their name to recognised rainfall types. Cyclonic or depression rainfall is formed in mid-latitude depressions in both hemispheres, and characteristic rainfall sequences can be identified in the associated frontal systems separating warm and cold air masses. More vigorous cyclonic rains occur in the tropical cyclones or hurricanes. Short-duration rainfalls, showers, are mainly produced in convective systems when moist rising air cools quickly. This situation operates widely in tropical regions and has been identified in frontal systems so that the classification of rainfall according to its formation is not always easy. Generalised values of rainfall intensities

Table 1.1 Rainfall type intensities, generalised (mm h^{-1}). (From Meteorological Office, 1969.)

Intensity	Rain Cyclonic/frontal	Showers Convectional
Slight	< 0.5	< 2.0
Moderate	0.5–4.0	2.0–10.0
Heavy	> 4.0	10.0–50.0
Violent	—	> 50.0

(mm h^{-1}) in continuous rainfall events and in showers are given in Table 1.1. To complete the rainfall types, there is a composite generic type, orographic, in which rainfalls with frontal or convective origins may be enhanced by the extra altitude effects of hills or mountain ranges. Orographic rain may also be formed when homogeneous moist air is obliged to rise over high land without being initiated by a dynamic meteorological situation.

These three most recognised types of rainfall, cyclonic/frontal, convective and orographic, can each play a part in producing excess rainfall. Persistent continuous rainfall from a slow-moving depression can saturate a catchment over a few days, while localised heavy showers lasting an hour or two can produce flood situations over saturated or impervious ground. Orographic rainfall plays a major role in increasing rainfall with altitude in the upper reaches of major catchments. For a more detailed account, a comprehensive treatment of precipitation formation is given by Sumner (1988).

1.2.2 *Measurement*

In order to make acceptable assessments of high rainfall values, good reliable records of rainfall measurements are invaluable. The most comprehensive assemblage of records derives from the regular reading of storage gauges, on a monthly basis in remote mountain areas but more widely on a daily basis. For shorter duration rainfalls, there is a variety of available instruments, the most common being the Dines tilting syphon rain recorder and the tipping bucket gauge. The former produces records on daily or monthly strip charts which need careful analysis, but the tipping bucket gauge can produce digital data recorded on a counter, on magnetic tape or directly onto a computer. Details of instruments, their siting and installation together with recommended operational practice can be obtained in standard texts (e.g. Shaw, 1988). Recent developments in precipitation measurements by radar and satellite imagery are more fully described by Sumner (1988).

For all measurements, the importance of quality control of data is being stressed increasingly. Errors in rainfall records can lead to serious misjudgments in adopting design values. However, the chance measurement of extreme falls by unconventional means should not be overlooked but

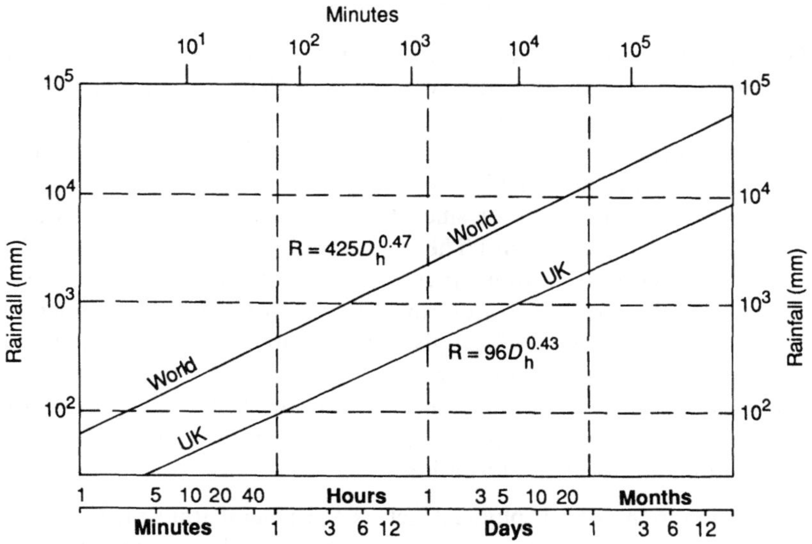

Figure 1.2 World and UK highest recorded rainfalls (from Shaw, 1988).

should be checked carefully with the nearest reputable gauges before the record is accepted. Failing any records at or near a problem site, the graphs of world and UK highest recorded rainfalls (R) related to duration (D) are given in Figure 1.2. These could be used as initial guidelines. Most countries have data archives in their hydrometeorological headquarters, and those with well-established raingauge networks have centralised meteorological services. Many rainfall records are published, and monthly totals are readily available. However, for rainfall intensities, it is usually necessary to obtain original charts and measurements.

1.3 Evapotranspiration

The combination of open-water evaporation and transpiration from vegetation results in a loss of water from drainage areas. When considering intense rainfalls on impervious surfaces, evaporation losses can be neglected, but on natural catchments and for irrigated areas evapotranspiration (E_t) on a daily or even seasonal basis may form a very significant proportion of the water balance equation:

$$P = R + E_t + \Delta S + G \tag{1.1}$$

where P = precipitation, R = runoff, ΔS = change in storage and G = seepage to groundwater.

The main factors affecting evapotranspiration are as follows:

(a) Solar radiation, resulting in direct short-wave and terrestrial long-wave radiation, provides latent heat to convert the water into vapour and is dependent on latitude and season.
(b) Air temperature and the temperature of the evaporating surface dependent on the available radiation.
(c) Vapour pressure of the air, since this is a measure of its vapour capacity at a given temperature (e_a). The saturation deficit given by $e_a - e_d$ (where e_d is the saturated vapour pressure at the dew point temperature) or $e_a - e_s$ (where e_s is the saturation vapour pressure at the temperature of the evaporating surface) gives a measure of the additional water vapour the air can hold at that air temperature.
(d) Wind speed at the evaporating surface affects the air's evaporating capacity. Saturated air is moved on and drier air replacement ensures continuation of the evaporation process.

In addition to these basic physical factors, the general atmospheric pressure with associated weather patterns and the character of the evaporating surface also influence evapotranspiration losses.

Transpiration is also governed by the available moisture in the soil. A very useful concept assumes a continuous supply of water, and thus potential evapotranspiration, PE, with unlimited water is the maximum possible loss rate resulting from the prevailing meteorological conditions.

1.3.1 *Evaluation*

The direct measurement of evapotranspiration in the volatile conditions of the atmosphere has provided a challenge to instrumental research, and to date hydrologists and others requiring quantification of losses or plant usage have made recourse to measurements by default or calculations using meteorological variables.

For open-water evaporation, the changes in volumes (or levels) over specific time periods have been measured. In reservoirs the change in storage is expressed as a change in depth over the surface area per week or per month and is assessed by taking into account inflows, outflows, consumption and possible seepage. Specially designed tanks or pans kept at climatological stations provide loss depths over a day. The latter need careful siting and installation, and the measurements are rarely directly representative of larger scale reservoir losses. Similarly, evapotranspiration can be evaluated from lysimeters, containers of soil bearing vegetation set in the ground, which may be operated on a water balance basis, inputs and outputs being measured at regular time intervals or by operating a weighing mechanism to record continuously the change in storage. Equivalent depths of evapotranspiration (mm) are obtained over a day or a week.

On the natural catchment scale, evapotranspiration is evaluated monthly by the water balance method, in which change in storage can be estimated from measured changes in soil moisture at selected representative sites.

1.3.2 *Formulae*

The calculations of open water evaporation E_o and evapotranspiration E_t are based on formulae either for vapour flux or for the energy budget (in which the heat used in evaporation is obtained) for a combination of these two physical approaches. Full explanations with examples are given in Shaw (1988), but the most pertinent methods of assessing loss for drainage design purposes are set out here.

From reservoirs, there is Penman's basic aerodynamic equation for the UK:

$$E_o = 0.35(0.5 + u_2/100)(e_s - e_d) \quad (\text{mm d}^{-1}) \tag{1.2}$$

where u_2 is wind speed in miles d^{-1} at 2 m above the water surface and the vapour pressures e_s and e_d are as previously defined in millimetres of mercury (mm Hg).

In the US, Harbeck (1962) incorporated a surface area factor for reservoirs up to 12 000 hectares:

$$E_o = 0.291A^{-0.05}u_2(e_s - e_d) \quad (\text{mm d}^{-1}) \tag{1.3}$$

with A in m^2, u_2 in m s^{-1} and vapour pressures in mb.

The Penman basic combination formula takes the form:

$$E_o = \frac{\Delta}{\gamma}H + E_a \bigg/ \left(\frac{\Delta}{\gamma} + 1\right) \tag{1.4}$$

where H is the available heat and E_a results from the aerodynamic equation based on the air humidity at air temperature T_a, Δ is the slope of the curve of saturated vapour pressure plotted against temperature, and γ is the hygrometric constant (0.15 mm Hg $^\circ\text{C}^{-1}$).

Empirical formulae provide expressions for H and E_a based on four measurements: T_a, mean air temperature; e_d, mean vapour pressure; n, hours of bright sunshine; and u_2, mean wind speed at 2 m above the surface. Tables give component parts of the formulae according to time periods and units of measurement used (Shaw, 1988). Values of E_o are finally obtained in mm d^{-1}. Measurements of net radiation where available may be used for H.

The calculation of potential evapotranspiration, PE, uses the same basic Penman formula, but the component formulae for H and E_a are modified to take into account the differing characteristics of a vegetated surface (short grass). The assumption of an unlimited water supply continues to be applied. Further modification of the formula taking into account transpiration gives an expression for actual evapotranspiration rate, E_t, the Penman–Monteith formula:

$$E_t = \frac{\Delta R_n + \rho c_p(e_a - e_d)/r_a}{\lambda\Delta + \gamma(r_s + r_a)/r_a} \quad (\mathrm{g\,m^{-2}\,s^{-1}}) \tag{1.5}$$

where R_n is net radiation ($\mathrm{W\,m^{-2}}$); r_s is net resistance to diffusion through the surfaces of the leaves and the soil ($\mathrm{s\,m^{-1}}$); r_a is net resistance to diffusion through the air from surfaces to the height of the measuring instrument ($\mathrm{s\,m^{-1}}$); ρ and c_p are density and specific heat of air respectively; λ is the latent heat of vaporisation of water; the vapour pressures (mb) are as previously defined and the air properties are in SI units (Shuttleworth, 1979).

Average values of r_s during daylight hours with unlimited water range between 40 and 50 $\mathrm{s\,m^{-1}}$ and r_a in low wind speeds ranges from 20 to 40 $\mathrm{s\,m^{-1}}$. Higher values of r_s operate for orchard trees and forests.

1.3.3 *Crop water requirements*

A reference crop evapotranspiration ET_o is first defined. Essentially equivalent to PE, this is the rate of evapotranspiration from an extensive, uniformly covered, grass surface with continuous water supply. To obtain ET_o, the Penman formula for PE may be used, but a simpler method using the Blaney–Criddle formula has been applied successfully in the United States. Over a specific period, usually a month or 10 days:

$$ET_o = p(0.46\,T + 8) \quad (\mathrm{mm\ d^{-1}}) \tag{1.6}$$

where T(°C) is the mean daily temperature and p the mean daily percentage of total annual daytime hours. Adjustment factors are required for both these estimates related to relative humidity, radiation or sunshine hours and wind speeds. ET_o may also be obtained from pan measurements:

$$ET_o = k_p E_{pan} \quad (\mathrm{mm\ d^{-1}})\ (\text{mean daily value}) \tag{1.7}$$

Pan coefficients, k_p, are available for the US class A pan.

Having determined monthly or 10-day period values of ET_o, a crop coefficient, k_c, is selected according to the timing within the growing season. Then:

$$ET_{crop} = k_c ET_o \tag{1.8}$$

for each of the monthly or 10-day periods during the growing season. These values are then compared with the expected rainfall to determine shortages or surpluses requiring irrigation or drainage provision. The designed drainage provision should normally ensure that the ground is never waterlogged even when water is not needed after the crop growth period. Good through-drainage of the soil is essential to prevent accumulation of harmful salts. For further details on this subject, the reader is referred to Doorenbos and Pruitt (1977), and Chapters 3 and 4.

1.4 River flow

Although knowledge of the hydrological elements, rainfall and transpiration, is important for many drainage problems, reliable information on river flows, particularly flood flows, is more often required as the basis of drainage design schemes. Unfortunately, it is rare to have stream or river discharges at the problem site, and the usual practice is to scale the nearest records according to the relative catchment or drainage areas.

1.4.1 *Measurement*

The establishment of a river gauging station is the first priority of a hydrometric scheme, and great care is taken in the choice of site. A straight-channel reach, preferably with uniform flow, provides the best results, and either a natural or constructed control is essential to ensure a constant relationship between a measured stage and the corresponding discharge. For the reliable measurement of high flows, a river gauging station should be designed to contain flood flows. However, there is not often sufficient knowledge of the extreme behaviour of a river to ensure total containment, and indeed this could be impracticable. Thus for in-bank flows, the measurements of stage, i.e. water level, recorded on charts, tapes and solid-state data loggers or transmitted via telytones give required discharges within the limits of calibration or from a carefully extrapolated stage–discharge relationship. For extreme events with the river out of its normal channel, levels may be obtained from special flood crest gauges or determined from debris or wrack marks after the event, taking care to omit spurious levels caused by surges and temporary blockages. Peak water levels on buildings identified immediately after a flood should be marked by paint. Field surveys across the flooded areas and of the slopes of the channel and flood plains are then carried out in order to calculate the several flow components, usually with the Manning formula (Table 4.7). For further details see Herschy (1978) and Chapter 7.

From careful research and detailed studies, a catalogue of historic flood events may be built up and related to a continuous river flow record. Most countries have such historic flood records for their major rivers, and a world catalogue of maximum observed floods has been compiled as a contribution to the International Hydrological Programme of UNESCO (Rodier and Roche, 1984). Reference to this publication is especially recommended to engineers working in developing countries. A general guidance to maximum floods related to drainage basin area is given in Figure 1.3.

1.4.2 *Derived flows*

Where there are limited or even no river flow records, discharges may be derived from rainfall, estimated losses and catchment characteristics. This

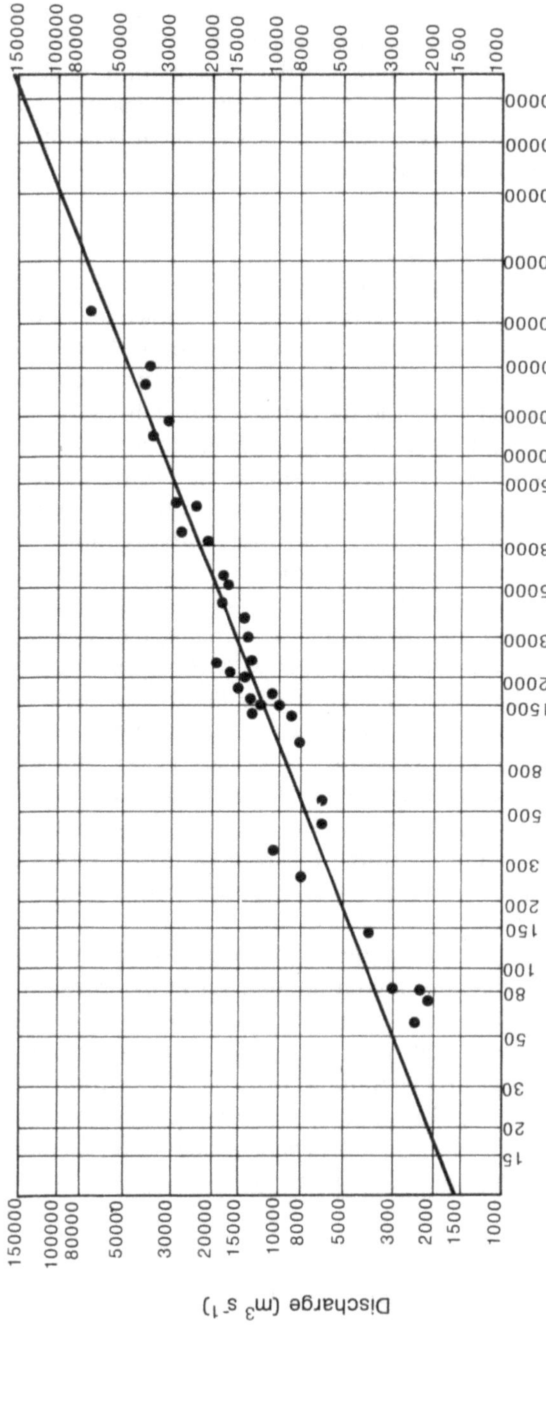

Basin Area (km^2)

Figure 1.3 Maximum floods in the world (up to 1982) (after Rodier and Roche, 1984).

Basin Area (km^2)

Figure 1.3 Maximum floods in the world (up to 1982) (after Rodier and Roche, 1984).

is the essence of surface hydrology. The choice from the many established techniques for any particular river site depends on the size of the drainage area and the degree of homogeneity of response to rainfall over the area. To synthesise a flood river flow sequence, it is usual to analyse a separate well-defined rainfall event which produces a distinctive river flow hydrograph, showing rising discharges, a single peak and a clear recession. For large catchment areas with varying characteristics and which are unlikely to experience a common rainstorm over the whole area, subcatchments are studied separately and the several flows are routed down to the problem site.

1.4.3 *Unit hydrograph*

The unit hydrograph, a concept attributed to Sherman in 1932, is the hydrograph of the surface runoff resulting from unit effective rainfall occurring in a unit of time and produced uniformly in time and space over the total catchment area. The derivation of the unit hydrograph is explained fully in most hydrological texts, and by taking the mean of several unit hydrographs from a number of storm events a characteristic catchment response is obtained for the particular drainage basin.

To identify the effective rainfall from the total storm profile, a constant loss rate or an initial loss with a continuing loss rate can be assumed. The losses are assessed so that the effective rainfall amount corresponds to the volume of the surface runoff under the recorded hydrograph from which a base flow has been deducted.

Failing adequate river flow records, a simple triangular unit hydrograph can be drawn using:

$$Q_p = 220/T_p \quad (\mathrm{m^3s^{-1}/10\,mm/100\,km^2}) \tag{1.9a}$$

and

$$\mathrm{TB} = 2.52\,T_p \quad (\text{hours}) \tag{1.9b}$$

where Q_p is the peak flow, T_p is the time to peak, i.e. basin lag time, and TB is the time base (Sutcliffe, 1978). T_p may be obtained from an equation derived from the multiple regression of UK Flood Studies data on catchment characteristics (NERC, 1975, Vol. 1).

In the United States, the derivation of a synthetic unit hydrograph by Snyder's method has long been recommended (Snyder, 1938). The time to peak, T_p, is related to basin size and shape:

$$T_p = C_t(L \times L_c)^{0.3} \quad (\text{hours}) \tag{1.10}$$

where L(km) is the main stream length from catchment head to the outfall and L_c (km) is the stream length from a point opposite the basin centroid to the outfall. The coefficient C_t varies from 1.4 to 1.7 and then the unit hydrograph peak Q_p is estimated from

$$Q_p = C_pA/T_p \quad (\mathrm{m^3s^{-1}}) \tag{1.11}$$

where A (km^2) is the drainage area and C_p is between 0.15 and 0.19. For the time base TB, Snyder used:

$$TB = 3 + 3T_p/24 \quad \text{(days)} \tag{1.12}$$

where the constants are dependent on the direct runoff–baseflow relationship (Linsley *et al.*, 1988). A fuller account of this method is to be found in Chow *et al.* (1988).

When a unit hydrograph (TUH) for a time period (T) appropriate to the drainage area has been determined, the T hour elements of a selected design rainfall profile are convoluted with TUH to give a simulated design hydrograph. For extreme events such as the estimation of a maximum flood it is generally assumed that the catchment area is saturated initially giving total surface runoff from the rainfall. For lesser events, such as the 30-year or 100-year flood, the initial state of the catchment and hence the amount of losses to the total rainfall must be assessed. In well-instrumented drainage basins of the developed world, monthly measurements of soil moisture content may be available, and from the soil moisture deficit (SMD, mm depth of water below field capacity; see section 3.2.4) an estimate of the effective rainfall can be made to give the surface runoff. However, for an immediate flood situation, a guide to the catchment state may be obtained from the daily antecedent precipitation index (API), which can be related to a constant loss rate to give the effective rainfall.

The application of the unit hydrograph method is readily carried out by computer once the requisite input information is available.

1.4.4 *Catchment models*

In this computer age, catchment models provide another means of deriving river flows. These range from theoretical developments of the unit hydrograph (Nash, 1960; Maddaus and Eagleson, 1969), through runoff-routing models (Laurenson, 1964; Price, 1978), to conceptual or deterministic models attempting to simulate the several land phases of the hydrological cycle by a sequence of storages. Many of the last-mentioned are described or mentioned in Fleming (1975) and Shaw (1988). With the increasing storage capacity of computers, component models are being developed. These seek to describe mathematically the water movements through the hydrological sequence of phases from rainfall to stream flow. Several researchers, notably in the United States, have produced single-phase and combined-phase flow models. This development of physically based components has resulted in the SHE model (Abbott *et al.*, 1986). The model takes into account spatial variations in hydrological inputs and catchment responses and, given the necessary data on inputs and catchment characteristics, has widespread future application.

For a single design problem, the unit hydrograph method or a runoff-routing catchment model is the simplest to use. However, in many authorities and consulting engineering firms, the derivation of a peak discharge or even a design flood hydrograph is only a beginning in major investigations. Composite repetitive operational catchment models have been assembled and are readily adaptable to different catchment and climatic conditions. Of these, the Stanford watershed model (Crawford and Linsley, 1966), the Wallingford procedure (NWC, 1981), RIBAMAN (Price, 1980) and ROSS (Simpson and Thorpe, 1982) are notable examples.

1.4.5 *Peak discharges*

Peak discharges have formed the basic tool of drainage design engineers for many years, and a large number of empirical formulae have evolved worldwide. These are essentially applicable only to the regions where they have been formulated, and it is not advisable to apply them elsewhere. However, one simple relationship, the rational formula, has stood the test of time and forms the basis of one of the methods of the Wallingford procedure (NWC, 1981). The original form:

$$Q_p = C \times i \times A \tag{1.13a}$$

becomes

$$Q_p(\mathrm{m^3 s^{-1}}) = 0.278C \times i(\mathrm{mm\ h^{-1}}) \times A(\mathrm{km^2}) \tag{1.13b}$$

in metric units, with i the mean rainfall intensity in the time of concentration of the catchment of area A (see section 9.5). Since the method assumes uniform rainfall intensity over the drainage area for the storm duration, the rational formula only gives satisfactory results for small urban catchments. The runoff coefficient C depends on the surface characteristics of the catchment, the degree of saturation and the rainfall intensity. In its simplest form, C ranges from 0.4 for flat residential areas 30% impervious to over 0.8 for moderately steep areas 70% impervious (Gray, 1970).

For many drainage problems, the flood volume of an extreme event is also required, and for this a flood hydrograph is necessary. The unit hydrograph method, a calibrated runoff-routing model, or a catchment model must be applied to give the flow sequence through the event. The probability of occurrence and the ordered magnitude of extreme events follow in the next section.

1.5 Extreme values

The existence of a long record, of rainfall or of river flow, at or near a problem site enables the application of another analytical method. Based on extreme value statistics, the evaluation of the return period or recurrence interval of specific rainfalls or river discharges can be made in addition to estimating extreme events. The return period of an event of given magnitude is the average number of years within which the event will be equalled or exceeded.

At least 10 years of records are necessary to give acceptable results. For rainfall, according to catchment response, a duration is selected such that for small catchments the annual maximum 1-hour falls may form a required series, while daily rainfall maxima may suffice elsewhere. For river flow, the annual maximum discharges form the most satisfactory series of data for analysis. However, if there are few years of records available, the peak-over-threshold series may be used, but care must be exercised in choosing the threshold to avoid undue dependence between successive peaks.

1.5.1 *Statistical analysis*

The statistical analysis, based on a series of N independent events X_1, $X_2 \cdots X_n$, gives the relation between X and its probability of occurrence by a cumulative distribution function, $F(X)$, so that $F(X)$ is the probability of an annual maximum $X_i \leqslant X$. Thus the probability of exceedence is $1 - F(X)$, and the return period $T = 1/[1 - F(X)]$. There are several statistical distributions applicable to extreme values, but for an annual maximum series of data the general extreme value distribution (GEV) is recommended. For the GEV:

$$F(X) = \exp\{-[1 - k(X - \mu)/\alpha]^{1/k}\} \tag{1.14}$$

If there is a good long record of over 25 years, this distribution may be fitted by estimating the three parameters, μ, α and k, by the method of moments or maximum likelihood (NERC, Vol. 1, 1975), and estimated values for return periods of twice the record length would be acceptable. For records of less than 25 years, the EV1 distribution with $k = 0$ (Gumbel type 1 distribution) should be used. For the EV1,

$$F(X) = \exp\{-\exp[-\mathrm{b}(X - a)]\} \tag{1.15a}$$

$$= \exp[-\exp(-y)] \tag{1.15b}$$

where the reduced variate $y = b(X - a)$.

The two parameters are related to the mean (μ_x) and the variance ($\sigma_x{}^2$) of the series:

$$a = \mu_x - \gamma/b, \text{ where } \gamma = 0.5772 \tag{1.16a}$$

and

$$b = \pi/\sigma_x\sqrt{6} \tag{1.16b}$$

For a more speedy graphical estimation of return periods, the annual maximum series may be ranked (i) in descending order of magnitude, and the probability values F_i calculated according to the Gringorten plotting formula:

$$F_i = (i - 0.44)/(N + 0.12) \tag{1.17}$$

where N is the number of years recorded.

These are then plotted on Gumbel probability paper where the x axis is calibrated in terms of reduced variate y or return period T. The points should approximate a straight line, thus simplifying extrapolation to values of higher return periods. However, such results from the analysis of a single record should be treated with great reserve.

The appreciation of the pattern of extreme discharge values is improved by the consideration of several records combined into a representative regional curve. A set of 11 regional curves has been established by the UK Flood Studies Report (NERC, 1975). These present the numerous analyses of countrywide records in the form of growth curves with $q_T = Q_T/\bar{Q}$ (where Q_T is the T-year flood, and $\bar{Q}$ is the mean annual flood) plotted against T and the reduced variate y. Ordinates for a selection of regional curves are given in Table 1.2. Once a mean annual flood has been established for a river in the UK (for a selection of methods, see the Flood Studies Report), values of flood peaks for required return periods can be obtained by applying the ratios (q_T) of the appropriate region.

The UK Flood Studies method is being applied worldwide. The annual maximum flood series are converted to the non-dimensional form $q_T = Q_T/\bar{Q}$ to simplify comparisons between stations and to help in defining regions. The analysis of combined q_T values in a region uses the GEV distribution chosen for its flexibility in varying climates. A sample of regional prediction growth curves is given for results considered 'good' or 'very good' according to data availability (Table 1.3).

1.5.2 *Data synthesis*

In an alternative approach to extreme value determination, the characteristics of the rainfall or river flow sequences may be identified by time series analysis. Given an acceptable river record, a suitable discrete time interval is selected for the data according to the size of catchment and the nature of the problem.

Table 1.2 Ordinates of regional growth curves (q_T). (From Sutcliffe, 1978.)

	Return periods (years)					
Region	2	5	10	25	50	100
NE England and Yorkshire	0.94	1.25	1.45	1.70	1.90	2.08
E Anglia and Lincolnshire	0.89	1.29	1.65	2.25	2.83	3.56
Great Britain	0.89	1.22	1.48	1.88	2.22	2.61
Ireland	0.95	1.20	1.37	1.60	1.77	1.96

Table 1.3 Worldwide growth curves (q_T). (From Farquharson *et al.*, 1987.)

Region	Return periods (years)		
	50	100	500
Europe			
Czechoslovakia	2.74	3.28	4.82
Denmark	2.08	2.33	2.92
Hungary and adjacent Yugoslavia	2.25	2.61	3.57
Americas			
Brazil (Rio Grande do Sul)	1.96	2.12	2.46
Africa			
Kenya	3.13	3.75	5.50
Malawi	3.13	3.81	5.80
South Africa and adjacent Botswana	4.45	6.06	12.06
Togo and Benin	2.02	2.17	2.45
Asia			
India (Kerala)	2.51	2.90	3.92
Indonesia (Java and Sumatra)	1.95	2.16	2.68
Jordan	4.07	5.28	9.28
Korea	2.31	2.60	3.29
Sri Lanka	3.25	4.17	7.32
Thailand	2.42	2.79	3.77

A series of annual runoffs will have no distinctive pattern, though a gradual trend may be discernible. A sequence of monthly values is very likely to show a seasonal pattern depending on the location and climate of the catchment area. Daily runoff values from medium or small catchments will show the hydrograph response to individual rainfall events. For the chosen time series, X_t, the trend (T_t) and periodic components (m_t and s_t) are identified, represented mathematically, and removed from the individual data. Several harmonics may be required to represent the periodic component. Then:

$$E_t = (X_t - T_t - m_t)/s_t \tag{1.18}$$

represents a residual stochastic component. This is standardised to give:

$$Z_t = (E_t - \bar{E})/s_E \tag{1.19}$$

which now represents a series of zero mean and unit standard deviation. The serial correlation coefficients of Z_t are calculated, and the resultant correlogram is inspected for a recognisable structure, e.g. a definable Markov process. When this has been removed the residual e_t is random and independent.

To synthesise a data series, a required number of random values of e_t is generated using a standard computer package. Then the Z_t values are obtained sequentially from a starting value Z_{t-1} and e_t and the analytical procedure is reversed to derive

$$E_t = Z_t s_E + \bar{E} \tag{1.20}$$

and

$$X_t - T_t = E_t s_t + m_t \tag{1.21}$$

In applying the time series method of data synthesis, a large number of data sequences can be generated with the same historic characteristics and used in the extreme value analysis to give a better estimate of required return period values than would be obtained from a single analysis of the historic data.

1.6 Design criteria

Before the drainage design engineer can settle down to the drawing board (or the computer-aided design facility), the scale of the remedial measures to solve the problem must be defined. The approach to this definition varies with the type of problem, but economics always play a large part, and nowadays the effects of a scheme on the natural environment are increasingly a cause for concern.

However, the initial design criteria are usually hydrological. The rainfall intensity, the quantity of surplus water or the magnitude of the river flood provides the first consideration. From the extreme value analysis, the chance of occurrence of a critical quantity and its estimated return period or average recurrence interval have been evaluated. For minor drainage works, standard criteria have often been accepted as general practice, but for expensive flood protection schemes more rigorous procedures are usually required.

1.6.1 *Agricultural land*

Conditions of climate, soil and agricultural practice provide the principal drainage design criteria. In any particular climate, the seasonal patterns of precipitation and evaporation govern the basic hydrological characteristics, to which are added the estimated occurrences of extremes. Thus for most climatic types, guidelines or 'codes of practice' can be established. Such standards for agricultural land drainage have been produced in the UK by the Ministry of Agriculture, Fisheries and Food (MAFF, 1974). Table 1.4 defines the classes of land potential related to soil quality and the degree of protection recommended for a range of land uses. The period of the year from March to November is critical for many crops such as high-valued

Table 1.4 Agricultural land drainage standards. (From MAFF, 1974.)

Land potential	Crops	Design flood frequency —not more than	
		Mar–Nov	Whole year
Very high	All agricultural land and horticultural crops	No flood allowed, say 1 in 100 years	
High	Root crops, cereals, grass	1 in 25 yrs	1 in 10 yrs
Medium	Cereals, grass	1 in 10 yrs	1 in 5 yrs
Low	Grass	1 in 5 yrs	1 in 2 yrs
Very low	Grazing land	1 in 3 yrs	1 in 1 yr

cereals and potatoes, but short-duration flooding of the fields during winter months would not be of great concern. However, the standard of protection should not fall below the minimum recommended for the whole year, which includes the winter flood events. Flood plains often left in rough pasture for grazing can be expected to be flooded on average once a year.

In a further helpful publication by the Agricultural Development and Advisory Service (MAFF, 1983), detailed daily rainfalls are provided for 52 agroclimatic areas in England and Wales with regard to the design of field drainage pipe systems. A sample of such information demonstrating the range of conditions in England and Wales is given in Table 1.5.

Where such detailed information is not available, the design engineer must consult the agricultural engineer for specialised knowledge of soils and crops in order to determine the surplus net rainfall requiring drainage. An agriculturalist should give guidance on the permissible duration of inundation applicable to the crop, as the temporary storage of flood water relates directly to the scale of alleviation measures.

Table 1.5 Daily rainfall for field drainage design ($mm\,d^{-1}$). (From MAFF, 1983.)

Agroclimatic areas	AAR (mm)	Mole drainage			Other schemes		
		Grass	Arable	Hort.	Grass	Arable	Hort.
England							
Essex	577	15	19	26	6	7	9
Lake District and N Pennines	1663	40	48	64	17	20	25
W Midlands	695	19	23	31	8	9	11
Wales							
Anglesey	1004	26	30	40	11	13	16
N mountains	1829	45	50	61	19	22	26
SW coastal	1258	32	36	47	13	15	19

1.6.2 *Urban areas*

In dealing with the drainage design for urban towns and cities, the areal extent to be considered may be comparable with that of agricultural land. However, the hydrological response to precipitation is modified considerably by the increased impervious surface areas. Groundwater recharge is reduced so that dry-weather flows are diminished, but higher peak flows result from the rapid runoff of intense rainfalls. Thus the urban catchment is less affected by antecedent conditions than a comparable rural catchment. The rapid response time also makes the urban catchment more sensitive to convective rainfall intensities than to the more prolonged depression rainfalls. Therefore, in contrast to agricultural areas, in the UK the flood risk season tends to be during the summer months.

With the contemporary expansion of urban areas and the overtaking of the design life of the sewerage systems of the major cities, considerable research into the design of urban storm drainage has been undertaken in the UK. This has culminated in the publication of the Wallingford procedure (NWC, 1981). The design recommendations have been built on the foundation of the Flood Studies Report (NERC, 1975). In practice, the design engineer needs the return period of flows rather than of rainfalls, but there is more information available on rainfalls than on flows in sewers. Therefore design criteria are dependent on good rainfall records. It is well appreciated that the rainfall with a T-year return period does not necessarily result in a T-year channel flow since the varying initial catchment conditions produce varying rainfall–runoff relationships. For rapid-response urban catchments, equal return periods for rainfall and derived discharge are acceptable if specific rainfall durations, storm profiles and antecedent conditions are used.

A summary of the recommended Wallingford design procedure is as follows:

(1) A series of rainfall durations, D, is defined, e.g. 15, 30, 60 and 120 minutes.
(2) The required return period is selected, T.
(3) The total depths of rainfall, $MT-D$ for return period T and durations D are determined.
(4) An areal reduction factor may be necessary for large areas where variations in the storm rainfall over the catchment are suspected.
(5) The shapes of the $MT-D$ storm profiles are required. The peakedness of a profile is the ratio of the maximum to mean intensity, and summer storms are more peaked than winter storms. Thus for storm sewer design the 50% summer profiles are recommended and then there is a final smoothing of the point rainfall to give a catchment average profile.
(6) A design value of an antecedent conditions index (UCWI) is taken from an average annual rainfall–UCWI relationship.

The four variables, the storm duration giving the maximum discharge, the return period, the 50% summer storm profile and the design value of UCWI, when used in the hydrograph computational method of the Wallingford procedure, should produce a good estimate of the complete synthetic flood frequency curve. Many of the requisite data are presented in map form or in the computer package, which takes care of data processing and analysis as well as pipe network design.

For an approach to design standards, the Wallingford procedure provides a decision matrix in which the return periods should be entered by the drainage authority. The nine-block matrix is defined by three levels of risk, normal, intermediate and high, and three flow conditions, pipe-full, manhole-full (surface flooding starts) and property flooding starts. The normal classification of risk includes normally sloping terrain, normal property values and road usage and no foul sewage. The high risk includes terrain liable to ponding, high property values and road use and foul sewage present. Individual responsible authorities have their own standards of protection for the several grades of risk according to their ability to provide the necessary works.

1.6.3 *Major flooding*

The widespread inundations of main rivers with the threat of flooding to large towns and industrial areas generally result in the design of expensive flood protection schemes. Some local government authorities, especially in developed regions of the world, have statutory standards of protection. For example, parts of Europe, individual states in the USA and responsible authorities in Australia have defined standards of protection to which their engineers are obliged to work. The greatest risk of all is of the serious failure of an impounding reservoir. The design criteria for a dam spillway require a series of critical assessments by the engineering hydrologist. Most clients now call for estimates of the probable maximum flood (PMF) which may result from the probable maximum precipitation falling on extremely sensitive catchments. These values have no statistical return period attached to them. The US Corps of Engineers defines a standard project flood which is about 50% of the PMF. Then the engineer has to evaluate a design flood, according to local conditions and cost–benefit considerations.

For main river flooding, a 100-year average recurrence interval (return period) is the usual design level in Australia for severe or rare events, but for major state road bridges a 1 in 2000 year annual exceedence probability design flood is required (Pilgrim, 1987). There are no set standards for such design criteria in the UK. Many alleviation schemes stimulated by the last occurring flood are guided by the maximum discharge reached in that event for their design flood. However, for such situations, it is now usual to design a range of alleviation measures according to the estimated return periods of two or three magnitudes. Then cost–benefit analyses of the proposed schemes are made after due consultation with the environmental experts before the plans are handed over to the clients, who are the final arbiters of the proposals. With the increasing value of land and property in developed countries, there is a tendency for an increase in the standard of protection and, in turn, this lays greater emphasis on the estimation of extreme values and their chance of occurrence.

1.7 Weather forecasting

The forecasting of the weather is one of the major functions of the professional meteorologist. Its operation is based on measurements of the current physical properties of the lower atmosphere and of the resultant elements at the ground surface, measured over specified time intervals. The relative importance of the two measured series is dependent on the lead time of the forecast and on the knowledge required of any particular element. Modern weather forecasting relies on supercomputers solving dynamic and thermodynamic equations by means of numerical weather prediction models operating on the regular updating of the atmospheric measurements of, for example, temperature, pressure and humidity. Such numerical models forecast the weather patterns up to 24 hours ahead, and by incorporating statistical analyses of model results may be extended up to 36 hours ahead. Weather forecasts for weeks or even a few months ahead are addressed to the more generalised form of average weather or climatic patterns and are made by the statistical analyses of the measurements of precipitation, temperature, wind, etc. It is these forecasts, or rather predictions since precise timing is not possible, that form the bases of design criteria for drainage works.

The potential of supercomputers is also being realised in the real-time forecasting of weather phenomena which affect the operation of drainage systems. The meterologists have made rapid advances in the past decade in the forecasting of weather events over immediate short-time periods. Such forecasts up to 2 hours ahead by extrapolation forwards from present weather conditions are known as nowcasting (Browning and Collier, 1989). These new short-lead forecasts result from the combination of the synoptic patterns from the numerical prediction models with added information from satellite data and continuous observations from ground-based radar. Mesoscale studies using weather radars across distances of less than, say, 100 km have explored the atmospheric processes in frontal systems and individual cumulonimbus clouds. Of special significance to the water engineer has been the careful development of precipitation measurement with weather radars. The UK Meteorological Office rainfall forecasting system FRONTIERS uses the combined satellite and radar data and expects to be able to forecast on a

5-km grid up to 6 hours ahead at half-hour intervals. The network of collaborating ground radars is shown in Figure 1.4.

The radar precipitation measurements are received by contributing regional river authorities and calibrated from ground rainfall measurements made over 15-minute durations by tipping bucket rain gauges. This automated information is displayed in the form of rainfall intensities over grid square areas using coloured codes on a visual display unit. By studying the mapped rainfall intensities, the flood warning engineer can assess the seriousness of a rainfall event. Areal values of rainfall over the sensitive river catchments are computed and fed into rainfall–runoff models to give estimated flood flows at the strategic points on the rivers.

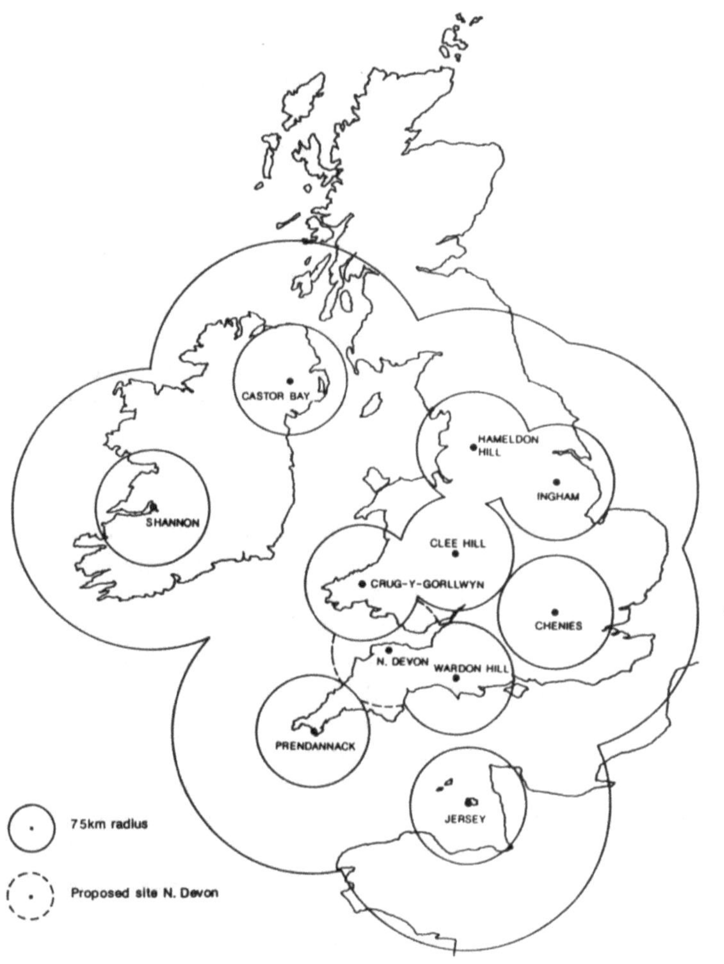

Figure 1.4 United Kingdom weather radar network, 1989 (from Collinge in BHS, 1989).

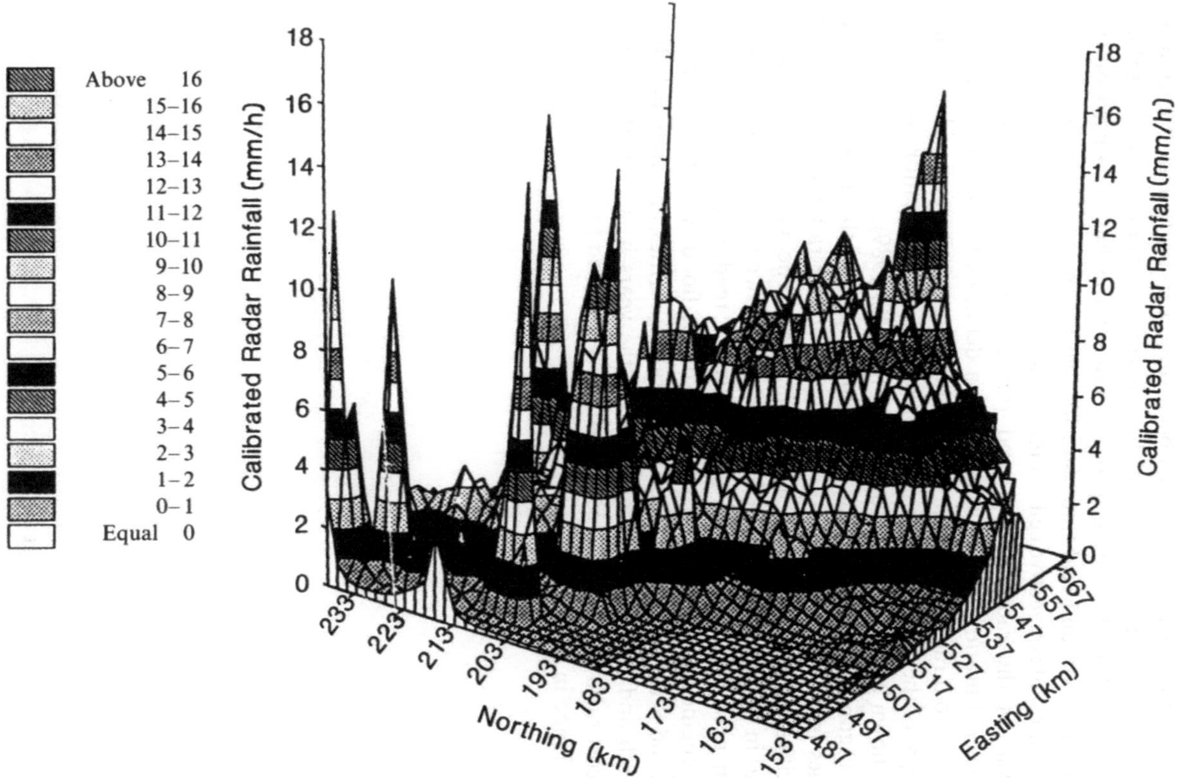

Figure 1.5 Calibrated radar rainfall. Parameters: time 03:30 08/05/88; number of gauges = 23(1, 2, 3, 4, 5, 6, 7, 8, 9, 10, 11, 13, 14, 16, 17, 18, 19, 20, 22, 24, 25, 27, 28); field minimum = 0.00; field maximum = 16.15 (from Moore *et al.* in BHS, 1989).

Considerable technical research has been necessary to assess the accuracy of the radar rainfall measurements and to overcome the problems of screening of the radar beam in hilly areas and of the varied radar sensing in different precipitation types, particularly in passing through the snow band. The calibration of the radar rainfalls has been subject to particular attention in the Thames catchment area, where there is concern about localised urban flooding in London. A reduced grid of 2-km squares has been used out to the range of 75 km and real-time data for every 5 minutes in order to give good resolution of convective cells. A recalibration system has been developed by analysis of the radar and ground rainfall measurements to define a continuous calibration factor surface over a delineated area. The surface is then applied to a radar field to produce a more accurate set of grid rainfalls. An example of the three-dimensional representation of a recalibrated rainfall event is shown in Figure 1.5 (Moore *et al.* in BHS, 1989).

From Figure 1.4, it can be seen that a major part of the area of England and Wales is covered by the 75-km radii around the radar sites, and most of the cities and industrial areas are included. The patterns of rainfall intensities in significant weather events are now shown regularly on the BBC television news broadcasts, and the details are readily available to flood warning engineers. Estimates of the value of the flood warning systems in England and Wales have been made by central authorities, and after including all research and development charges over the years it is estimated that a benefit–cost ratio of 3.0 to 3.5 results, with this expected to increase in future years (Collinge in BHS, 1989).

2 Soil physical principles

E.G. YOUNGS

2.1 Introduction

The purpose of installing land drains in soils is to remove water in order to improve soil physical conditions for agricultural production and for engineering operations. The problem facing the drainage engineer is therefore one of the physics of water flow through both saturated and unsaturated soils, caused by physical conditions at the soil surface and at the drain peripheries.

The specific objectives of land drainage are not always the same. In temperate regions of the world drainage is used in agriculture to desaturate the soil so as to create more favourable conditions in the root zone for plant growth and near the surface for cultivation. Without drainage installations, excess rainfall or foreign water entering the region would cause the soil to be excessively wet, producing anaerobic conditions and preventing timely cultivation because of unsuitable soil mechanical properties. On the other hand, in arid regions where agriculture depends on irrigation, land drainage is necessary in order to allow percolation of water through the soil profile to leach salts and thus avoid toxic accumulation of these salts near the soil surface. For civil engineering purposes, besides the obvious use of drainage for dewatering construction sites, drainage is required to increase the strength of soil for traffic and foundations, and also to reduce seepage pressures to avoid slope failures.

The objectives of installing a land drainage system are therefore known in terms of the required soil conditions. The attainment of such conditions is determined by the laws of soil physics.

2.2 Physical state of soil water

Soils are complex porous materials made up of solid particles of varying sizes and shapes, packed together to form a tortuous interconnecting pore space in which soil water resides and moves. When the pore space between granular soil particles is not completely saturated and contains both water and air, water in the pores is drawn into the smaller interstices, with the interfaces between the water and the air forming curved menisci as a result of surface tension forces. In fine-textured clay soils, water is held between charged plates, giving rise to swelling and shrinking that affect the size of the larger pores between aggregates. Water is also absorbed onto the surfaces of soil particles, held by van der Waals' forces.

The ease of water movement through soils depends on the size and distribution of the interconnecting pore channels containing water, and so becomes less as the water-filled pore space is reduced by saturation. While the movement of water in the pore space takes place according to the laws of hydrodynamics in the microscopic pore channels, it is generally only possible to make macroscopic measurements that provide measures of some average state of the water in the soil pores. Calculations of soil-water movement are based on theory developed from macroscopic studies of water movement in porous materials, although a consideration of the microscopic behaviour of water in the soil pores leads to an understanding of the physical processes involved.

2.2.1 *Soil-water pressure*

If a pipe with a small filtered opening at its base is inserted into a saturated soil (Figure 2.1a), water enters the pipe until the bulk water in the pipe is in equilibrium with the water in the soil pores near the filter. The level of water

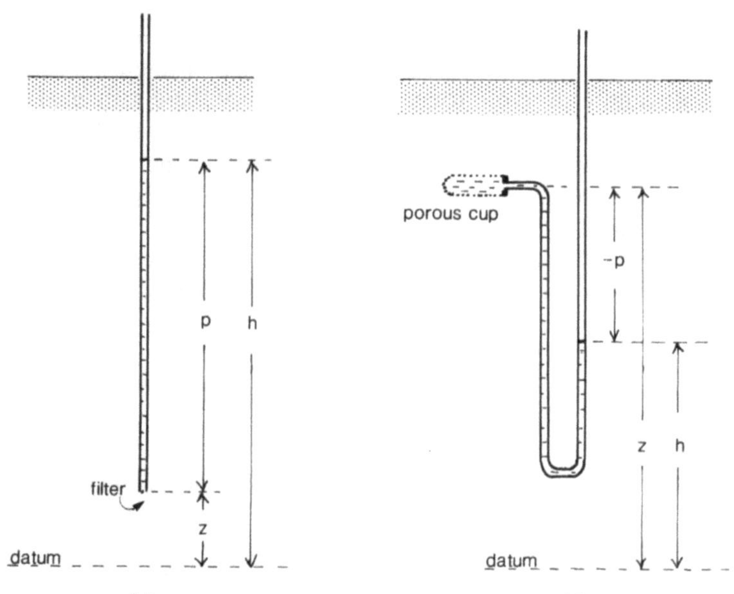

Figure 2.1 The measurement of soil-water pressures (a) with piezometers (p positive) and (b) with tensiometers (p negative).

in the pipe then is at a height p above the opening at its base and at a height h above some datum level. The soil water is therefore at a pressure in excess of the atmospheric pressure. If the opening is at a height z above the datum:

$$h = p + z \tag{2.1}$$

where p is the *soil-water pressure head* and h is the *hydraulic head* measured relative to the datum level. Both are potentials expressed in units of work per unit weight of soil water, the *pressure potential* and the *hydraulic potential* respectively; h is sometimes referred to as the *piezometric head,* and pipes used in this way are known as *piezometers.* If, on the other hand, a piezometer is inserted into an unsaturated soil, no water will enter it, indicating that the water in the pores of such soils is at a pressure less than atmospheric. However, if a manometer capable of registering negative pressure heads relative to atmospheric is in communication with the soil water via a porous membrane that can hold a negative pressure without air bubbling through it, the equilibrium head in the manometer will be below the level of the porous membrane in contact with the soil (Figure 2.1b). The soil water in unsaturated soils is therefore held at a pressure less than atmospheric. Instruments that measure negative soil-water pressure heads via porous membranes are known as *tensiometers.* Again the hydraulic head is given by eqn 2.1 as the sum of the soil-water pressure head p (in this case a negative quantity) and the height z of the position of the porous membrane in contact with the soil; p is sometimes referred to as the *matric potential,* and, to avoid the negative sign, $-p$ referred to as the *matric suction.*

2.2.2 *Soil-moisture characteristics*

The pressure-head drop Δp across the curved menisci of the lenses of water held between soil particles in unsaturated soils, causing tensiometers to record negative pressures, is given by the Laplace–Young equation:

$$\Delta p = \frac{\sigma}{\rho g}\left(\frac{1}{r_1} + \frac{1}{r_2}\right) \tag{2.2}$$

where σ is the surface tension and ρ the density of water, g the acceleration due to gravity, and r_1 and r_2 are the principal radii of curvature of the surface of the air–water meniscus. As soils become less saturated with the water drawn into the smaller pores and interstices between the soil particles, the curvature of the menisci becomes smaller, resulting in larger values of Δp. In the case of water held in fine-textured clay soils, the force required to keep the charged clay plates together increases as the plate separation decreases, so that again the soil-water pressure difference increases with decrease in water content. Δp is the soil-water pressure head $-p$ as registered by a tensiometer. The relationship between the soil-water content and the soil-water pressure is a characteristic of the soil, reflecting the pore-size distribution on account of eqn 2.2, and is often referred to as the *soil-moisture characteristic*. However, this is not a simple monotonic relationship but is hysteretic. The reason for this is the complex geometry of the pore space that does not allow large pores to drain until Δp becomes large enough to draw the menisci through smaller channels connecting larger pores, and conversely does not allow water to fill smaller pores via larger ones until Δp becomes small enough. Thus, water in the pore space is contained in different configurations, depending on the past history of wetting and draining. In field drainage work, the drainage arm of the moisture characteristic is the most important and is often referred to as the *soil-water retention curve*.

The measurement of the soil moisture characteristics (Klute, 1986; Smith and Mullins, 1991) is usually done on soil cores removed from the field with minimum disturbance. The cores can be conveniently placed on tension tables and in soil-water pressure apparatuses, and the equilibrium soil-water

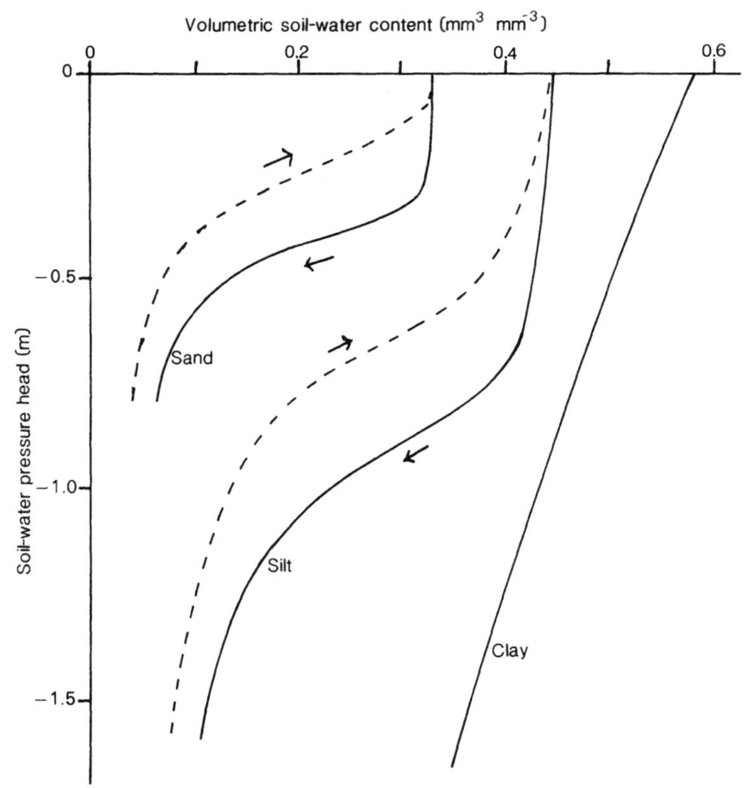

Figure 2.2 Moisture characteristic curves for various soils.

contents determined at the applied soil-water pressure. Alternatively, measurements of the soil-water content and soil-water pressure down the soil profile in the field when the soil is draining enable field measurements of the soil-water retention curve to be made on different soil layers. Examples of moisture characteristics are shown in Figure 2.2.

2.2.3 *The water table*

Piezometers and tensiometers in the field record the soil-water pressure heads at their particular locations. When piezometers operate, showing positive soil-water pressures relative to atmospheric pressure, they are located in the groundwater zone where the soil is saturated except perhaps for small air bubbles in the water. Tensiometers record soil-water pressures less than atmospheric in unsaturated soil. The boundary between the groundwater and unsaturated soil-water zones where the soil-water pressure is atmospheric ($p = 0$) is known as the *water table* or *phreatic surface*. This boundary is an arbitrary division as far as the soil-water flow is concerned, since the flow region includes both the saturated and unsaturated zones with the flow continuous across the boundary between the two. However, the water table does have a great significance in land drainage, since water will only discharge into drain pipes when the soil-water pressure is greater than atmospheric. Drain pipes installed in unsaturated soils cannot run and are ineffectual.

2.3 Water flow in soils

If piezometers and tensiometers installed in a soil register different heads of water at different positions, water moves from positions where the head is high to those where it is low. In Figure 2.3 are shown some situations that occur in the field. The movement of water caused by differences in head is resisted by viscous forces that increase with the decrease in size of the complex tortuous pore channels. In the case of unsaturated soils, the pore channels containing air are non-conducting so that the remaining smaller more tortuous channels offer greater resistance to flow.

2.3.1 *Darcy's law—saturated soils*

In 1856 Darcy published the results of experiments on water flow down columns of sand. These showed that the rate of flow Q was directly proportional to the head difference, Δh, causing the flow and the cross-sectional area A of the column, and inversely proportional to its length L. Thus:

$$Q = kA\Delta h/L \tag{2.3}$$

where the proportionality constant k has units of velocity and is known as

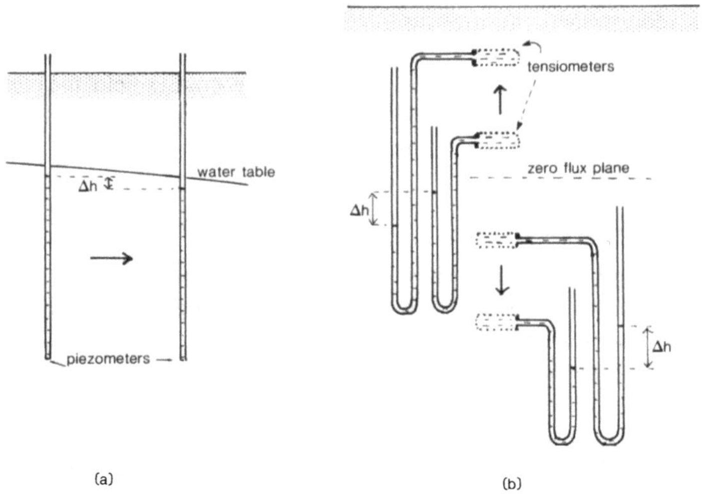

Figure 2.3 Soil-water movement caused by hydraulic head gradients. (a) Lateral groundwater movement; (b) vertical soil-water movement, showing upward movement near the soil surface and downward movement at depth, separated by a zero-flux plane.

the *hydraulic conductivity* of the porous material. Equation 2.3 is Darcy's law, which can be written in terms of the flow velocity v per unit area as:

$$v = -k \operatorname{grad} h \tag{2.4}$$

The negative sign in eqn 2.4 shows that the flow is in the direction of decreasing head. Since with flow in saturated non-shrinking soils there can be no increase or decrease of water content:

$$\operatorname{div} v = 0 \tag{2.5}$$

and since k in such soils is a constant:

$$\nabla^2 h = 0 \tag{2.6}$$

which is Laplace's equation. Equation 2.6 can be used to obtain distributions of h with given boundary conditions and then eqn 2.4 used to obtain the flow pattern.

Various methods are used to determine the hydraulic conductivity of saturated soils (Klute, 1986; Smith and Mullins, 1991). In the laboratory measurements are made using permeameters containing soil cores, removed carefully from the field, that essentially repeat Darcy's experiments. *In situ* field determinations use a variety of techniques that measure the rate of flow of water taken up or removed from the soil under known boundary conditions that allow the hydraulic conductivity to be obtained from solutions of eqn 2.6. Since hydraulic conductivity values are very sensitive to any cracks and fissures that can form during core collection, field measurements that minimise soil disturbances are preferable.

By analogy with flow in bundles of capillary tubes, a model of soil used in many early studies of soil-water flow, the contribution to the hydraulic conductivity of a pore of radius r would be proportional to r^2, so that generally it may be concluded that the finer the soil texture the smaller the hydraulic conductivity. However, the structures of soils found in the field often have larger pore channels surrounding soil aggregates, and this precludes any general relationship between hydraulic conductivity and particle size distribution. Because of this macrostructure found in many soils, it is important that measurements of hydraulic conductivity are done on samples large enough to encompass a volume of soil that is representative, that is on a sample larger than the *representative elementary volume* that includes these larger pore channels. Drainage installations themselves can act as large permeameters that sample the large volume of soil between drain lines. Typical values for hydraulic conductivity range from 10 m d^{-1} or more for saturated coarse-textured and well-structured soils down to 10 mm d^{-1} or less for fine-textured unstructured soils.

2.3.2 *Richards' equation—unsaturated soils*

Richards (1931) argued that the flow of water in unsaturated soils was similar to that in saturated soils except that there were fewer conducting pores. Thus Darcy's law would be obeyed with a hydraulic conductivity value greatly reduced because of the absence of the larger pores that empty first. Richards also recognised that the wetting and draining of the soils provide a component of flow. In an inert porous material that does not swell and shrink:

$$\frac{\partial \theta}{\partial t} = -\operatorname{div} v \tag{2.7}$$

where θ is volumetric moisture content. Since v is given by Darcy's law (eqn 2.4), it follows that:

$$\frac{\partial \theta}{\partial t} = \operatorname{div}(k \operatorname{grad} h) = \operatorname{div}(k \operatorname{grad} p) + \frac{\partial k}{\partial z} \tag{2.8}$$

where k is now the hydraulic conductivity of the unsaturated soil. Equation 2.8 is a form of the equation derived by Richards. In this equation the relationship between θ and p is given by the moisture characteristic: the hydraulic conductivity k decreases rapidly as the soil desaturates, and can be given as a function of either θ or p; the $k(\theta)$ function shows little hysteresis, whereas the $k(p)$ function shows more, as illustrated in the examples of relationships shown in Figure 2.4. The measurement of the hydraulic conductivity of

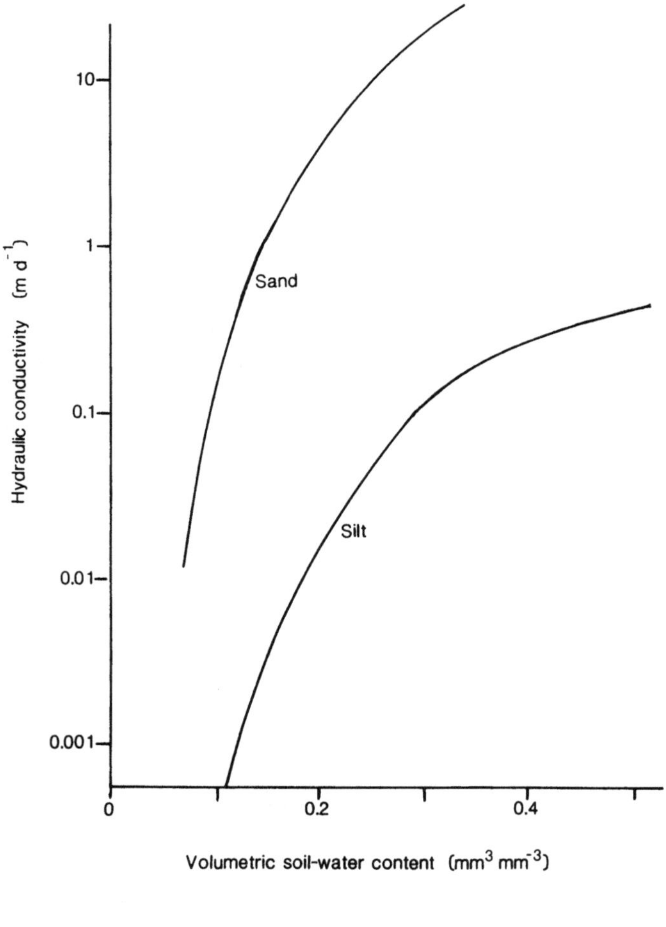

Figure 2.4 The variation of hydraulic conductivity with (a) soil-water content.

unsaturated soils is not easy, particularly in the field. Both steady-state and non-steady-state methods are used (Klute, 1986; Smith and Mullins, 1991).

For steady-state conditions when θ and h do not change with time, eqn 2.8 becomes:

$$\operatorname{div}(k \operatorname{grad} h) = 0 \tag{2.9}$$

It is seen that Laplace's equation (eqn 2.6) is a special case of eqn 2.9 with k a constant.

The accurate relationships between θ, p and k have to be given in graphical, as in Figure 2.4, or numerical form. However, various empirical relationships for $k(\theta)$ and $k(p)$ as well as those for $p(\theta)$, usually for the draining relationships,

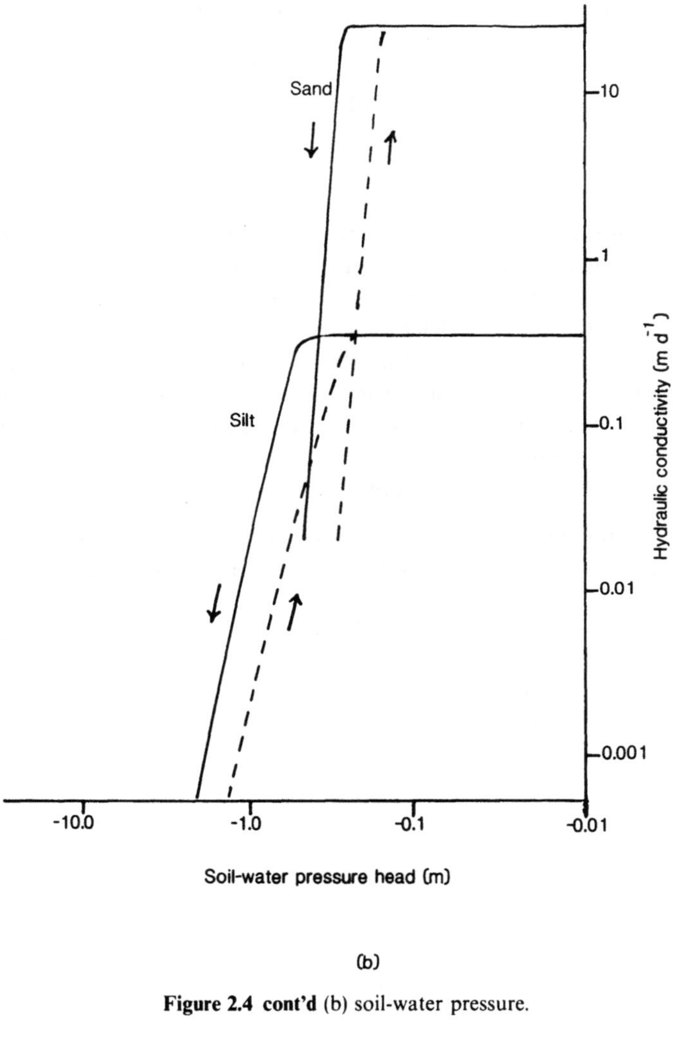

(b)

Figure 2.4 cont'd (b) soil-water pressure.

are often used to facilitate solutions of eqns 2.8 and 2.9. For example, $k(p)$ is often found to be well represented by an exponential relationship:

$$k(p) = k_0 \exp(cp) \tag{2.10}$$

where k_0 is the hydraulic conductivity of the saturated soil and c is a constant, that allows analytical solutions to many two- and three-dimensional steady-state problems; or a power-law relationship:

$$k(p) = a'/[1 + b'(-p)^{c'}] \tag{2.11}$$

where a', b' and c' are constants. $k(\theta)$ is often described by:

$$k(\theta) = k_0 \theta^{c''} \tag{2.12}$$

and the moisture release curve $p(\theta)$ by a simple power law equation:

$$p(\theta) = a''(\theta_0 - \theta)^n/\theta^m \qquad (2.13)$$

where c'', a'', m and n are constants, and θ_0 is the saturated soil-water content.

2.3.3 *Boundary conditions*

The pattern of soil-water flow is determined by the values of hydraulic head that occur at the boundaries of the given soil region, and by the soil–water relationships in unsaturated soils. The boundary values are used in solving the general flow equation (Richards' equation [eqn 2.8], which becomes Laplace's equation [eqn 2.6] for steady groundwater flow) to obtain distributions of p or h and θ, and of the flow using eqn 2.4, for a given situation. The hydraulic head value itself may be imposed or may be the result of an imposed flux that produces a gradient of the head h. Figure 2.5 illustrates various types of boundary conditions involved in soil-water flow problems:

(a) On a ponded soil surface, as for ponded surface infiltration and ponded surface drainage, $p = 0$ and $h = 0$ if the head is measured from the soil surface.
(b) For constant-rate infiltration through the soil surface at a rate F that does not saturate the soil so that $p < 0$, the prescribed flux gives $\partial h/\partial z = -F/k$ through the surface.
(c) At a water table there is a mixed boundary condition with $p = 0$ and

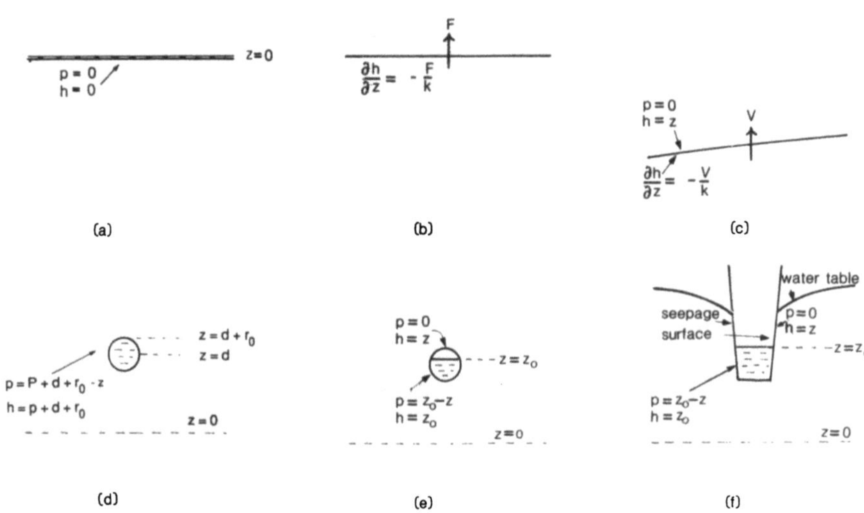

Figure 2.5 Boundary condition to soil-water flow problems. (a) Ponded surface; (b) flux condition at the surface; (c) water table condition; (d) drain running full; (e) drain running partially full; (f) surface of seepage above water levels in ditches.

$h = z$, and with the prescribed flux V between the groundwater region and unsaturated soil-water region giving $\partial h/\partial z = -V/k$.

(d) On the walls of a drain installed below a water table and running full so that $p = P$ at its top ($P > 0$), $p = P + d + r_0 - z$ and $h = P + d + r_0$, where d is the height of the drain axis and r_0 is the radius of the drain.

(e) On the walls of a drain installed below a water table but not running full, a seepage surface where $p = 0$ and $h = z$ exists above the water level. Below the water level, $p = z_0 - z$ and $h = z_0$, where z_0 is the height of the water level.

(f) On the walls of a water-filled ditch, water seeps out of the saturated soil above the ditch-water level at height z_0 through a surface of seepage where $p = 0$ and $h = z$. Below the water level, $p = z_0 - z$ and $h = z_0$.

2.3.4 *Saturated groundwater and unsaturated soil-water regions*

In the field situation involving both saturated groundwater and unsaturated soil-water regions, eqn 2.8 can be used to determine the non-steady-state flow behaviour throughout the complete flow region when the boundary conditions are known. Generally, however, this is difficult and the flows in the two regions are treated separately, with the water table being a common boundary, as illustrated in Figure 2.6. In the unsaturated region above the water table, the decrease in hydraulic conductivity accompanying the decrease in soil-water content with height causes the flow to be almost vertical (Childs, 1945), so that the soil-water behaviour can be obtained from solutions of the one-dimensional Richards' equation:

$$\frac{\partial \theta}{\partial t} = \frac{\partial}{\partial z}\left(k\frac{\partial p}{\partial z}\right) + \frac{\partial k}{\partial z} \tag{2.14}$$

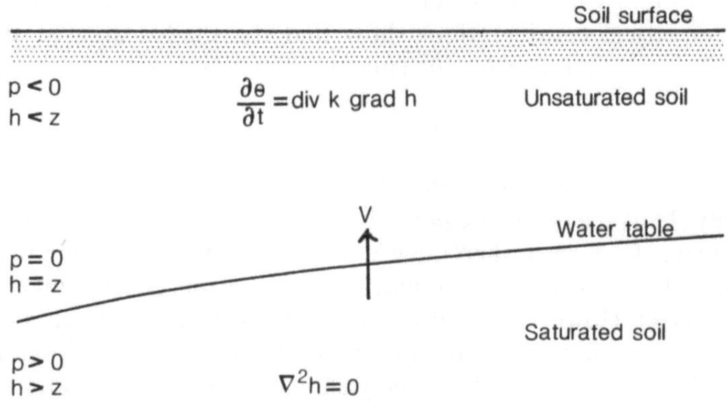

Figure 2.6 The complete flow region, including both saturated and usaturated zones.

instead of the more complicated three-dimensional form of eqn 2.8. In the groundwater region there is generally a lateral component of flow, so that the two- or three-dimensional Laplace equation (eqn 2.6) has to be solved.

The common boundary condition at the water table is the mixed boundary condition (c) of section 2.3.3 with $p = 0$ and the given flux passing between the unsaturated zone and groundwater region. This flux is given by the product of the hydraulic conductivity and head gradient, which is generally not easily determined. It may, however, be considered to be made up of a component arising from the flux through the soil surface caused by surface precipitation and evaporation less any runoff, and a component arising from any draining or wetting of the unsaturated zone that is usually accompanied by a change in the water table height. Use can then be made of the concept of *specific yield*, which is defined as the amount of water draining per unit area from the unsaturated zone per unit fall of the water table height. The flux V_H through the water table as a result of changes in the soil-water content is thus given by:

$$V_H = S\frac{\partial H}{\partial t} \tag{2.15}$$

where S is the specific yield and H the water table height at time t.

The specific yield is often equated to the *drainable porosity*, i.e. the amount of water drained from a soil profile, initially in equilibrium with the water table, when the water table falls a unit distance and the profile is again restored to an equilibrium condition. The drainable porosity is dependent on the proximity of the water table to the soil surface. This is illustrated in Figure 2.7, which shows the equilibrium soil-water profiles with a steady surface flux when the water table is lowered from a depth H below the soil surface to a depth $H + \delta H$. The shaded area is the water released from the soil profile through the water table for this water table fall. Since the profiles are in equilibrium with a water table, they are the same (see section 2.4.1). Simple geometrical considerations show that the shaded area is equal to $(\theta_0 - \theta_s)\delta H$ in the limit as $\delta H \to 0$. Thus:

$$S = \theta_0 - \theta_s \tag{2.16}$$

where θ_0 and θ_s are the water contents at saturation and at the soil surface respectively. Thus the drainable porosity is the air content at the soil surface, which increases from zero when the water table is close to it and approaches a constant value for deep water tables; this latter value is often taken to be the specific yield. However, because in practice the water table does not fall slowly enough to maintain the equilibrium soil-water profile, the development of the profiles is complex, and specific yield values have been found to vary between zero and very large values (dos Santos Jùnior and Youngs, 1969). In the field, values of the specific yield may be obtained from observations on the

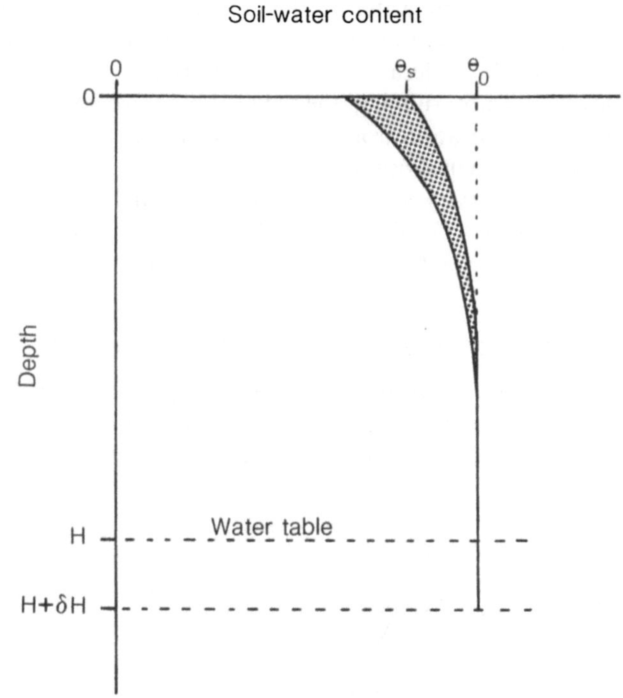

Figure 2.7 Equilibrium soil-water profiles above a shallow water table.

water table behaviour and drain discharge by observing the rate of discharge at the same time as the rate of fall of the water table.

2.4 Soil-water movement above water tables

The water movement in the unsaturated soil-water region above a water table depends on the conditions imposed at the surface by meteorological conditions, in the root zone by the water abstraction by plants, and at the water table, that are themselves interdependent. In particular, the position and shape of the water table develop depending on the distributed flux across this surface, caused by soil-water changes, meteorological conditions and plant-water use, as well as on the sinks and sources in the groundwater region. With the water movement almost vertical above water tables, so that the soil-water behaviour is described by the one-dimensional form of Richards' equation (eqn 2.14), estimates of the soil-water profile development can be obtained in principle if the water table position is known together with the boundary conditions.

When rainfall rates are high, water tables build up to near the surface and drains run fast. After the cessation of such periods of heavy rainfall, water tables fall and the soil above desaturates, and the drain discharge decreases. When the drains finally stop running, the water table throughout is at drain level, and, provided evaporation from the surface is negligible, the water in the unsaturated soil is in equilibrium with the water table. The soil is then said to be at *field capacity*. The soil can then lose water further through evaporation and plant use. The decrease in the amount of water held in the soil profile below the state of field capacity is termed the *soil-water deficit*.

2.4.1 *Steady-state flow between soil surface and water table*

With steady one-dimensional vertical flow, the flow per unit area V is given everywhere by Darcy's law as the product of the hydraulic conductivity at the prevailing soil-water content and the hydraulic potential gradient at the

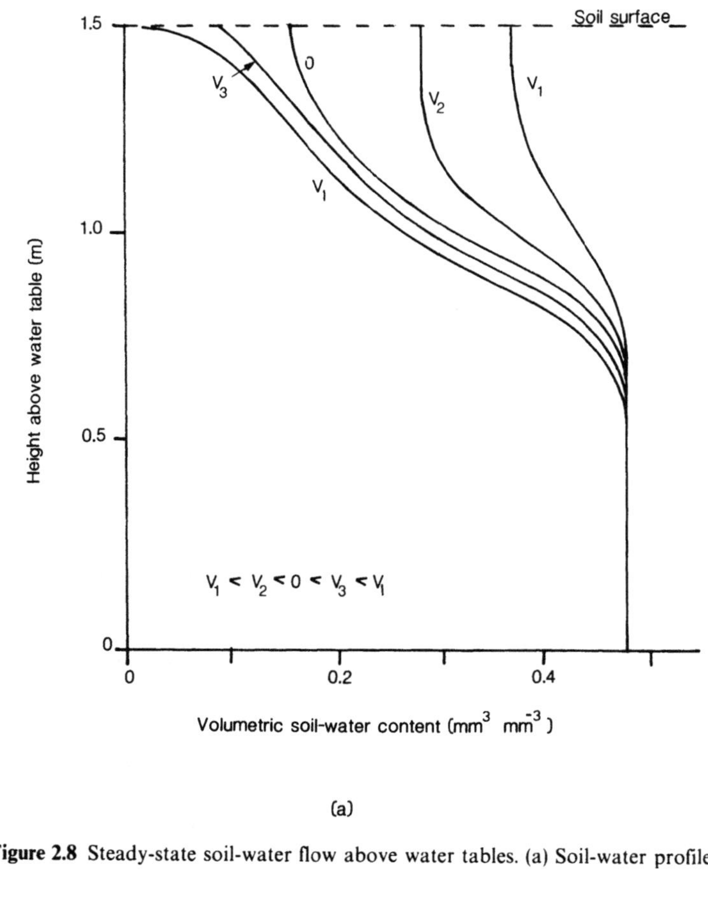

Figure 2.8 Steady-state soil-water flow above water tables. (a) Soil-water profiles.

given position. Thus:

$$V = -k\frac{\partial p}{\partial z} = -k\left(\frac{\partial h}{\partial z} + 1\right) \qquad (2.17)$$

Since at the water table $p = 0$, integration of eqn 2.17 gives the height above the water table z where the soil-water pressure has the value p:

$$z = -\int_0^p \frac{\mathrm{d}p}{1 + V/k(p)} \qquad (2.18)$$

This can be integrated numerically for any $k(p)$ relationship, or analytically if $k(p)$ is given in a simple algebraic form such as eqn 2.10. For a steady-state rainfall rate (V negative), this gives soil-water pressures and soil-water

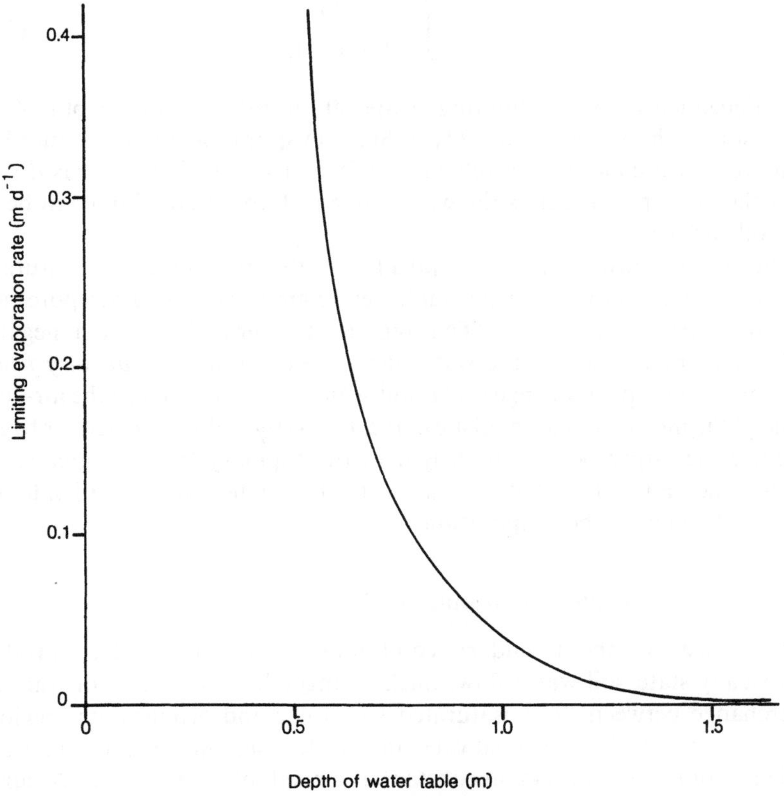

Figure 2.8 cont'd (b) the limiting evaporation rate plotted against the depth of the water table below the soil surface.

contents that approach constant values as the height above the water table becomes large, as illustrated in Figure 2.8(a); the constant values are those corresponding to a hydraulic conductivity equal to the steady rainfall rate. When there is no flow so that the profile is at field capacity, with $V=0$ in eqn 2.18, $z=-p$ everywhere. Thus the profile corresponds to the moisture characteristic curve. With steady upward flow, often termed *capillary rise*, from a water table to the soil surface where it is removed by plant use or evaporation (V positive), the profiles are below field capacity. In this case there is a maximum flow rate V_l that can be sustained for a given depth of water table below the soil surface before the soil-water pressure approaches a large negative value and the soil properties, rather than meteorological conditions, limit the capillary rise. The depth Z for which the soil becomes limiting for the flux V_l is.

$$Z = -\int_0^\infty \frac{\mathrm{d}p}{1 + V_l/k(p)} \tag{2.19}$$

The dependence of the limiting evaporation rate on the depth Z for a silt soil is shown in Figure 2.8(b). Since evaporation rates produced by meteorological conditions rarely exceed $10\,\mathrm{mm\,d^{-1}}$, soil conditions do not limit the evaporation unless the water table is deeper than about 1 m below the soil surface.

The profiles shown in Figure 2.8(a) all show that the soil remains saturated for some height above the water table before air enters the larger pores and the soil starts to desaturate. This region of saturated soil at a negative soil-water pressure above the water table is known as the *capillary fringe*. The top of the capillary fringe is at a soil-water pressure equal to the air-entry value of the moisture characteristic curve, that is the value at which air begins to enter the larger pores. The height of the capillary fringe is greater the smaller the value of V, that is it is greater the higher the rainfall rate and smaller the greater the evaporation rate.

2.4.2 *Non-steady-state flow to water tables*

Any changes in the boundary conditions at the soil surface produce non-steady-state soil-water flow. Such changes have an effect on the flux interchange between the unsaturated soil-water and groundwater regions. Since the extent of the groundwater region depends on this flux, the water table position does not remain constant as a result of such changes. Accurate simulations can be made using numerical procedures to solve eqn 2.14. However, using approximations based on the concept of specific yield, the water table movement can be more simply computed as a result of changing meteorological conditions (see section 2.7), with the non-steady-state profiles assumed to be a succession of average steady-state ones.

2.4.3 *Infiltration and runoff*

Infiltration is the downward entry of water into soils through the soil surface. It is thus given by the product of the hydraulic conductivity and the hydraulic head gradient at the soil surface. If the incident rate is such that the soil-water pressure at the surface becomes positive, the surface will pond and runoff, that is the difference between the incident rainfall rate and the infiltration rate, will occur. Infiltration and runoff are therefore controlled by the hydraulic soil properties of the surface layer of the soil.

Infiltration equations that relate the cumulative infiltration and time generally refer to the water absorption from a ponded surface into soil that is relatively dry to an appreciable depth, and do not consider the situation of the presence of a water table. They give an upper limit to the amount of water the soil can accept. The problem is well posed for the solution of Richards' equation when the soil is uniform. The simplest equation which is physically based is Philip's (1957) two-term equation:

$$i = A\sqrt{t} + Bt \tag{2.20}$$

where i is the cumulative infiltration at time t, A is the *sorptivity* (the proportionality constant between the cumulative infiltration and the square root of time at early times) and B is the infiltration rate at large times that is identified with the hydraulic conductivity k_0 of the saturated soil. An early physically based infiltration equation was that of Green and Ampt (1911):

$$i - a \ln(1 + i/a) = bt \tag{2.21}$$

where $a = -h_f \Delta\theta$ and $b = k_0$ where h_f is the soil-water pressure head at the wetting front and $\Delta\theta$ is the difference in water content between the saturated and initial state of the soil.

When water infiltrates into a soil at a constant rate, the surface will not pond until the infiltration has gone on for some time. The time to ponding t_p is related to the hydraulic properties of the soil by the equation:

$$t_p = -\frac{h_f \Delta\theta}{F_0(F_0/k_0 - 1)} = \frac{A^2}{2F_0(F_0 - k_0)} \tag{2.22}$$

where F_0 is the steady infiltration rate, which has to be greater than k_0 for ponding to occur.

If a water table is present, the advancing infiltration front meets the top of the capillary fringe of saturated soil above the water table after some time. When this occurs, the water table, which up until this point has shown negligible response to the surface infiltration, responds with a rapid rise in level. The time delay in water table response is very dependent on initial soil conditions.

2.5 Steady-state groundwater flow beneath a water table

2.5.1 *Exact solutions by potential theory*

By solving Laplace's equation (eqn 2.6) with the boundary conditions of the groundwater region, exact solutions to steady-state groundwater flow problems can be obtained. A ponded surface presents a relatively simple situation whose solution is common to many other branches of physics and can be found, for example, by the method of images. However, the potential problem presented by the groundwater situation with a water table is unique to groundwater hydrology with its mixed boundary conditions at the water table whose position and shape emerge as part of the solution. In this case, solutions for two-dimensional flows can often be found using the hodograph method and employing conformal transformations.

Instead of using mathematical methods to solve Laplace's equation, groundwater problems, as with other problems that are described by the equation, can be solved with electric analogues (those using either graphited paper, conducting liquids or resistance networks) or Hele–Shaw viscous flow parallel plate analogues (Karplus, 1958). Also, numerical solutions using finite difference methods (see, for example, Roache, 1972) that are analogous to resistance networks or finite element methods (see, for example, Zienkiewicz, 1971) can often be obtained easily.

2.5.2 *Dupuit–Forchheimer approximate analysis*

The flow in shallow, unconfined groundwater regions that overlie a horizontal impermeable barrier is predominantly horizontal. This implies that the equipotentials in the groundwater region are almost vertical and that the potential gradient causing this predominantly lateral flow is given by the gradient of the water table. These are the assumptions that are used in the Dupuit–Forchheimer analysis of groundwater flow in unconfined shallow aquifers.

If the water table height measured from the horizontal impermeable barrier at the position (x, y) is H, then the gradients of the head over the whole depth of the groundwater region at (x, y) in the x and y directions are $\partial H/\partial x$ and $\partial H/\partial y$ respectively, so that the components of flow Q_x and Q_y are from Darcy's law:

$$Q_x = -kH\frac{\partial H}{\partial x}, \qquad Q_y = -kH\frac{\partial H}{\partial y} \tag{2.23}$$

If there is a flux V measured positive upwards through the water table at (x, y), then:

$$\frac{\partial Q_x}{\partial x} + \frac{\partial Q_y}{\partial y} = -V \tag{2.24}$$

and therefore:

$$\frac{\partial}{\partial x}\left(kH\frac{\partial H}{\partial x}\right)+\frac{\partial}{\partial y}\left(kH\frac{\partial H}{\partial y}\right)=V \tag{2.25}$$

Thus, given the boundary values of H on a given region, the water table height over the whole region can be estimated from solutions of eqn 2.25 and the horizontal seepage of groundwater determined using eqn 2.23, knowing the hydraulic conductivity k of the saturated soil.

The assumptions in the Dupuit–Forchheimer analysis are not self-consistent, since the flow cannot be truly horizontal with a water table having a gradient to cause the flow. Also, in using the analysis, water tables are assumed to be drawn down to the levels of free water in channels acting as sinks and the existence of surfaces of seepage are ignored. However, the concern expressed by Muskat (1937) concerning the 'widespread and indiscriminate use' of the Dupuit–Forchheimer analysis is not so great today since in many cases the analysis does give exact horizontal seepage rates.

2.5.3 *Seepage analysis*

Instead of making the assumption of horizontal flow as in the Dupuit–Forchheimer analysis, the horizontal components of flow can be exactly expressed by:

$$Q_x=-\frac{\partial E}{\partial x},\quad Q_y=-\frac{\partial E}{\partial y} \tag{2.26}$$

where E is the seepage potential defined by:

$$E=\int_0^H k(h-z)\,\mathrm{d}z=\int_0^H kp\,\mathrm{d}z \tag{2.27}$$

where h is the hydraulic head at (x, y, z) measured with the datum at $z=0$ on the impermeable barrier, and p is the soil-water pressure at (x, y, z). Thus, using eqn 2.24:

$$\frac{\partial^2 E}{\partial x^2}+\frac{\partial^2 E}{\partial y^2}=V \tag{2.28}$$

Solutions of eqn 2.28 with the boundary values for a given flow problem give exact values of E over the region. Exact horizontal seepage rates are given by eqns 2.26. On both entrance and exit vertical faces of vertical channels that extend down to an impermeable barrier, the seepage potential E is equal to $kH^2/2$, even taking into account the seepage surface where $p=0$ on exit faces. For a flux boundary condition, $\partial E/\partial n$ is given, where n is the direction of the normal to the boundary. Thus at a watershed, $\partial E/\partial n=0$, whereas at the periphery of a well being pumped at a rate Q, $\partial E/\partial r=Q/2\pi r_0$, where r_0 is the radius of the well. The seepage analysis, however, does not give the water table height over the groundwater region, although physical arguments can often be used to locate this surface between limits (Youngs, 1965; 1980).

It is seen that the approximate Dupuit–Forchheimer equation (eqn 2.25) becomes the same as the seepage equation (eqn 2.28) if $kH^2/2 = E$. Thus for situations where boundary values of $E = kH^2/2$, as on vertically sided channels extending in depth to an impermeable barrier, values of $kH^2/2$ given by the Dupuit–Forchheimer solutions are exact values of E. Since from eqn 2.26 the exact horizontal seepage rate is the gradient of E and that given by the Dupuit–Forchheimer analysis is the gradient of $kH^2/2$ (see eqn 2.23), the approximate analysis gives correct horizontal seepage rates. The approximate analysis therefore often gives fortuitously exact flow rates, just as the seepage analysis does, for example that through earth banks (Youngs, 1980). It can also give estimates of the water table height with a high precision except in the vicinity of exit faces (Youngs, 1990).

2.6 Steady-state groundwater flow to drains

Land-drainage installations are used to alleviate various groundwater problems that occur in the field. The boundary conditions for the groundwater flow for different steady-state situations allow particular solutions of Laplace's equation (eqn 2.6) which can be used for the engineering design of optimum drainage installations.

2.6.1 *Ponded surface drainage*

In arid regions where irrigation is necessary for agriculture, land surfaces are often kept ponded for periods of time in order to leach salts that have accumulated near the soil surface as a result of water moving upwards through the soil profile to supply the water lost to the atmosphere by evaporation. Also, in humid areas high rainfall rates will pond the surface of drained lands.

The situation of groundwater flow in an infinitely deep soil from a ponded surface to a horizontal cylindrical drain of radius r_0 at depth d below the soil surface is the same as if the flow originated from a cylindrical source of radius r_0 located in a fictitious semi-infinite soil region above the ponded surface as the mirror image of the drain sink (see Figure 2.9a). The cylindrical sink and source can be regarded as a line sink and source that each produce a potential (or head) at some point P, at a distance r from the centre of the drain and r' from that of the fictitious source, given by $Q/2\pi k \ln(r/r_0)$ and $-Q/2\pi k \ln(r'/r_0)$ respectively, where Q is the flow rate into unit length of drain. The potential h_P at the point P as a result of the combination of the

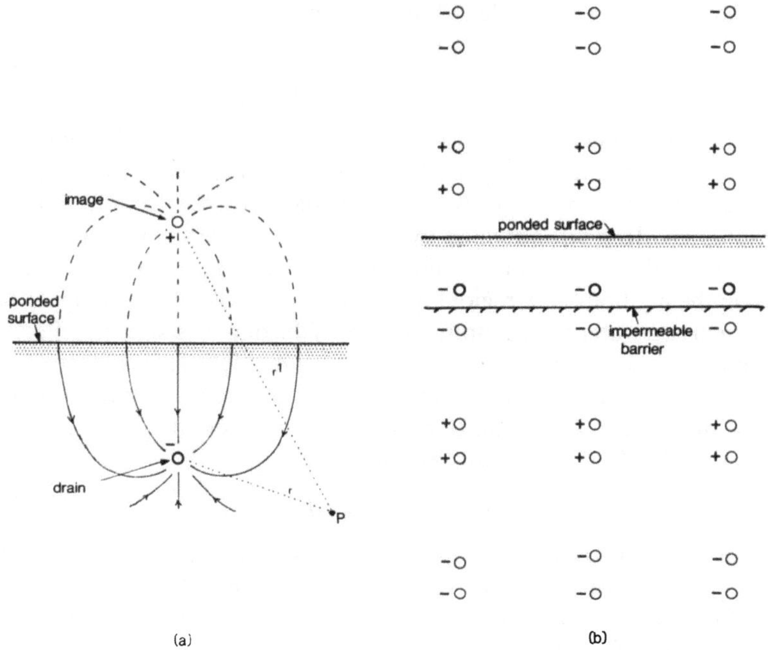

Figure 2.9 Ponded surface drainage. (a) Flow to a single cylindrical drain; (b) array of image sources and sinks to calculate flow to a parallel system of pipe drains from a ponded surface in a soil bounded below by a horizontal impermeable barrier.

sink and source is the sum of the potentials produced individually, so that:

$$h_P = \frac{Q}{2\pi k}\ln\left(\frac{r}{r_0}\right) - \frac{Q}{2\pi k}\ln\left(\frac{r'}{r_0}\right) + C \tag{2.29}$$

The constant C in eqn 2.29 depends on the datum level, which can be taken as the drain axis. Since at the ponded surface the water pressure is atmospheric so that the head is the height d above the datum level, we have:

$$d = \frac{Q}{2\pi k}\ln\left(\frac{d}{r_0}\right) - \frac{Q}{2\pi k}\ln\left(\frac{d}{r_0}\right) + C \tag{2.30}$$

so that $C = d$. If the drain is running just full so that the pressure of the water at the top of the drain is atmospheric, then the head at this point is r_0 so that:

$$r_0 = -\frac{Q}{2\pi k}\ln\left(\frac{2d - r_0}{r_0}\right) + d \tag{2.31}$$

giving the flow rate per unit length of drain as:

$$Q = \frac{2\pi k(d - r_0)}{\ln(2d/r_0 - 1)} \simeq \frac{2\pi kd}{\ln(2d/r_0)} \quad (2.32)$$

An array of parallel drain pipes can be treated in exactly the same way with the potential at a point given by the sum of potentials of all the sinks and image sources considered as line sinks and sources. If the flow region is not infinitely deep but bounded by a lower impermeable barrier, the flow is then exactly the same as in an infinite region with image sources and sinks located in the fictitious flow regions above and below. While an equipotential surface such as a water table requires images of the opposite sign on reflection, an impermeable barrier requires images of the same sign. This is illustrated in Figure 2.9(b). For the situation of an array of drain pipes of radius r_0 spaced $2D$ apart at a depth d in a soil terminated by an impermeable barrier at a depth s, then the flow Q per unit length of pipe is:

$$Q = 4\pi k(d - r_0)/f \quad (2.33)$$

where f is a factor given by an infinite series of terms involving r_0/D, d/D and s/D that converges rapidly (Kirkham, 1949; Luthin, 1957). The problem of ponded water drainage is also easily solved using the method of conformal transformations. Then the factor f in eqn 2.33 is given in terms of elliptic functions (Youngs, 1982).

2.6.2. *Water table drainage*

When drains are installed in lands to control water table heights that would otherwise be unacceptably high over long periods of time because of rainfall incident on the surface, the water table is highest at the watershed between drains, being drawn down towards the drains. There are two points to note concerning the control of the soil-water regime by such drainage installations. First, although the water table at the watershed is lowered as the spacing between drains decreases, no drainage installation, however intense, can prevent the water table rising to the soil surface and ponding if the rainfall rate is sufficiently high. Secondly, the soil-water pressure head at the surface can only be reduced by the drains themselves to that given by the depth of the water table, and this is usually not sufficient for the soil to have sufficient strength for traffic. The drains can only remove water in excess of field capacity. Meteorological conditions have to be relied on to remove extra water by evaporation and thereby reduce further the soil-water pressure at the surface.

2.6.2.1 *Drains laid on impermeable barrier.* The steady-state water movement in lands intersected by drainage ditches dug to an underlying horizontal impermeable barrier is simply analysed using the seepage analysis for the case of steady rainfall incident on the soil surface. For parallel ditches spaced $2D$ apart with a ditch-water level H_0 above the impermeable barrier (Figure 2.10a), $E = kH_0^2/2$ at the ditch and $\partial E/\partial x = 0$ at the watershed midway between ditches, so that solving eqn 2.28 with a steady rainfall rate q ($q = -V$):

$$E_m - E_0 = qD^2/2 \tag{2.34}$$

where the subscripts m and 0 refer to values midway between and at the ditches, respectively. The seepage analysis does not allow E_m to be given simply in terms of the maximum water table height H_m. However, the vertical component of the downward flow on the plane midway between ditches decreases from the rainfall rate q at the water table to zero at the impermeable barrier. Thus $q > k\,\partial h_m/\partial z > 0$, which can be used in eqn 2.27 to give eqn 2.34 in the form of the inequality:

$$\frac{q/k}{1 - q/k} > \frac{H_m^2 - H_0^2}{D^2} > \frac{q}{k} \tag{2.35}$$

The left-hand side of this inequality is the exact result of the groundwater problem obtained from potential theory for horizontal drains at the level of the impermeable barrier (Engelund, 1951) (which obviously gives a water table higher than for the case of water draining through the sides of a ditch).

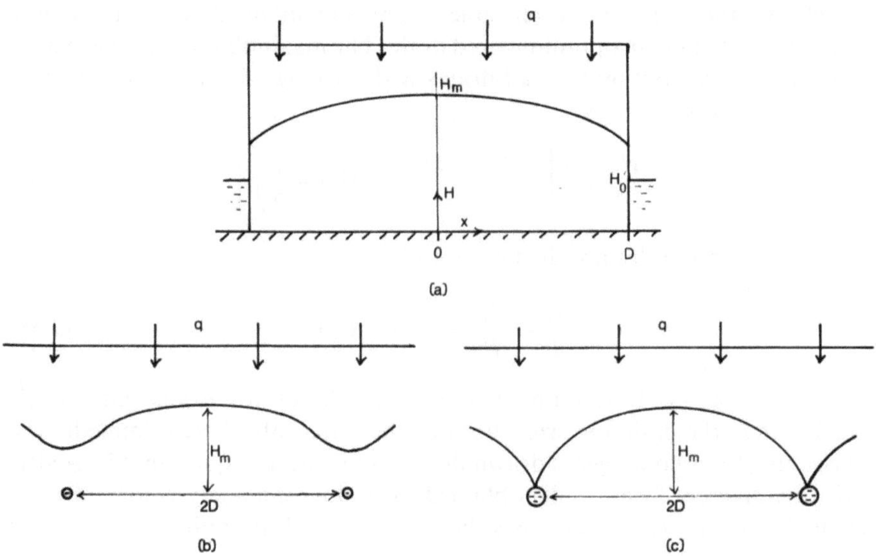

Figure 2.10 Water table drainage. (a) Drainage to ditches dug to a horizontal impermeable barrier; (b) water tables in infinitely deep soils above parallel rows of pipe drains of sub-optimum size; (c) water table shape in infinitely deep soils above parallel rows of pipe drains of optimum size.

The right-hand side is that derived by the Dupuit–Forchheimer analysis and first published by Colding in 1862. This approximate analysis also gives the water table height at any position x measured from midway between the drains:

$$H^2 = H_0{}^2 + (D^2 - x^2)\,q/k \tag{2.36}$$

For small values of q/k it has been shown (Youngs, 1990) that the water table height H is given with a fairly high precision by eqn 2.36 except in the vicinity of the ditch; for example, for $q/k = 0.02$, the precision is within 5% of the exact value at $x/D = 0.9$.

2.6.2.2 *Drains laid in infinitely deep soil.* The solution of the groundwater problem for the drainage of steady incident rainfall to parallel rows of sinks in an infinitely deep soil can be found by conformal transformations using the hodograph method (van Deemter, 1950; Childs, 1969). For cylindrical drains of radius less than some optimum size running just full so that the pressure of the water at the top of the drain is atmospheric, the water table has the shape shown in Figure 2.10(b) with the water table height overall, and particularly over the drain, becoming higher as the drain becomes smaller. For a drain of optimum size the water table is drawn down to the top of the drain as shown in Figure (2.10c) and the water table height is the minimum for the given rainfall rate. Drains of greater size maintained just full of water will produce higher water tables. However, drains may not run full, in which case the maximum water table height is maintained at approximately the same as that for an optimum-sized drain. The maximum water table height midway between optimum-sized drains with spacing $2D$ for the steady-state rainfall rate q is given by:

$$\frac{H_{\mathrm{m}}}{D} = \frac{1}{\pi}\left[\ln\left(1 + \frac{2}{\gamma}\right) + \frac{2}{\gamma}\ln\left(1 + \frac{\gamma}{2}\right)\right] \tag{2.37}$$

with the optimum drain radius r_0 given by:

$$\frac{r_0}{D} = \frac{H_{\mathrm{m}}}{D} - \frac{2}{\pi\gamma}\ln(1 + \gamma) \tag{2.38}$$

where $\gamma = k/q - 1$. It is found that eqn 2.37 holds for drain radii much smaller than the optimum size, although the water table height immediately above the drain no longer is drawn down to the drain. Equation 2.37 is also not very different from results obtained by hodograph analysis for drainage to ditches with ditch-water levels the same as the drain radius.

2.6.2.3 *Intermediate depths of impermeable barrier.* The presence of an impermeable barrier below the drain restricts the flow to the drain so that the water table is higher for a given rainfall rate than it would be if the soil were infinitely deep. This is recognised in Hooghoudt's (1940) equivalent depth equation, which considers the flow to be radial in the vicinity of the drain and horizontal in the central region between drains:

$$\frac{H_m}{D} = -\frac{d_e}{D} + \left[\left(\frac{d_e}{D}\right)^2 + \frac{q}{k}\right]^{1/2} \tag{2.39}$$

where the 'equivalent depth' d_e is defined in terms of the depth d below the drain to the impermeable barrier, the drain spacing $2D$ and the drain radius r_0 (or the wetted perimeter of the drain u in place of $2\pi r_0$) by:

$$\frac{d_e}{D} = 1 \Big/ \left[\frac{(\sqrt{2}D - d)^2}{2dD} + \frac{4}{\pi}\ln\left(\frac{d}{\sqrt{2}r_0}\right)\right] \tag{2.40}$$

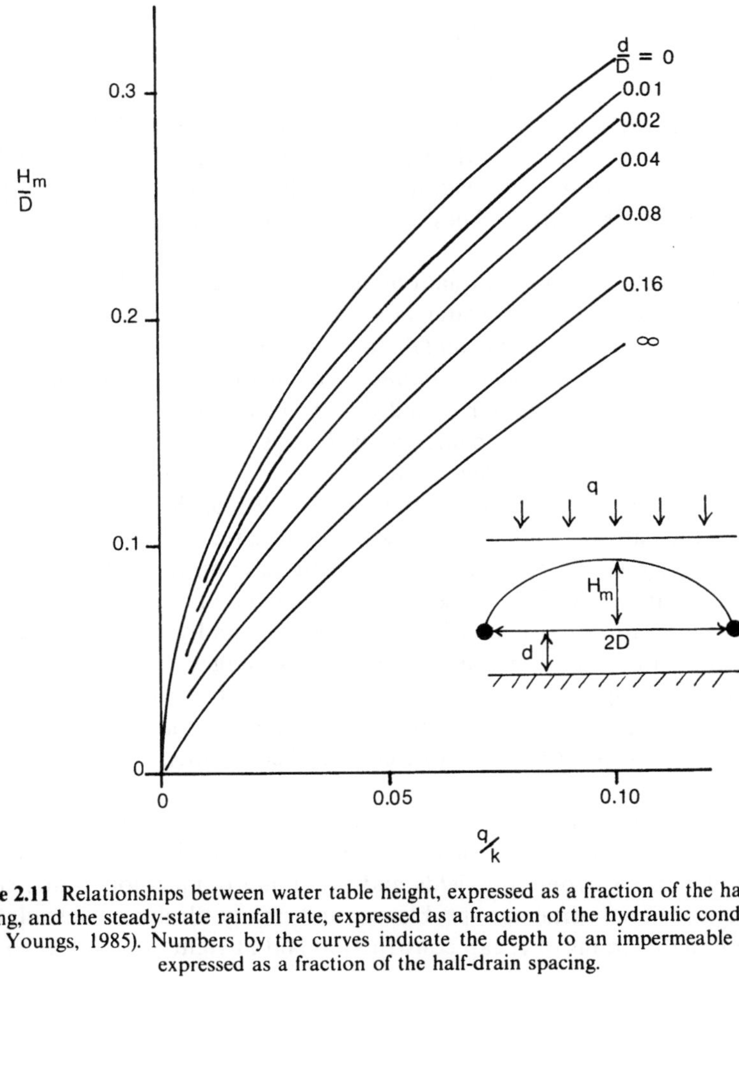

Figure 2.11 Relationships between water table height, expressed as a fraction of the half-drain spacing, and the steady-state rainfall rate, expressed as a fraction of the hydraulic conductivity (after Youngs, 1985). Numbers by the curves indicate the depth to an impermeable barrier, expressed as a fraction of the half-drain spacing.

or given in tables. Although this equation is widely used, it requires a knowledge of the drain radius r_0 or wetted perimeter u, which are not well defined in drains installed in the field. The flow into field drains is through narrow gaps between tiles or through small peripheral openings in plastic pipes, further complicated by soil disturbance and gravel backfilling during installation. These permeable surrounds generally allow the drain pipes to be considered to be of a size greater than optimum as defined in the hodograph analysis for infinitely deep soil. Then the maximum water-table height can be simply described by Youngs' (1985) empirical formula:

$$\frac{H_m}{D} = \left(\frac{q}{k}\right)^{1/\alpha} \tag{2.41}$$

where:

$$\begin{aligned} \alpha &= 2(d/D)^{d/D}, \quad 0 < d/D < 0.368 \\ \alpha &= 1.384, \qquad d/D > 0.368 \end{aligned} \tag{2.42}$$

which for values of q/k less than 0.1 fits the extreme cases of $d/D = 0$ ($\alpha = 2.0$) and $d/D \to \infty$ ($\alpha = 1.368$), and the intermediate values of d/D applying Houghoudt's equation with a drain radius that of the optimum size given by the hodograph analysis. These results are shown in Figure 2.13.

2.6.2.4 *Drainage equations.* Equations such as eqns 2.35, 2.37, 2.39 and 2.41, which relate the maximum water table height midway between drain lines to the drain spacing, steady rainfall rate and the hydraulic conductivity of the soil, are know as *drainage equations.* Because of the difficulties associated with solving the flow equation (eqn 2.9) with the boundary conditions of the flow region that properly includes both the unsaturated soil-water and the saturated groundwater regions, all derivations of drainage equations make physical and often mathematical assumptions. While the derived equations differ mathematically, numerically they should agree if the assumptions are acceptable. However, because of the varying assumptions, there is a wide discrepancy in results from these equations (Lovell and Youngs, 1984). The power-law relationship (eqn 2.41) agrees with soundly based theoretically derived equations and experiment, and has advantages over other equations because of its simplicity. Also, if there are departures from the ideal conditions of optimum drain size and uniform soil hydraulic conductivity, a power-law relationship can be fitted with little error to field results.

2.6.2.5 *Three-dimensional drainage.* Drainage systems only approximate to the two-dimensional situations considered commonly in land-drainage theory. Ditches surrounding fields and providing outfalls for drains create three-dimensional drainage problems, and many drainage installations employ minor drains of cheap construction laid at right angles over majors that act as main conduits. The water table control in such three-dimensional systems can be investigated by solving the seepage equation (eqn 2.28) with the conditions imposed at the two-dimensional boundary of the flow region (Youngs, 1980; 1984). Results are summarised in Figure 2.12(a), in which the maximum water table height at the central watershed position, relative to that for a parallel drainage system, is plotted against the ratio of the length of the rectangular sides for different heights of the minor drains above the majors, expressed relative to the water table height in the centre of the parallel system. These results show that the water table height at the centre of such mesh systems approaches that of a parallel system when the ratio of the side lengths becomes greater than about 2.0. Whilst Figure 2.12(a) is for rectangular systems, other geometries often occur and can be treated in the same way.

2.6.2.6 *Drainage by wells.* Another three-dimensional drainage situation that requires special mention is the use of wells for drainage purposes. While in humid regions pipe and ditch drainage are the most commonly used methods of agricultural drainage, in irrigated lands and in many civil engineering dewatering schemes wells are employed to lower water tables. The seepage analysis can be used to consider the flow into wells. The catchment area of one well in a hexagonal array of wells of radius r_0 spaced $2a$ apart, as shown in Figure 2.12(b), can be approximated to a circular area so that $\partial E/\partial r = 0$ at $r = a$. If the wells are sunk to an impermeable barrier and the water level in the wells maintained at a height H_0 with a uniform flux q over the soil surface, in the steady state the solution to the seepage equation is:

$$E_m - E_0 = q[a^2 \ln(a/r_0) - (a^2 - r_0^2)/2]/2 \tag{2.43}$$

where E_m and E_0 are the values of the seepage potential at the watershed and at the well surface respectively. Applying the same reasoning as with the parallel drainage problem regarding the head distribution down the plane at the watershed, we obtain the inequality:

$$H_m^2 - H_0^2 < (q/k)[a^2 \ln(a/r_0) - (a^2 - r_0^2)/2] < H_m^2(1 - q/k) - H_0^2 \tag{2.44}$$

the left-hand side of which is the Dupuit–Forchheimer result.

2.6.3 *Interception drainage*

While all drains intercept water flowing through the soil, the term *interception drainage* is used to describe drainage installations that are designed to remove water flowing into the soil region and originating some distance away. It is generally associated with the geological formation of the land.

2.6.3.1 *Foreign water interception on a slope.* Groundwater originating

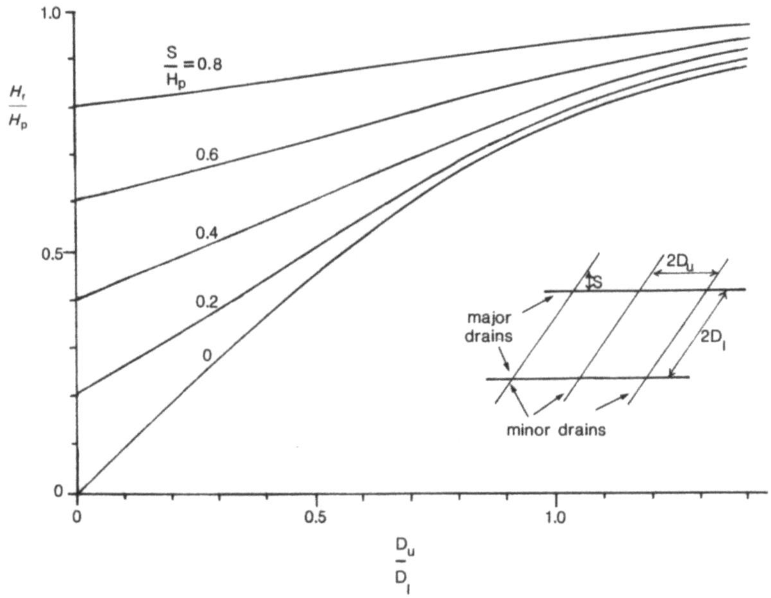

(a)

Figure 2.12 Three-dimensional drainage. (a) Mesh drainage (after Youngs, 1984). The water-table height H_r in the centre of the mesh, expressed as a fraction of the water-table height H_p in the absence of the minor drains, is shown plotted against the ratio D_u/D_l of the half-spacings of the upper minor drains and lower major drains for different heights S of the minor drains above the majors expressed as a fraction of H_p.

upslope and moving downwards over an inclined impermeable barrier can cause springlines to develop unless drains are installed to intercept the seepage. The reduction in the water table height is shown schematically in Figure 2.13(a) for water flow down a slope inclined at an angle β to the horizontal. For steady flow some distance upslope from the drain, where the depth of groundwater is H_u measured perpendicular to the barrier, the flow is parallel to the slope and equal to $kH_u \sin\beta$ per unit width. At some distance below the drain where the groundwater thickness is H_b, the flow down the slope is $kH_b \sin\beta$. Thus, the water removed per unit length of drain is:

$$Q = (H_u - H_b)k \sin\beta \tag{2.45}$$

2.6.3.2 *Interception of artesian flow.* High water tables and ponding of the soil surface can occur as a result of upward flow of water through the soil from a permeable substratum under an artesian head. The problem can be alleviated by installing interceptor drains, for example a system of ditches as illustrated in Figure 2.13(b). The boundary conditions of this problem allow Laplace's equation to be solved using conformal transformations with

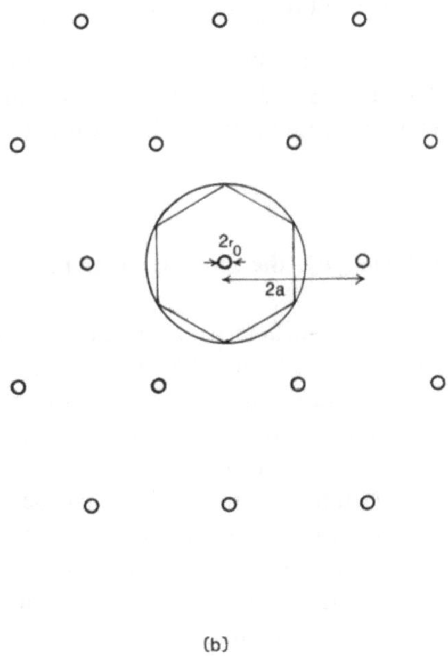

Figure 2.12 cont'd (b) well drainage.

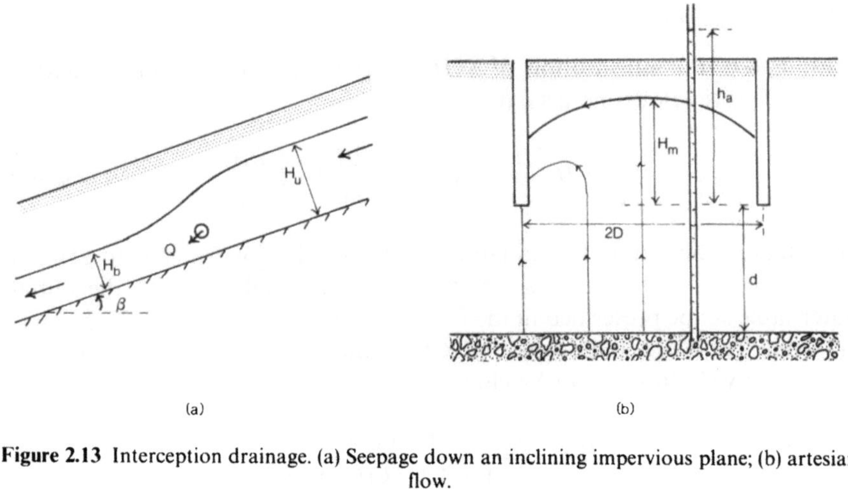

Figure 2.13 Interception drainage. (a) Seepage down an inclining impervious plane; (b) artesian flow.

Zhukovsky's function (Youngs, 1986a). The results fit the empirical equation:

$$D = 0.606(h_a + d)\ln(1 - H_m/h_a) \tag{2.46}$$

where h_a, measured relative to the bottom of the ditches, is the artesian head in the substratum. The analysis also gives the drain discharge rate, which becomes very large as the bottom of the ditch becomes close to the permeable substratum.

2.7 Non-steady-state drainage—the moving water table

Changes of flux at the soil surface as a result of changing rainfall and evaporation rates cause changes in the state of the soil water in the unsaturated zone and the water table to move up and down. The exact analysis of this non-steady-state drainage problem requires the solution of Richards' equation (eqn 2.8) over the whole flow region, noting that $\partial\theta/\partial t = 0$ in the saturated zone. Numerical methods must be employed. Usually, however, approximate methods of analysis are used, making use of the concept of the specific yield to give an estimate of the flux through the water table caused by the changing water content of the unsaturated soil zone. With the movement of water in the unsaturated zone assumed to be vertical, the flux across the water table V is then:

$$V = V_s + S\frac{\partial H}{\partial t} \tag{2.47}$$

where V_s is the flux across the soil surface. Three approaches to this problem are considered below; Chapter 10 discusses deep drainage.

2.7.1 *Boussinesq's equation*

With $V_s = 0$, the substitution of $S\partial H/\partial t$ for V in Forchheimer's equation (eqn 2.25) gives Boussinesq's equation:

$$k\frac{\partial}{\partial x}\left(H\frac{\partial H}{\partial x}\right) + k\frac{\partial}{\partial y}\left(H\frac{\partial H}{\partial y}\right) = S\frac{\partial H}{\partial t} \tag{2.48}$$

Boussinesq's solution to this equation for the problem of drainage to parallel empty ditches is obtained by the separation of variables. With the initial water table shape prescribed in the form of a special function $f(x/D)$ that has the value 0 at $x = 0$ and 1.0 at $x = D$, the water table height $H(x, t)$ at time t is given by (Polubarinova-Kochina, 1962):

$$H(x, t) = \frac{H_0 f(x/D)}{1 + 1.115kH_0t/SD^2} \tag{2.49}$$

where H_0 is the maximum water table height midway between drains at time $t = 0$.

A commonly used drawdown equation is Glover-Dumm's linearised solution of Boussinesq's equation (Luthin, 1957; van Schilfgaarde, 1974) for the maximum water table height $m(t)$ above the ditch-water level midway between parallel ditches at time t when the latter is lowered a height m_0 at zero time:

$$m(t) = \frac{4m_0}{\pi} \sum_{n=1,3,5\ldots}^{\infty} \left[\frac{(-1)^{(n-1)/2}}{n} \exp\left(-\frac{n^2\pi^2 k\bar{m}t}{4SD^2} \right) \right] \tag{2.50}$$

where $\bar{m} = d + H_0 + m_0/2$, the average initial depth of the aquifer if d is the depth of an impermeable barrier below the bottom of the ditch and H_0 is the maintained ditch-water level.

2.7.2 *Assumption of continuous succession of steady states*

If non-steady-state water tables in drained lands can be considered as a continuous succession of steady states (Muskat, 1937; van Schilfgaarde, 1974), drainage equations can be used to give the water table height for an equivalent steady rainfall rate equal to $-V$ given by eqn 2.47. This implies that water tables fall without change of shape, so that there is a further physical assumption using this approach. With Youngs' empirical drainage equation (eqn 2.41), we have:

$$\frac{V_s}{k} + \frac{S}{k}\frac{\partial H}{\partial T} = \left(\frac{H_m}{D}\right)^{\alpha} \tag{2.51}$$

Integration of this gives the water table recession from a height H_0 with no rainfall as:

$$H(D, t) = \frac{H_0}{[1 + (\alpha - 1)kH_0^{\alpha-1}t/SD^{\alpha}]^{1/(\alpha-1)}} \tag{2.52}$$

Thus, for the situation with drains sunk to the impermeable barrier when $\alpha = 2$:

$$H(D, t) = \frac{H_0}{1 + kH_0 t/SD^2} \tag{2.53}$$

which is not very different from Boussinesq's result.

2.7.3 *Drain hydrographs*

Drain hydrographs give the response of the drain discharge to the rain input on the land surface. Since the driving force for the discharge is the height of the water table, they also provide an indication of the water table behaviour.

Conversely, the water table response, for example the water table recessions given by eqns 2.49, 2.50, 2.52 and 2.53, reflects the drain discharge. For example, with drains laid on an impermeable barrier with the water table recession given by eqn 2.53, the drain discharge $q = k(H_m/D)^2$ so that at time t:

$$q = q_0[1 + \sqrt{(q_0 k)}t/SD]^{-2} \tag{2.54}$$

where q_0 is the drain discharge at zero time. Similar expressions are obtained with other drainage equations. These expressions show the dependency of the drain discharge on the hydraulic soil properties and on the drain spacing. From eqn 2.53 it is seen that the time taken for the water table to fall a given distance from some initial level is inversely proportional to the square of the drain spacing; that is, halving the spacing quarters the time.

The water table recession from high water table levels is an important feature in the design of drainage installations, since it is often the time that the soil remains excessively wet or even ponded on the surface that is detrimental to agricultural production and delays civil engineering operations. With no rainfall, these recession curves can be simply estimated and are found to fit field results. When there is rainfall, a more difficult situation arises. The flux through the water table is given by eqn 2.47. The difficulty in using this equation with a drainage equation, as in eqn 2.51, is that the specific yield S has to be known, and this is not easily estimated when the soil-water profile is far from an equilibrium state as is the case when

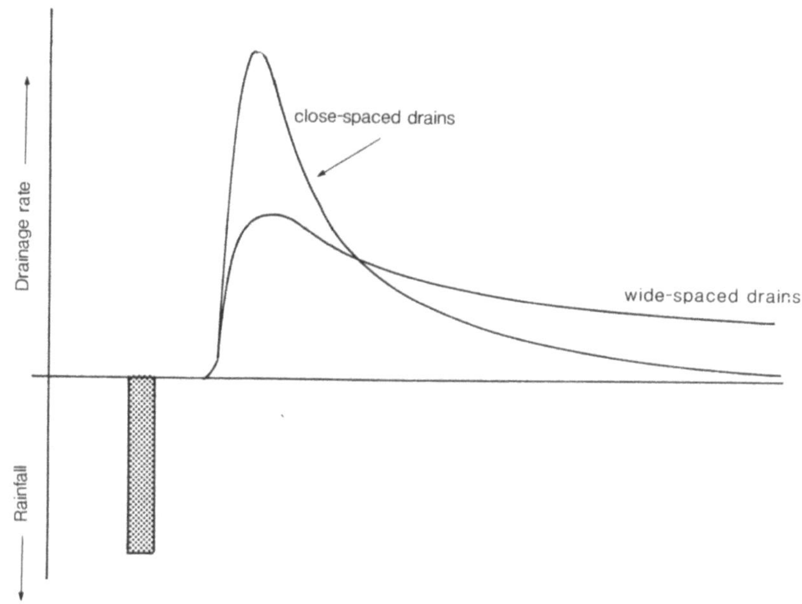

Figure 2.14 Drain hydrographs.

the profile is wetting up. There is a delay in communication being made between the water infiltrating through the soil surface and arriving at the water table. Thus the drain does not react immediately to a rain input and usually it takes some hours before it starts running after a rainstorm. Figure 2.14 illustrates the form of drain hydrographs and their dependency on drain spacing.

Equation 2.51 is therefore not easily applied to show the short-term drain response to surface infiltration caused by rainstorms. However, on a long-term basis the seasonal change of the water table level can be adequately modelled using this equation, since then the profiles, averaged over a period of 1 or 2 days, approximate to an equilibrium state (Youngs *et al.*, 1989). This approach to modelling water table behaviour allows the numerical integration of eqn 2.51 using any drainage equation with variable rainfall and evaporation through the soil surface. The specific yield need not be assumed to be constant; for example, it can be related to the depth of water table below the soil surface, and values of $S(H)$, obtained from the moisture characteristic curve and the average flow rate down the soil profile (dos Santos Jùnior and Youngs, 1969) used in the numerical integration.

2.8 Complicating factors

Concepts in soil physics have developed by considering soils to be inert, homogeneous and uniform, from which the continuum theory of soil-water movement has been derived. However, this theory has not been readily applied in the field because of complicating factors (Towner, 1989). Land-drainage theory based on this classical approach to soil-water movement to sinks of simple geometry, while providing an insight into groundwater behaviour and an understanding of soil-water regimes, often requires further development to take into account these complicating factors that include soil anisotropy, heterogeneity, aggregation as a result of cultivation and natural cracking through shrinkage, and instability, as well as considering the nature of the drain channel (Youngs, 1984).

2.8.1 *Nature of the drain channel*

Without a permeable surround to commonly used land drains where water entry is between butted clay tile pipes or through perforations in plastic pipes, water flow in the soil around such pipes converges to openings that are spaced at intervals along the drain lines. The equipotentials and flow pattern around a pipe system are illustrated in Figure 2.15(a), where it is seen that at some radial distance the equipotentials become almost cylindrical. These cylindrical equipotentials coincide with those for the radial flow to a smaller, ideal, completely permeable drain, as shown in Figure 2.15(b). The

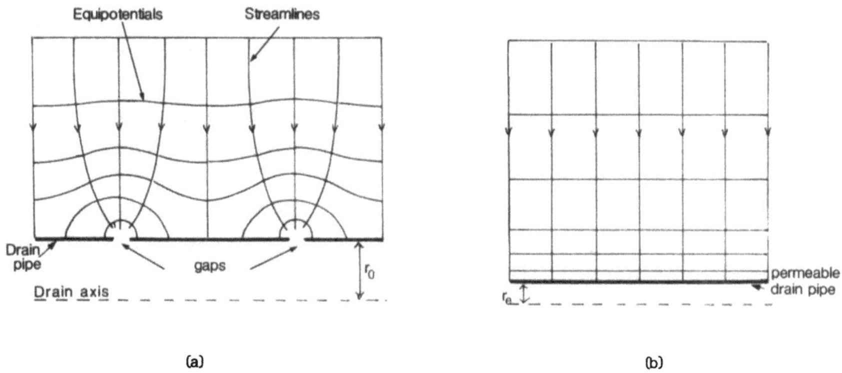

Figure 2.15 Equipotentials and streamlines in soils around (a) a gappy non-ideal drain and (b) an ideal cylindrical drain (after Youngs, 1984).

non-ideal drains can thus be considered as having an equivalent drain radius of an ideal drain with much smaller radius than that of the pipes themselves. Alternatively, they may be considered as having a drain resistance. If the actual radius of the drain is r_0 and that of the equivalent ideal drain is r_e, then the resistance W to the flow Q from a radial distance R where the head is h_R is:

$$W = h_R/Q = (1/2\pi k)\ln(R/r_e) = (1/2\pi k)[\ln(R/r_0) + \ln(r_0/r_e)]$$
$$= (1/2\pi k)\ln(R/r_0) + W_e \quad (2.55)$$

W_e is the additional resistance, or *entrance resistance*, resulting from the equivalent drain radius being r_e because of the convergence of the streamlines to the gaps, instead of the actual radius r_0.

In order to overcome the entrance resistance, as well as to afford some protection to silting up of drain pipes, filter materials such as gravel backfill or porous matting are often used to surround clay tile pipes and plastic drain pipe, thereby increasing the equivalent drain radius. The latter is thus an unknown quantity, and this prevents the reliable use of drainage equations that include the drain radius as one of the factors. With the equivalent drain made sufficiently large with filter surrounds so that it approaches the optimum size, maximum possible drawdown with the particular drain spacing and depth is achieved as given by eqn 2.41, and hence the drain radius need not enter into design criteria in this respect.

2.8.2 *Soil anisotropy*

Soil formation processes often impart to soils a different hydraulic conductivity in the vertical direction than in the horizontal. The effect of this anisotropy is to distort the flownet and flow region associated with the same groundwater problem in isotropic soil. This has the effect on drainage equations of the replacement of the dimensionless vertical heights H_m/D and d/D appearing in these equations by the parameters $H_m/\surd(A)D$ and $d/\surd(A)D$ respectively, where A is the ratio of the vertical to horizontal hydraulic conductivities k_z/k_x, with the dimensionless rainfall rate given by $q/k_z = q/Ak_x$ (Luthin, 1957; Youngs, 1986b).

2.8.3 *Soil heterogeneity*

With water flow in composite porous materials there is continuity of flux and continuity of soil-water pressure (and therefore hydraulic head) throughout the whole of the flow region. This means that, when two soils with different moisture characteristic curves are contiguous, abrupt soil-water content changes can occur across the boundaries, since the relationships between soil-water content and soil-water pressure differ. At the interface, the streamlines are refracted according to the cotangent law:

$$k_1 \cot \alpha_1 = k_2 \cot \alpha_2 \tag{2.56}$$

where k_1 and k_2 are the hydraulic conductivities of the two adjoining soils and α_1 and α_2 are the angles to the normal that the streamlines make.

Generally, to obtain complete solutions, numerical methods of solution of the flow equation have to be employed, such as the finite difference method or the finite element method, which is particularly useful in these situations.

Another approach that gives the horizontal groundwater flow is the use of the seepage analysis (Youngs, 1965; 1980). The seepage potential is defined by eqn 2.27 for soils whose conductivity varies with height, not just for uniform soils. Values of the seepage potential E at the face of a vertical drainage ditch that extends down to a horizontal impermeable barrier is (Youngs, 1980):

$$E_0 = \int_0^{H_0} \left[\int_0^H k(z)\, \mathrm{d}z \right] \mathrm{d}H \tag{2.57}$$

where H_0 is the ditch-water level. The value of E can be determined at the watershed of the ditch-drainage system by solving eqn 2.28. The water table height there can be obtained with known precision by noting that the head gradient decreases from a value to accommodate the rainfall rate at the water table to zero at the impermeable barrier, just as in the case of uniform soils. In this way it is found that the water table height is known with greater precision the greater the vertical increase of hydraulic conductivity. The lower bound obtained using this approach is that given by the Girinsky potential Γ, defined by:

$$\Gamma = \int_0^H (H - z) k(z)\, \mathrm{d}z \tag{2.58}$$

that makes the same assumptions as the Dupuit–Forchheimer analysis.

While the seepage analysis is particularly useful for soils in which the hydraulic conductivity varies with depth, it can be used in the consideration of some situations where there are variations in both vertical and horizontal directions. Analyses show that water table heights are more sensitive to variations of hydraulic conductivity in the neighbourhood of the ditches than near the watershed. Low values of hydraulic conductivity near the ditch have the effect of raising the water table height overall.

2.8.4. *Soil aggregation*

Cracks and fissures in fine-textured soils, created either by natural shrinkage or by tillage operations such as subsoiling and mole draining, are important in the drainage of heavy soils. They form a network of macropores that surround regions of micropores that are formed by aggregates of soil particles, and give the soil a large hydraulic conductivity value when they are full of water. However, above the water table, the aggregate regions can become isolated when the macropores empty, and then water flow becomes restricted. When dry, the aggregates imbibe water from the surfaces of the aggregate regions bounded by the macropores. Bypass flow, which gives a rapid drain response to heavy rainstorms, occurs when the sorptivity value of the micropore space is too small for all water to infiltrate (Beven and Germann, 1982; Youngs and Leeds-Harrison, 1990).

2.8.5 *Soil instability*

Capping of silty soils by the impact of raindrops on the soil surface reduces infiltration and increases the occurrences of runoff, and is often a cause of poor seed germination. Such soils give rise to eluviation of soil particles with the consequent silting up of drainpipes, making necessary the provision of filter surrounds to the drains to prevent drains in such soils having a short life.

As well as the breakdown of the soil structure of silty soils, the macrostructure, which imparts to clay soils their conductivity, can deteriorate because of slaking. This is of particular concern in obtaining stable mole-drain channels and also in the drainage of saline clay soils in coastal areas. Many methods are available to determine the stability of soils to wetting (Klute, 1986; Matkin and Smart, 1987; Smith and Mullins, 1991). One method for determining the stability of soils for mole drainage is Childs' moisture characteristic method that compares the draining moisture characteristic of rapidly wetted and slowly wetted soil crumbs (Rycroft and Thorburn, 1974). Since the moisture characteristic reflects the pore size distribution, the deterioration of the soil structure is easily detected if the soil breaks down during quick wetting.

3 Field drainage in temperate climates

W.C. HENDERSON and E. FARR

3.1 Objectives

Much of the world's supply of food is produced in the northern temperate climatic zone, which includes the cleared deciduous forest lands of western Europe, the equivalent region in eastern North America and the steppes and prairies of the continental interiors. The equivalent zone in the southern hemisphere is much more restricted in area but is equally productive. The soils of the prairies and steppes usually do not need drainage works because of their location in regions where annual precipitation rarely exceeds evapotranspiration. Field drainage is an important feature of agricultural production mainly in the maritime temperate regions, the former deciduous forest lands, where annual precipitation usually exceeds evapotranspiration, sometimes by a considerable amount. This results in an excess of soil water, at least during a part of the year, and experience has shown that soil productivity can be improved by removing excess soil water. The main objective of field drainage is to maintain or improve soil productivity but, as a secondary benefit, it also improves trafficability.

Civil engineers, in the normal run of projects, tend to look upon soil as just part of the overburden and, as often as not, use it as readily available inert fill. Even when planning consent requires separate storage for site restoration purposes, it is not treated in a manner which preserves its fertility. It is moved in all weathers by heavy scraper/dumpers, which constantly run over the storage heap as it is built up to the maximum possible height, thereby minimising the storage area. Any subsequent delay in restoration beyond a single growing season results in a loss of fertility in deeply buried anaerobic layers. It must be emphasised that fertile soil is the result of biological activity working on the surface layer of rock waste in aerobic conditions over many years. Fertility is by no means a permanent condition, and it is easily lost or diminished by poor management. Field drainage is an investment intended to maintain or improve productivity, but the hoped-for benefits may not be obtained if any part of the drainage operations impairs some other aspect of productivity. For this reason the basic needs of conserving soil productivity will be described briefly as an essential component of successful field drainage.

3.2 Soil properties

3.2.1 *Soil productivity*

Soil productivity is a measure of the ease by which plants, particularly crop plants, can establish themselves in a soil coupled with their subsequent rate of growth. To achieve good results, plants need a soil that is sufficiently friable and provides balanced quantities of water, dissolved nutrients (such as nitrate, phosphate and potassium) and oxygen. Developing root systems branch out to explore every part of the soil mass where the finest branches, the root hairs, absorb water by osmotic pressure through delicate cell walls. In order to remain active and viable, the cells of the root tissue must respire, and for this a supply of oxygen is required. For most crop plants, this must be derived directly from the airoccupying voids in the soil mass. Soil compaction or soil saturation can cause anaerobic zones in the soil where roots cannot survive for any length of time and, of course, compaction directly inhibits plant growth. Conversely, in exceptionally loose soils with a large proportion of air-filled pore spaces, plants may suffer from a lack of water during a dry season. The length of time that plants can endure soil saturation in the rooting zone without damage depends on the stage of growth and the species of plant. It is usually somewhere between 2 and 20 days and is an important concept with regard to drainage design.

In natural conditions, soil fertility is maintained by a complex process of recycling. Green plants are able to convert the energy of sunlight into an available form in the process of *photosynthesis.* Atmospheric carbon dioxide absorbed through the leaf tissue and water taken in through the roots are converted to carbohydrate according to the much simplified equation:

$$6CO_2 + 6H_2O + \text{energy (sunlight)} \rightarrow C_6H_{12}O_6 + 6O_2$$

The plant, or any animal or micro-organism consuming plant tissue in its diet can then acquire energy in the process of *respiration*, according to the general equation:

$$C_6H_{12}O_6 + 6O_2 \rightarrow 6CO_2 + 6H_2O + \text{energy}$$

All organic debris such as discarded plant tissue, animal bodies, excrement and waste is incorporated into the soil by the concerted action of earthworms, other soil invertebrates and micro-organisms. The constituent carbohydrates, fats, proteins and other molecules are broken down as follows:

$$\text{Organic molecule} + O_2 \rightarrow CO_2 + H_2O + \text{nutrients} + \text{humus} + \text{energy}$$

These processes underpin the 'cycle of life' upon which terrestrial activity is based. It should be noted that management activities such as continuous arable cropping and stubble burning tend to interrupt the natural cycle. Fertility can be bolstered by using inorganic fertilisers derived from fossil fuel and mineral deposits, but they become progressively less effective as the organic content of soil diminishes. Long-term fertility depends on keeping the organic residues at a satisfactory level to support the vast array of living organisms which have a crucial role in soil processes. This helps to explain why rock waste from the overburden, spread on the surface to replace soil removed for engineering works, often does not support the expected plant population, no matter how much chemical fertiliser is added.

3.2.2 *Soil composition*

Soils vary in their level of fertility, partly as a result of environment and of their inherent properties derived from the original soil-forming processes, and partly as a consequence of their management and use. Mature soils, in the broadest terms, can be divided into four basic components:

Mineral matter. Most soils are composed mainly of mineral particles such as sand, silt and clay together with larger rock fragments like gravel, stones and boulders. Such materials contain a wide range of elements, but the great bulk of their mass is formed from silicon, aluminium and oxygen. Sand and silt particles are chemically inert, being derived from the rock-forming mineral silica (SiO_2). Clay particles are much more chemically active and appear as a wide range of secondary minerals, produced by the chemical weathering of many different parent materials, mainly aluminosilicates but sometimes from ferromagnesium silicates.

Organic matter. Amongst the mineral particles, there exist the living and dead roots of plants, plant and animal debris, humus, earthworms, ants, millipedes and many other living species, with special importance attached to the microbiological populations (bacteria, fungi, etc.) responsible for humification and the release of available plant nutrients. A fertile soil is literally teeming with life, numbered in millions of organisms per gram of soil.

Soil air. This contains oxygen, nitrogen and carbon dioxide whose proportions can vary markedly compared with the atmosphere above the soil. Depending also on the conditions, other gases such as hydrogen sulphide, acetylene and methane may be present in the mixture. Not only may the composition of soil air fluctuate with time, it is often very heterogeneous, with significant differences occurring over short distances.

Soil water. This shares the intergrain spaces and other voids in the soil with soil air. For the drainage engineer, the most important properties of soil are the amount of contained water, the way the amount of water varies and its relationship with soil air.

The amount of water in a soil, at any given time, is defined as the moisture content (%), where:

$$\text{Moisture content} = \frac{\text{weight of moisture in the soil}}{\text{weight of the oven dry (106°C) soil}} \times 100$$

It can vary markedly from time to time, depending on additions to and losses from the soil by the natural processes that constitute the hydrological cycle. In a maritime temperate region, precipitation tends to be evenly distributed throughout the year while evapotranspiration peaks during the summer months so that soils tend to dry out during the summer and become wetter in winter. Evapotranspiration has a maximum of about 600 mm of equivalent rainfall per year and, in the most productive areas, annual precipitation ranges from about 500 to 750 mm. In wetter areas it can reach 2000 mm with 1000–1500 mm being common in areas where hill farming predominates. To a large extent the kind of farming possible in any area is determined by the amount of excess rainfall.

The behaviour of water within soil is a fundamental factor of productivity and must be understood by a drainage engineer. When viewed in cross-section, the soil profile is seen to consist of three main layers—the topsoil, the subsoil and the parent material. The composition of the smaller particles forming the soil mass is both a stable and an important property of the soil:

Soil texture is defined as the percentage of sand, silt and clay in the soil where particles are classified according to their size. Details of one agricultural classification are given in Table 3.1.

Table 3.1

Soil type	Effective diameter (mm)
Stones and gravel	>2
Coarse sand	2.00–0.20
Sand	0.20–0.10
Fine sand	0.10–0.06
Very fine sand	0.06–0.02
Silt	0.02–0.002
Clay	<0.002

It is instructive to visualise the range of particle sizes, for it can be seen that the average diameter of a grain of coarse sand is a hundred times larger than a grain of silt. This difference must be cubed when comparing the relative volumes of the two size fractions. It follows that, for an even distribution of particles, soil voids will have a volume which relates to soil texture.

3.2.3 *Soil structure*

In many soils the particles are aggregated and may form a coherent mass, in which case the profile is said to be *massive* or structureless. This may be a natural condition or it may be the result of compaction by traffic. Cultivation of the topsoil can break it up into the familiar clods, and frost shatter can further break the aggregates down into crumbs, which is the friable state required by plants. Fissuring of the subsoil may occur naturally as a result of the shrinking and swelling of clay minerals whose vertical columns and blocks can be found separated by distinct fractures in the soil mass. This phenomenon is called *soil structure* and the structural units are called *peds*. Soil structure in the subsoil can produce a much higher value of permeability for a soil profile than might be expected from soil texture. Structure is most strongly developed in certain stable clay soils which have been subjected to a marked drying out cycle in summer. It is less well developed where clay minerals are not so stable and where summers are cooler and wetter. In the wettest areas good soil structure may not occur at all. Soil traffic may cause *induration* or *compaction*, and where it is restricted to a single layer it is called a *pan*. Soils composed mainly of sand particles, and especially those low in organic matter, may lack effective structure because the grains do not readily aggregate.

3.2.4 *Soil water*

Rainfall landing on the surface of a dry soil begins the wetting up process as water forms a film around soil particles on the ground surface. This film of water gets progressively thicker until it can hold no more and further addition of water moves down the profile, building up a film on the drier particles below. In this manner soil is wetted progressively from the surface downwards until downwards flow reaches a level below which all the soil voids are completely filled with water. This is called the *groundwater table*. If rainfall continues, added water may cause the groundwater table to rise through the profile and, eventually, to reach the surface at which point the soil is *saturated*. Further rainfall then ponds or becomes *surface flow*. The entry of water into a soil is called the *infiltration rate* and, if the rate of precipitation exceeds this value, ponding or surface flow can occur over a non-saturated soil. The speed with which water in the topsoil passes into the subsoil is called the *percolation rate*, and when this value is less than the infiltration rate the topsoil can be saturated over a non-saturated subsoil. Where conditions of this general description have any degree of permanence, as they would have over an indurated subsoil or pan, the soil is said to have a *perched water table*. Any resultant flow laterally through the profile is called *interflow*. Water passing downwards below the rooting zone of plants is called *deep seepage*, and any lateral flow at depth is called *groundwater flow*.

When rainfall stops, a freely draining soil immediately begins to lose water, and the process is of such importance for soil productivity that it must be considered in detail. What happens as a soil loses water is determined largely by the size of the soil pores or voids found in the profile and these should be considered as shown in Table 3.2.

Table 3.2

	Diameter (mm)
macropores	>0.05
mesopores	0.05–0.002
micropores	<0.002

Water forms a film around a soil particle because it adheres to the surface and because of its own surface tension. It can be removed by a suction force, which must increase as the film becomes thinner. Beginning with a saturated soil, water drains out under the force of gravity and is lost from ground level downwards as macropores are emptied to the maximum thickness of water film around soil particles. The space created is filled with air, but all mesopores and micropores remain filled with water. In this condition, when the effect of gravity ceases to remove water, the soil is said to be at *field capacity* or *water-holding capacity*. During the growing season plants absorb water from the water film, causing it to become thinner, thereby creating a *soil moisture deficit* which increases as the film size diminishes. Most crop plants continue to obtain water by this means until the remaining water is held at a tension of about 15 atmospheres. At this stage, all the mesopores have emptied apart from their residual water film, but the micropores remain filled with water. Without further rainfall, plants begin to wilt and the soil has reached *wilting point*. Therefore, water surrounding soil particles to a film thickness which fills mesopores is *available water* (for plants). Thinner films, sufficient only to fill micropores, are *unavailable water*. Air drying can reduce the moisture content of soil further, to a limiting tension of about 30 atmospheres. The wilting point need not be reached in practice if roots are able to penetrate as far as the groundwater table, but this picture accurately describes the condition of the soil in the normal rooting zone.

3.2.5 *Soil pores*

Pore size distribution is a major factor in soil productivity. The classification of particle size in Table 3.1 should be compared with that of pore size in Table 3.2. It will be noted that, for homogeneous soils, only fine sands or larger particles can have intergrain pore spaces of macropore size. Very fine sands and silts have spaces of mesopore size, whilst clays have only micropores. Soils composed mainly of sand drain freely but have very small reserves of available water unless their organic content is high. Humus acts like a sponge and greatly increases the quantity of available water in a profile. Very fine sand and silt have a large reservoir of available water but drain slowly because the profile is composed of unstable particles which run together and lose structure when the profile is saturated. This condition can be improved by the addition of humus, which helps to promote aggregation, binding particles together. Massive clay profiles present difficulties for crop growth but can be drained and rendered fertile when organic material is incorporated, creating and preserving structures with a network of macropores and mesopores. Most profiles are not uniformly homogeneous but possess mixed textures which tend to one or other of these characteristics, depending on the predominant particle size. Standard reference works on soils or field drainage should be consulted for more detailed information on soil texture, soil structure, terminology, methods of assessment and other aspects.

Pore size distribution is also crucial in determining the drainage characteristics of a soil profile. Assuming in all cases that the site is potentially free-draining, and referring again to Tables 3.1 and 3.2, it can be seen that only profiles with interconnecting macropores of either textural or structural origin can be drained by deep seepage under the influence of gravity. Furthermore, only those profiles can have a groundwater table. Profiles lacking macropores in the subsoil cannot drain by gravity and in wet periods will be affected by a perched water table. They can be drained only by creating fissures and, if successful, the dewatering process deep in the subsoil for the first time may initiate the natural formation of stable structures. Such operations do not create a groundwater table in the true sense, they only deepen the zone in which a perched water table may be found, but, for practical purposes, as long as the network of macropores persists in the subsoil, it has the same effect as a groundwater table as far as the plant is concerned. For drainage design purposes, the term 'water table' should be avoided because it is not precise enough. When assessing soils for drainage design, as a first step structure should be ignored and, based on textural assessment, soil should be considered either as a *surface aquifer* or a *surface aquiclude.* For this purpose, all heavy soils (such as clay, clay loam, silty clay, sandy clay and sandy clay loam) should be assigned to the latter category. Detailed design thereafter should take account of any natural structures present, but the basic design requirements are necessarily considered separately.

3.3 Effects of poor drainage conditions

Even the best-drained and naturally freely draining land can become saturated under severe climatic conditions, whilst land with the most inadequate drainage can appear to be quite dry at the height of a drought. In practical terms, the assessment of the need for improved field drainage is based on the speed with which soil recovers from total saturation, coupled with an evaluation of the adverse effect that an extended period of waterlogging has on crop plants, the soil and, in particular, its management and use.

Soil saturation for an extended period—waterlogging—renders the land unsuitable for any kind of agricultural activity other than extensive rough grazing, and the natural vegetation reflects the soil drainage status. In the wettest conditions, where precipitation is a major factor, the soil will have a cover of peat and drainage is usually not worthwhile. In less extreme conditions, drainage works may be feasible but land clearance or reclamation projects to convert rough grazing land to more productive use are not common because of the uncertainty of financial return. The majority of projects are for the benefit of land that has already been in use for more intensive forms of agricultural production.

Waterlogging has a marked effect on the plants that can grow on a site, particularly crop plants like cereals, roots and pulses, which need an aerobic rooting zone. Waterlogged soils are low in oxygen, they are colder and take longer to warm up when the growing season begins. The combination of retarded germination and restricted respiration results in poor, stunted and patchy growth. Anaerobic conditions also inhibit beneficial soil organisms, with the result that essential processes are impaired, the most noticeable being humification as plant debris accumulates in or on the soil. At the same time other soil organisms flourish, producing toxic substances like hydrogen sulphide, converting nitrates into gaseous nitrogen, which is lost to the atmosphere, and rendering other nutrients ineffective. In addition, poor crop growth allows competing weeds to proliferate and wet soil encourages plant diseases like take-all and club root. Thus poor drainage conditions can have a multiple effect on soil fertility.

Once established, grassland plants are more tolerant of soil saturation and, as a consequence, grassland farms are more common in lowland areas with high rainfall. Nevertheless, grass is affected in the same way as other plants by wet, anaerobic soils which restrict root development, reduce soil temperature and cause loss of plant nutrients. The production of stem and leaf tissue is reduced, and during long periods of waterlogging the most productive species are suppressed and replaced by competing weed species. Growing roots cannot tolerate a persistent zone of saturation and the developing roots tend to form near to the soil surface where oxygen is more available. For some types of soil, however, this top layer is susceptible to the trampling effect of grazing animals and forms a churned-up slurry (poaching) in wet conditions. Under drying conditions, this slurried layer forms a hard crusty mass which restricts root development just at the time when available water in the topsoil is diminishing, so that the plants are further stressed by lack of moisture. In addition to reducing the amount of grazing material, soil waterlogging provides a suitable habitat for animal disease organisms like liver fluke, parasitic worms and foot rot, and it harbours populations of irritant flies.

The amount of water found in a soil at any time can influence the physical properties which control its workability and trafficability, factors which in turn can affect fertility. Sandy soils are least influenced by soil water content and tend to remain friable because the soil particles lack cohesion. Such soils are therefore favoured for root crops like carrots, potatoes and sugar beet, for which harvest involves heavy field traffic and the separation of crop and soil. Clay soils behave very differently, and in this respect it is useful to keep in mind the valuable properties of puddled clay for the construction of reservoirs. Loams and other mixed soils have intermediate properties.

The physical properties of clay are well known. It forms a hard resistant mass when dry, becomes soft, pliable and cohesive when sufficiently wet to reach the plastic limit, and changes into a slurry at its liquid limit. Great care is needed to form and preserve the friable structure required by plants. Dry soil can support traffic easily, but cultivation can be difficult because of the inherent strength of the dried mass. Some degree of wetting can help make cultivation easier but any attempt at traffic or cultivation when the soil is at its plastic limit simply causes smearing and compaction. Most damage is done usually at harvest time when crops must be removed irrespective of soil conditions. All traffic in unsuitable conditions causes compaction of the soil or rutting, and sometimes traffic becomes impossible when the topsoil approaches the liquid limit. In addition, civil engineering plant may be so heavy as to compact wet subsoil underlying dry topsoil. All compaction results in loss of structure, and subsequent drying out produces the formation of an impervious topsoil. The relationship between the soil water status and its physical properties can be complex, but for clay soils it should be noted that a soil moisture deficit may be concurrent with plastic limit conditions.

There are many reasons for impermeability in a soil profile. Sedimentary clay subsoils can be *impermeable* if lacking in structure because macropores are absent from the undisturbed material. Drift, laid down by glaciation, can be *naturally indurated* throughout and can be impermeable even when the percentage clay content is not high. Natural processes can form an *iron pan* or a *clay pan* in an otherwise permeable subsoil, while the smearing effects of cultivation blades and tines and of spinning tractor wheels can form a *plough pan* at the top of the subsoil. Pressure from vehicles or animals can cause a *topsoil pan* as described above, and intense rainfall on a friable topsoil can cause *soil capping*. All of these conditions prevent deep seepage of incident rainfall and inhibit the deep penetration of roots so that there is a perched water table in wet conditions and meagre reserves of available water in dry conditions.

Soil drainage characteristics are of similar importance for the management of land used for other purposes. Natural or specially enhanced soil fertility is a basic requirement for the activities which require a surface of good-quality turf. For turf growing on a surface aquifer the main problem, usually, is to supply sufficient soil water in dry weather, but for other kinds of drainage situation the difficulties are exactly as described for agricultural lands. Winter sports grounds are worst affected, but soil damage can occur at any time. The most obvious damage is seen on sports fields or race tracks where the surface is poached by heavy traffic and can become slurried in the worst conditions. It is less obvious on greens and lawns if the soil is subject to pressure whilst in a plastic condition. In all circumstances the damaged topsoil becomes indurated and loses fertility when drying conditions return. The provision of a specially mixed topsoil layer can help if the natural subsoil is effectively drained as a preliminary step, otherwise the topsoil remains saturated by virtue of a perched water table in wet weather.

3.4 Strategy

To be successful, field drainage works must relate closely to the basic drainage problem or problems affecting the site; must take account of the inherent soil properties; and require to be carried out in suitable soil conditions. It is necessary to identify the characteristics of the soil profile in the field and to select a time when further soil damage will not result from the drainage operations. The factors causing the prolonged presence of excess soil water can fall into four distinct groups, and it will be noted that the traditional concept of 'lowering the water table' is true only for a proportion of projects.

A widespread drainage problem for any kind of land use is the *disposal of rainfall* and, for land that must support plant growth, the excess soil water is the result of interaction between precipitation, evapotranspiration and soil permeability. In general terms, the greater the amount of rainfall, the cooler the climate, the lower the soil permeability, the greater will be the soil drainage problem. Every permutation of these highly variable factors can occur, and in the temperate zone the extremes are identified by semidesert scrub and by blanket peat mire at sea level, with agricultural land in its various forms falling somewhere in between. The most common manifestation of the problem is *surface ponding* or a *perched water table*. Drainage works must involve actions to improve profile permeability in addition to providing channels to remove excess water, and it will be noted that where precipitation is persistently high a practical drainage improvement may not be possible.

Incident rainfall, in excess of that lost by evapotranspiration, is the source of all natural drainage systems, which it may enter directly as surface flow or indirectly as groundwater flow. Natural drainage may or may not be effective in removing excess water, depending on the *topography* of the site or general area. For sites with a surface aquifer, any restriction in natural drainage results in a persistently *high groundwater table*; this is the classic drainage problem. For surface aquicludes, any topographical problems simply add to the difficulty of clearing a perched water table. A necessary first step is to provide outlet channels for the excess water and, for the most difficult sites, this may involve the installation of a pumping system.

Thereafter, field drainage works require regularly spaced drains to control the groundwater table in aquifers and improvement of profile permeability in aquicludes.

As a further consequence of the local topography, some sites are affected by *inflows from other areas.* Where inflowing water cannot be controlled in its source area, as is the case for land in a valley near to local steep hill slopes, it is necessary to design drainage works accordingly. Protection of the site involves interception and diversion of the inflowing water.

Soils can remain wet, irrespective of weather conditions, if located on a site where *groundwater flow* reaches the surface. *Gravity spring seepage* is the most common cause of localised poor drainage in non-glaciated regions where the pattern of wet areas in the landscape reflects the outcrop of aquifers contained in the local rock formations. Careful planning of interceptor drains is the essential remedy. Areas with a surface formed on glacial till can have *artesian springs*, particularly where it overlies permeable rocks in undulating countryside. The glacial till acts as a confining layer, and at certain points, where the groundwater is under sufficient pressure, it can force its way upwards through the confining layer, either as a diffuse seepage or through a distinct narrow and vertical channel. The required control strategy is to dewater the supplying aquifer.

These four basic drainage problems may be encountered singly or in any combination. As an example, the impermeable glacial till which forms the confining layer of an artesian structure is also the parent material of local soil and will act as a surface aquiclude to incident rainfall. Where both factors are significant for field drainage improvement, the chosen design must cater for each problem in an effective but integrated manner to minimise costs. Where a combination of drainage problems occurs, particular mention must be made of river flood plains, which are valued by farmers because of their inherent fertility, but which can present a drainage engineer with formidable problems. A cross-section of a floodplain in a once glaciated region is shown in Figure 3.1. Possible drainage problems include a high groundwater table, impermeability and instability in the soil-forming alluvium, lateral groundwater flow from river to drainage channels, groundwater flow from an up-valley source confined by the alluvial layer, lack of gradient across the flood plain and surface inflow from the marginal bluffs and beyond. All this, of course, takes no account of the construction of flood banks where there is a piecemeal need to prevent further flooding. Much depends on the level of the flood plain surface relative to the level of water in the river and, in the most difficult circumstances, drainage investments are probably not worthwhile.

Removing excess soil water is in fact the last stage in the construction of a drainage system. The scale of a project is usually dependent on local topography with schemes initiated by a single farm business for individual fields in undulating countryside while regional developments, organised on

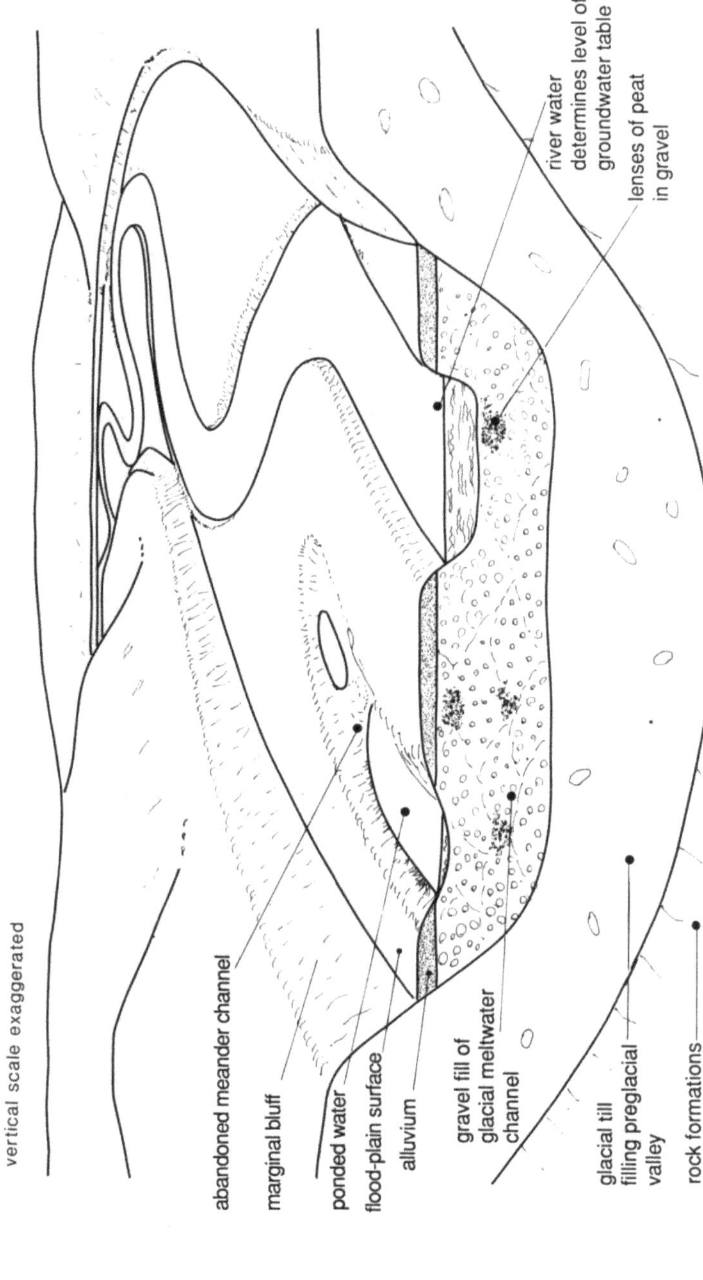

Figure 3.1 Cross-section of a river flood plain in a glaciated landscape.

a community basis, may be essential for wide plains not greatly elevated above sea level. However, all projects require carrier channels to remove drainage water to the nearest available outlet, and design criteria are not different in principle. As described in section 3.5, there are advantages in using piped channels for the smaller carriers and open channels for the larger arterial discharges.

The majority of farm ditches and the smaller arterial channels tend to have a discharge that is insufficient to clear weeds, sediment or other obstructions and require regular maintenance. For this reason, the channel must have a smooth, regular cross-section with a precise, uniform gradient for the best possible flow velocity and minimum maintenance costs. However, for greater discharge values, there is some tolerance of variation in the channel, which can then be modified for other purposes provided that the primary drainage function is not impaired. The specialist structures required for navigation canals are outwith the scope of land drainage design, but general capacity and flow requirements are identical. This applies also to irrigation channels, drinking water supplies and mill races, and they share with navigation canals the need to avoid excessive leakage from the channel if the primary function is to be achieved.

River systems and their man-made extensions are important wildlife habitats which can be damaged or enhanced by the effect of engineering works. The benefits to be obtained by sympathetic measures apply equally to fishing, wildfowling and other sporting interests as well as to conservation of wild species, because the requirements are identical in terms of a suitable environment. Surface drainage systems are valuable wildlife habitats because they traverse a wide range of land environments and act as corridors for wildlife activity as well as providing direct support for a multitude of species. The most valued systems are varied and range from cascading mountain streams to wide, meandering, lowland rivers. Ideally, the channel should have, from place to place, protruding boulders, flanking rocks, gravel banks, islands, alternating deep and shallow sections, rapids and still pools. The banks should range from vertical bare soil to steep vegetated banks with overhanging trees to gently sloping grassy banks providing easy access to the water. This is, of course, the very opposite of the smooth, idealised, trapezoidal cross-section which drainage works seek to achieve, but compromise is often possible. Suitable variations to the standard engineering design are described in detail in Newbold *et al.* (1983).

3.5 Modern drainage systems

Field drainage design can involve various combinations of open channels, buried pipe systems collectively known as *underdrainage* and a number of operations referred to as *soil treatment* or *secondary treatment*. The appropriate action for a particular project depends on the drainage problems at the site and on other factors such as the presence of earlier drainage investments and the availability of a suitable network of outlet channels. Correct selection demands a good understanding of the characteristics and installation requirements of the different kinds of drainage improvement works.

3.5.1 *Open channels*

Open channels are variously called ditches, dykes, cuts, drains or canals and can have a variety of functions in addition to land drainage. However, none of this is of any significance in terms of design criteria for land drainage works and the term '*ditch*' is used here to represent all open channels. Ditches can be used for the following drainage purposes:

To act directly as land drains in surface aquicludes.
To control the groundwater table in surface aquifers.
To intercept surface flow, interflow or groundwater flow.
To collect water from underdrainage systems.
To carry water to the outlet channel.
To act as reservoirs for drainage pumps.

The merits of these various functions can be discussed in turn, but it is necessary, first, to consider the general characteristics of open channels. *Ditches* have the advantage of allowing easy entry of surface flow or interflow water into the channel. They can be very effective even with slight gradients and have a very good overload capacity to cope with storm conditions. The open channel permits easy access to the outlets of associated underdrainage systems for maintenance purposes. They also have some disadvantages. Open channels permanently occupy land and restrict field traffic. They often require protective/safety fencing and crossing points, while the channel efficiency can deteriorate rapidly as weeds grow, silt accumulates and obstructions occur. Regular maintenance work is always required to keep the channel clear and free-flowing. The net effect is that ditches are chosen only for specific purposes, and each farm generally retains the minimum length which will remove excess water efficiently at an acceptable cost.

Land drainage ditches cut at intervals across the land can be quite effective. Carefully graded from an outlet and set at appropriate and regular intervals, they can control the groundwater table in an aquifer and remove excess water from the surface of an aquiclude. This breaks up the land into small parcels and is unacceptable for most productive farms except in special circumstances where land grading is employed in association with open channels (see Chapter 4). A cheap and long-established alternative is found in moorland and other areas of low-value grazing land where open channels are cut with a special plough through the existing turf. They are called moorland grips, hill drains or sheep drains. Although they help to remove surface water, the economic justification of such activity is at best only marginal. Somewhat similar drains are used in forestry for establishing a crop and in reclamation for the initial dewatering of saturated soil.

Well-placed *interceptor ditches* can collect and direct incoming surface flow and interflow where access to the source area is not available. All that is required is a small-scale ditch graded across the slope along the upper margin of the site to be protected. Interceptor ditches are less valuable for the control of groundwater flow because the seepage tends to cause instability in the ditch bank, which can slump and block the channel.

The *collector ditch* is by far the most common type on farms and is nearly always found along field margins where it acts as an outlet point for field underdrainage systems. In aquifers it will act as a land drain for adjacent land, and for very permeable aquifers the field margin ditches may achieve satisfactory control of the groundwater table across the whole area. This, however, is unusual unless the fields are very small, and the collection of underdrainage water is the primary function of most farm ditches. For this purpose, obviously, the ditch must be deeper than drain outlets, and it is desirable to have sufficient freeboard between outlets and ditch-water level at design discharge values. The *carrier ditch* is an extension of the collector ditch system and carries drainage water to the major outlet channel. It will be noted, therefore, that there is no clear distinction between these various functions, and design requirements are identical.

3.5.2 *Underdrainage*

Underdrainage is the basis of the great majority of field drainage works and involves the creation of permanent drainage channels by means of buried pipes. The pipes are usually either short-length, butt-jointed, clayware tiles which permit water entry at the joints, or continuous-length, perforated and flexible plastic piping. For most projects, one type or the other will be used exclusively, based on customer/contractor preference, but both types are effective if installed correctly. For larger capacity drains the normal range of cast concrete or fibre cement pipes can be used, and, where the pipes need not be sealed and will not be under pressure in use, it is quite satisfactory to use sound, outgrade sewerage pipes.

The buried channels of underdrainage can remove excess water without occupying land. They do not restrict field traffic and are protected from the general accumulation of rubbish. There is no weed growth in the channel, and the system can remain effective for many years with little need for maintenance. However, buried channels are not immune from siltation and blockage, and where maintenance is required it can be expensive and troublesome, sometimes requiring considerable remedial attention or even complete replacement of the whole system. Installation costs of new systems are more expensive than for an equivalent open-channel system. Pipes have very little overload capacity and, without special provision for regular maintenance, they require a greater gradient than open channels to remain effective. The most common limiting factor, however, is that excess water is prevented from flowing into the drainage channel by a poorly permeable soil profile.

Regularly spaced *field drains* can be used to control a high groundwater table or a perched water table (Figures 3.2 and 3.3). Such drains constitute the bulk of most projects and are called *minor* or *lateral drains* (Figure 3.3). The laterals may discharge directly into a ditch or they may connect to a single *collector drain*, which is called a *main* or *leader drain*. Leaders usually discharge into a ditch, but for large schemes several collector drains may connect to a single larger capacity leader, in which case the collector drains are called *submain* or *subleader drains*. Leader drains may connect with a *carrier drain* when the outlet channel is some distance away. All subleaders and leaders can act as field drains to nearby land, while all except the extremities of the laterals act also as carriers to a greater or lesser extent. True carrier drains do not act as field drains and do not require to allow entry of additional soil water, so that any solid-walled pipe of sufficient capacity may be used. Well-sited field drains can be *interceptors* for groundwater flow seepage if laid at appropriate depth, but their effectiveness against surface flow or interflow is less satisfactory unless the trench is filled to the surface with permeable material to form a *French drain*. Even then, the surface must be kept clear of vegetation and sediments if the interceptor is to remain effective.

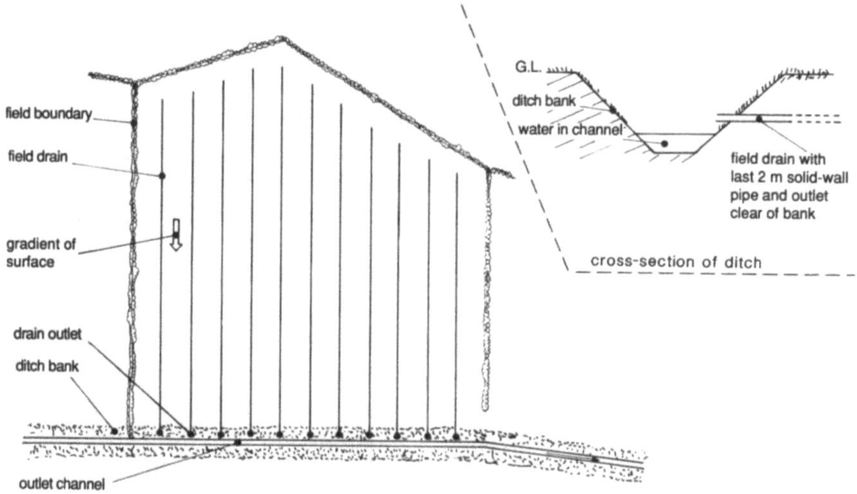

Figure 3.2 Underdrainage system with fen layout.

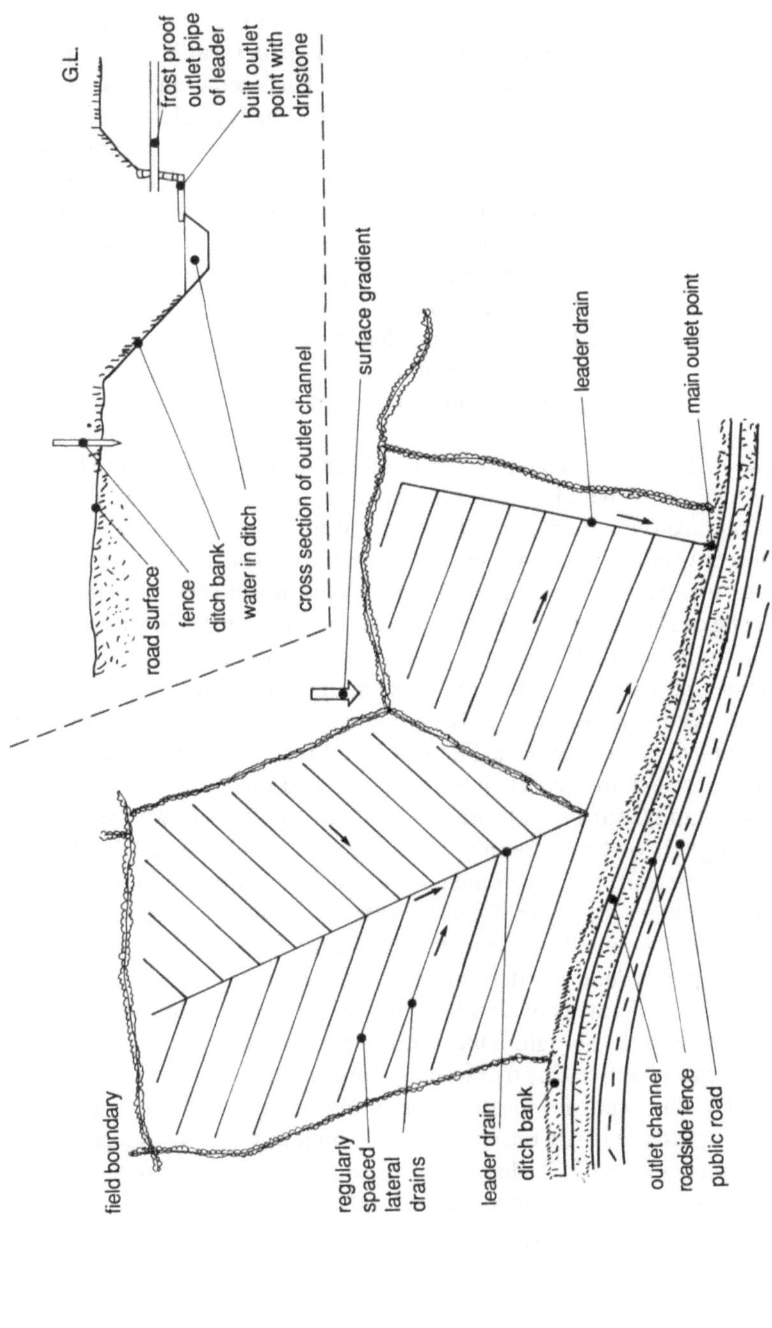

Figure 3.3 Underdrainage system with herringbone layout.

3.5.3 *Secondary drainage treatments*

Impermeable profiles usually do not respond well to drainage works when field drains only are installed. Interflow through permeable topsoil can cause some degree of dewatering for a time, until soil in the excavated trench settles and loses the macropores created by excavation. Structural improvement of this nature may not occur if a trenchless machine had been used. Loss of drain trench permeability is speeded up by the passage of heavy field traffic, and as this happens the profile drainage status tends to return to its predrained condition unless steps are taken to improve soil structure. The traditional response in this situation has been to adopt closely spaced drainage systems with adjacent drains installed at as little as 5-m intervals across the site. Theoretical calculations suggest that, with very low hydraulic conductivity values, spacings should be even closer. Very close spacings are neither practical nor economically sensible, and the situation must be tackled by the use of what have been termed *soil treatments* or *secondary treatments*. These include the use of permeable fill, subsoiling, mole drainage, gravelled mole drainage and gravel-filled slots.

Permeable fill is the name given to a range of materials, of which the best are washed gravel, small pebbles or graded broken rock, set on top of new field drains to replace the natural soil. Its main purpose is to act as a permanent permeable connection between new drains and the topsoil, or the zone affected by soil treatments, or old drains set higher in the soil profile. The materials used must be durable and resist decay, slaking or collapse, with the result that traditional materials such as straw, peat or brushwood are useful only for a time. Particle size can vary from 5 mm to 5 cm diameter, but it is preferable to have uniformity in size to prevent bridging in the hopper and to allow easy flow through delivery chutes. The fill must rest directly on top of the pipe and be piled high enough in the trench to make good connection with old drains, mole channels and fissuring, or topsoil as required, making allowance for up to 15 cm settling. In order to reduce costs, drains should be as shallow as circumstances permit and the trench should be as narrow as possible. The general arrangement for gravel-filled trenches is shown in Figure 3.4.

Mole drainage is usually the most effective method for draining soils in which profile permeability is determined by a dense clay subsoil. The mole drains are unlined channels of circular cross-section created in the subsoil by the passage of a mole plough, which consists essentially of a bullet-shaped share on the end of a tine. The method depends on the plastic cohesive nature of clay and works well in subsoils containing at least 30% of stable clay minerals which do not easily become slurried when wet. It is not successful for soil containing less than 25% clay, and difficulty is experienced with unstable clay minerals, particularly when moled for the first time. Experience has shown that the dewatering effect of repeated treatments often improves their stability. The disadvantage of mole drainage is that the unsupported channels will

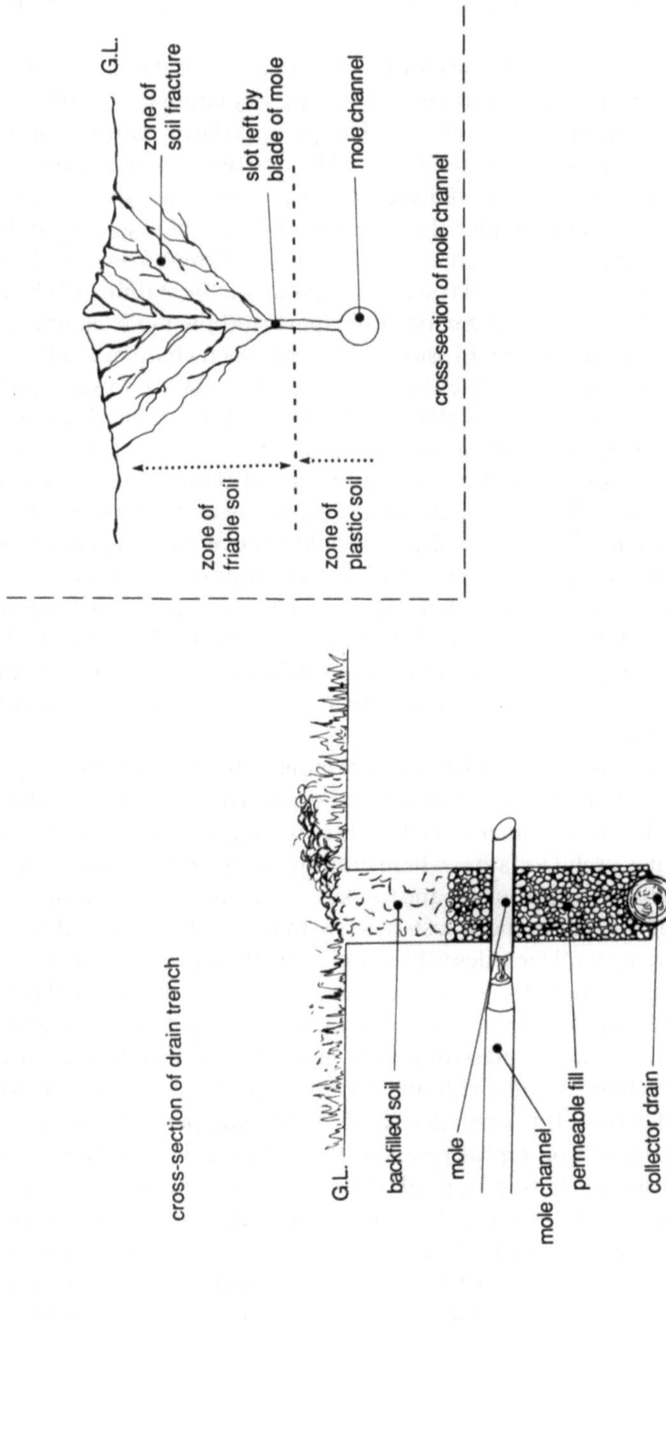

Figure 3.4 Mole dranage.

collapse, sooner or later, and the work must be repeated at regular intervals. Nevertheless, even where drainage must be carried out every few years, it is still cheaper and ultimately more effective than a closely spaced field drainage system.

The most favourable conditions for moling occur when the profile at mole depth is in a plastic condition but the soil above is dry enough to shatter when disturbed by the tine of the mole plough. This permits the formation of a clean, stable mole channel connected to the topsoil by a network of macropores (see Figure 3.4). Moling in wet conditions leaves only the tine slot above the mole, and this is quickly closed under the pressure of field traffic and by natural collapse. The gradient of mole channels cannot be different from the slope of the surface along the direction of travel. Depending on the stability of clay, the mole runs may be from 1 m to 5 m or more apart, and the mole channel from 45 to 60 cm below the surface. Erosion is reduced when channel gradients lie in the range 4–6‰, smaller values being selected for clays of lower stability. The collector drains should be as close as 20 m for the least stable clays, usually around 40 m spacing for more stable clay and, for the most satisfactory clay soils with an even surface and natural gradient, collector drains may not be needed at all. This is often the case in those areas where mole drainage has been a traditional activity. All collector drains should be covered with permeable fill to mole depth as illustrated in Figure 3.4. The technique of *mini-moling* is useful for draining sports fields and lawns. It should have similar but temporary benefits for pasture land and involves small-scale mole channels at about 30 cm depth, usually with several tines on a single frame set at 30 cm or more apart, but it should be considered as a cultivation activity rather than drainage for farm conditions.

Gravel tunnel drains or *gravelled moles* are mole channels formed by a special mole plough which delivers carefully graded pea-gravel into the mole channel as it is formed. The requirements and benefits are exactly as described for mole drainage, and it is useful for areas where mole draining presents difficulty. The gravel keeps the channels open and makes it much more expensive than moling but still likely to be more cost-effective than closely spaced field drains.

Subsoiling is a general term describing soil cultivation at depths greater than normal field cultivations. As a drainage improvement, it is more suited to non-clay soil profiles. Thus, it applies to potential surface aquifers with a perched water table over a pan or massive profile induration. Subsoilers are heavy-duty cultivation tines, usually with side plates, which lift and shatter the whole soil mass as they pass. It is very effective for shattering pans, but with deeper induration in the subsoil repeat passes with heavy tackle may be needed to achieve penetration. This is typical of restoration works on the site of completed engineering projects. After a pan has been broken up the profile may be restored to its natural permeability and any field drains present can be reactivated. In all other circumstances the provision of new collector drains is an important prerequisite for success. Subsoiling an indurated or impermeable profile without field drains to remove the excess soil water simply deepens the zone of saturation and makes cropping operations more difficult.

Subsoiling clay soils requires special consideration. There is a tendency to attempt subsoiling in heavy clay soils when there is reason to believe that moling will not be satisfactory. In order to achieve benefit, the profile should be reasonably dry and friable down to the required depth of subsoiling. This is an unlikely situation in the wetter maritime regions where such soils are common. Attempts to subsoil a plastic profile simply creates a rough square-section channel which is less stable even than a mole channel. Progress may be achieved by progressively deepening the depth of subsoiling in a sequence of operations. It is essential that the work is carried out over collector drains covered with permeable fill up to the base of the topsoil, thereby ensuring the immediate dewatering of any zone recently disrupted by the cultivation.

Subsoiling is a disruptive process, and one not concerned with the formation of channels or with precise gradients. The effects of subsoiling are shown in Figure 3.5. In the best conditions soil disruption creates a network of macropores, and ideally the adjacent zones of shattering should meet at the surface. For aquicludes, collector drains are needed for fast dewatering.

Gravel slotting involves cutting a narrow trench in the soil surface and filling it with gravel. It is cut by a machine that looks like the blade of a circular saw and can be quite narrow, something in the range 2–3 cm. It affects the topsoil only and is useful for dewatering sports fields or golf courses. It could also be used for permanent pasture for it is cheap to instal and causes little disruption

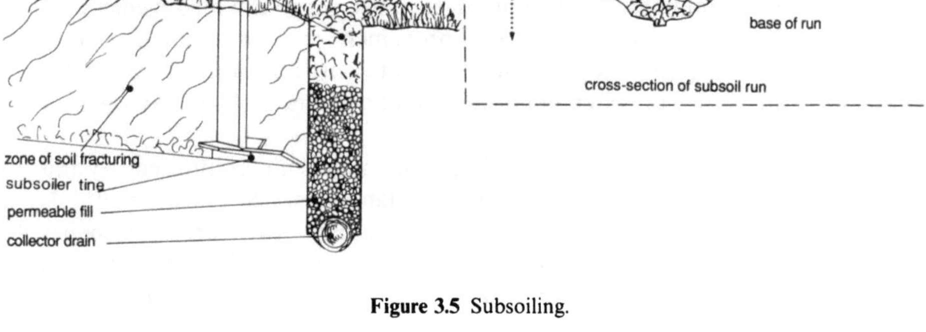

Figure 3.5 Subsoiling.

of the surface. But it is not more effective than other methods for permanent drainage works.

Unstable soil particles such as silt and very fine sand present particular drainage problems where they constitute a large part of the soil profile. They are carried into the drainage channel by flowing water, where they accumulate and block the pipe. *Filter-wrapped pipes* have been used to resolve this difficulty, but when the filter material is fine enough to prevent the entry of such small particles it quickly becomes clogged by them and rendered impermeable. The use of filter pads laid on top of field drains presents the possibility, albeit an expensive one, of replacing clogged filters, but this is feasible only if all drainage water enters the pipe via the drain trench. It ignores the pattern of flow towards drains through an aquifer.

3.6 Old drainage systems

The benefits of land drainage have long been known to farmers, and in the established temperate farming areas it is unusual to find an enclosed field that does not show signs of past attempts to improve the drainage characteristics of the soil. Records of drainage improvement going back as far as Roman times are essentially engineering projects to gain new land. Evidence of in-field drainage improvement is more recent.

The open field, strip-farming system operated by Saxon, Norman and later Medieval societies involved allocation of land in the form of long narrow strips which were convenient for ploughing with a team of oxen. With this system, it was a minor or perhaps inadvertent development to turn the furrow towards the centre of the strip for a sufficient number of years to create a central ridge and marginal furrows. Similar management of all the strips gave the land a ribbed appearance, and drainage improved as surface water was shed from each strip into the furrows. The strip system with its ridge and furrow drainage was lost as a result of the oft-repeated cross-cultivations made possible by the enclosures, which dated from about 1500; and now only remnants survive in areas of old pasture. Some of these have been underdrained more recently, with drains laid along the line of the wet furrows. New drainage and levelling cultivations are inhibited by the uneven surfaces, which are inconvenient for modern machinery. Comprehensive improvement in a one-stage operation would require storage of topsoil. In addition to cost restraints, the old ridge and furrow pastures are often important wildlife habitats which may warrant conservation.

Underdrainage did not become widespread until the nineteenth century and was initiated mostly by the improvers of great landed estates. Various methods were tried, including stepped trench walls capped with turf or trenches partially filled with peat, straw, brushwood or stone collected nearby. Of these, only the stone filled, or rubble drains persisted. Improved techniques employed channels constructed with slotted boards, slates or masoned stones. Clayware products became the most successful. At first, bricks with longitudinal cavities were followed by U-sectioned slabs developed from roofing tiles. Finally, true pipes of varing shape and dimension were manufactured and have been used ever since, but the term 'tile' has remained. Government assistance for drainage improvement began in the nineteenth century and has survived until the present day, which largly explains the widespread, almost comprehensive distribution of underdrainage. At an early stage, financial assistance depended upon adherence to specified design criteria, which may not have always been appropriate for the site or problem. Generally for assistance today in the form of a grant or low-interest loan, sound design and good standards of workmanship are required. Old underdrainage systems often are still partially active or have the capacity to become active if provided with a good outlet. As a general rule it may be assumed that old systems on level sites, when set deeper than the new scheme, may be ignored. On the other hand, very shallow systems may be disrupted by deep cultivation. In all other circumstances, every existing drain should be connected to the new system, either by a band of permeable fill or by special collector drains.

3.7 Systematic design

Detailed design criteria, methods of installation and standards of workmanship may be obtained from published texts (van Schilfgaarde, 1974; Hillel, 1982; Newbold *et al.*, 1983; Smedema and Rycroft, 1983; Farr and Henderson, 1986). However, it is important for engineers to be acquainted with the basic requirements of field drainage in order to provide satisfactory outlet channels. Sound design requires a systematic approach based on scientific principles so that the various stages are tackled logically and in the correct sequence.

The first requirement is to identify the drainage problems present, and this requires detailed examination of the soil profile and assessment of the influence of local and perhaps regional topography, the local geology and climate and the intended land use. The next step is to establish an outlet for the drainage water and where comprehensive natural gradients are not obviously available it will be necessary to carry out a levels survey. On very flat sites with only minor undulations it may be necessary to prepare a detailed contour map for drainage purposes. It is important at an early stage to identify the need for pump drainage. In the following paragraphs it is assumed that drainage by gravity flow is possible, either directly to the outlet channel or to the reservoir of a pumped drainage system.

It is convenient to begin discussion of field drainage design by considering a high groundwater table in a surface aquifer, as this land drainage condition is the basis of theoretical concepts. Drainage improvement demands only regularly spaced field drains and suitable outlet channels. The first limitation with design is that drains with a cover of less than 60 cm are liable to be damaged by field traffic. This may have a profound effect on gradient and, on the flattest sites, it may be necessary to set the drains absolutely level so that flow occurs by hydraulic gradient only. Levelling in these circumstances must be very accurate, and each drain should discharge directly into an outlet channel, thereby permitting regular jetting to remove the build-up of silt and other particles which can obstruct water flow in the drain. With deeper outlets into a ditch, gradient is possible, but when the values are less than 0.25% it is necessary to retain individual outlets. All such systems, based on a series of single parallel drains with individual outlets, are called *fen layout* (Figure 3.2). Where greater gradients are available the inconvenience of numerous outlet pipes along the ditch bank can be eliminated by connecting all field (lateral) drains to a leader drain, and if the connections are made at right angles the system is called a *grid layout*. Where drainage involves gradients greater than 2% it becomes necessary to align the laterals across the major slope to intercept any lateral flow and to avoid erosive flow velocities. Such systems, usually not associated with a high groundwater table, have lateral drains meeting the leader at an angle less than 90° and are called *herringbone layouts* (Figure 3.3). Where aquifers occur in an undulating surface, wet land may be confined to the hollows requiring an *irregular* or *natural layout*. Layouts with leader drains are not easily cleaned out by jetting, and the system can remain effective at minimum cost only if gradients are accurately and evenly maintained. Any section with a flatter gradient reduces flow velocity and causes siltation, which can lead to channel blockage.

In aquifers the drain spacing is a function of profile permeability and drain depth. Where gradients allow, the drains should be set as deep as possible. Spacings may be determined by any suitable formula based on steady-state or non-steady-state conditions (see section 5.1.7 and Chapter 2). It is commonly the case that the traditional drain spacing for a district is not very different from the theoretical value. All of this assumes that it is possible to measure the crucial hydraulic conductivity values in the profile. This is unlikely, and it is often better to assess profile permeability from soil texture and structural characteristics (See Table 4.2). Drain spacings usually lie between 10 and 80 m, the smallest values being suitable for aquifers composed of silt or very fine sand formations.

Having established gradient and drain spacing it is possible to calculate pipe size. The *design rainfall rate* should be obtained from average daily precipitation during the critical season multiplied by a factor which is based on 5-day storm events. The return frequencies range from once per year to once per 25 years depending on the crops to be grown. *Design drainage rate* is calculated from these figures, with allowance made for the effects of water-gathering surfaces, water-spreading surfaces, deep seepage and incoming groundwater flow. A margin of safety should be provided for pipe rugosity, siltation, entry resistance and concentration losses. Drainage design rate is converted to discharge for a given area of land which, with gradient, determines the internal diameter of the pipe.

Outlet ditches must be able to clear the drainage water, and for agricultural catchments the discharge may be based on design rainfall rate, the area of catchment, the channel gradient and any known additional inflows. Thereafter:

Ditch bottom width must match the discharge and provide a satisfactory ratio of depth of flow to width of flow at design discharge.
Ditch depth should be sufficient to provide a minimum of 15 cm freeboard between drain outlets and ditch-water level at design discharge flow rates.
Ditch batter must be sufficient to provide stable banks.
Ditch width follows from the other factors.

As a general rule it is better to reduce ditch gradient rather than field drain gradient where margins are limited. Ditches can flow satisfactorily down to about 0.01% gradient if kept clean. This completes the design work for controlling a groundwater table in an aquifer and, of course, the work must proceed in the opposite direction starting at the outlet and proceeding to the end of the lateral drains. Design for other drainage problems, though similar, differs in technique as described below.

Elimination of a perched water table in an aquifer involves subsoiling to disrupt the indurated layer. This may be sufficient to reactivate the existing drains, but where new drains are needed they should be installed first, as described above.

Much drainage work is concerned with alleviating the effects of a perched water table in a surface aquiclude. Whenever drain-spacing assessments indicate a value of less than 10 m the land should be considered as an aquiclude. Drainage improvement is essentially achieved by the creation of macropores in the profile by subsoiling or mole draining under the optimum conditions. A skeletal system of underdrains is required beforehand to act as collector drains for the water now able to move through the soil profile. Drain spacing is a function of soil stability: 20 m is satisfactory on the less stable soils, whilst the majority of sites respond well to a spacing of 40 m or more. In the most stable soils, mole drainage alone may produce effective results. In all circumstances, collector drains must be provided with permeable fill to a depth which intercepts the mole channels, the zone of subsoiling disruption or existing old drains as appropriate. It may be necessary to execute repeat treatments of the soil cultivation to reform channels or voids with the passage of time. The drains need not be any deeper than gradient and adequate cover require, and the trench should be as narrow as possible for economical use of permeable fill. It is an important requirement for secondary treatments that the soil voids so created are not left full of standing water for any length of time.

This will help to avoid slaking, collapse and premature loss of macropores. For this reason, the design rainfall rate should be based on 1-day storm events with the appropriate return frequency.

Appreciable quantities of surface flow or interflow reaching a site may be controlled by an interceptor ditch (or drain) aligned across the line of flow. Where lesser inflows occur, normal underdrainage for the site may be sufficient.

Control of groundwater flow requires interceptor drains located in a pattern as determined by the distribution of spring seepage. Gravity springs require one or more drains aligned across the slope and set into the supplying aquifer at a depth and spacing needed to divert groundwater from the soil. Artesian springs indicate the need to reduce groundwater pressure, and this is most easily achieved if drains graded from the outlet can be set into the aquifer. Where this is not possible the drain must be connected to the underlying aquifer by means of stone-filled sumps or by wells depending on the depth involved. Drainflow can be assessed by normal methods, but for minor seepages this may not be justified. Good results are usually achieved by selecting pipes of adequate capacity such as 10- or 15-cm diameter tiles.

The various drainage strategies can be complicated from site to site by the occurrence of difficult soils. The most widespread of these will be discussed in turn, and it will be noted that they need not be found in isolation from each other.

Flood plains. The special difficulties of river flood plains have already been mentioned in section 3.4 and include general lack of gradient, risk of inundation, leakage of river water into drainage channels, arterial seepage from underlying gravel, poorly permeable soil and inflows from marginal bluffs. Another factor is that the soil in the floodplain, usually river alluvium, is composed mainly of silt particles which are unstable in flowing water. Any disturbance of floodplain soil arising from drainage works or main channel improvement can disturb a sufficient quantity of silt to pollute river ecosystems or fish farms downstream.

Peat. Comprehensive drainage of an all-organic soil profile can be difficult to achieve and the degree of success uncertain. Unimproved peat is very soft when wet and may not support heavy drainage machinery without preliminary dewatering. Even after drainage is installed, the removal of surplus water causes loss of bulk in the profile and initiates decay of organic matter by creating aerobic conditions. The net result is that the soil mass shrinks to a remarkable extent and loses permeability. Shrinkage can occur both above and below the field drains and is often uneven. To counteract this and maintain alignment in the drains, tiles were often laid on boards, but plastic piping solved the problem and loss of gradient by sagging is less damaging when the pipes are covered with permeable fill, allowing continuation of flow through the gravel. Drains in peat should not be less than 1 m deep, which provides adequate cover. A further difficulty arises from the fact that, when drained, organic soils often give rise to the rapid formation of iron ochre. Most of these difficulties, apart from shrinkage, have been solved in long-cultivated peatlands, where new drainage can be quite straightforward, but reclamation projects should be considered with care since the benefits are uncertain and, even where successful, drainage may seriously damage a valuable wetland habitat for wildlife.

Iron ochre. Many soils contain appreciable amounts of water-soluble compounds of iron which can be oxidised to insoluble ferric oxide after drainage introduces aerobic conditions deep in the soil profile. The iron ochre may remain in the soil mass, it may form a scale on pipes, gravel, filters and trench walls or it may appear as a floating red–brown gelatinous material in the drainage water. Drainage should be of the fen layout design, which permits regular jetting to flush out the ochre in the pipes. Remedial flushing should be carried out before the ochre has time to dry out and harden in or on the pipes. Once it is allowed to dry it forms a scale which cannot be removed and, if the water entry points become blocked, the pipes have to be replaced. The amount of ochre which does form depends on the original iron content in the soil. After the initial period of flush, the amount released tends to reduce with time so that, once again, reclamation projects are potentially the most troublesome. Regular subsoiling at an early stage after drains have been installed may encourage ochre formation within the soil mass, reducing the amount reaching the drainage system. Significant amounts of ochre in drainage water is a polluting material which may require containment in settling ponds.

Unstable silt. Any loose soil not protected by vegetation can be eroded by flowing water such that the greater the flowing velocity the larger the size of particles that can be removed. The natural cohesion of clay minerals gives them a degree of stability not possessed by silt and very fine sand which are the least stable of soil particles. They can be moved through the soil body by water flowing towards drains and, when present in quantity, can cause such siltation in the pipe that blockage occurs. Measures to alleviate the problem include adopting a fen layout to facilitate low-pressure jetting (jetting can erode the soil outside the pipe) and the use of silt traps which must be emptied at regular intervals. Filters are not normally very satisfactory. With regard to ditches, the normal methods of bank stabilisation can be used, and structures to reduce flow velocity may be necessary. In the worst situations, very flat gravel bankings should be considered when revetment would not be justified.

Acid sulphate soils. When drain pipes, etc., are to be made from cement, it is prudent to test the soil water for its acidity and sulphate content. Where subsoils are more acid than pH 6.5 or groundwater contains more than 0.06% dissolved sulphate, ordinary Portland cement is corroded and pipe life, especially the porous types, is shortened. Sulphate-resistant cement should be specified where the use of concrete materials cannot be avoided.

3.8 Reinstatement of field drains

Engineering works crossing agricultural land, particularly pipelines, nearly always disrupt drainage systems and may also interfere with outlet channels. Reinstatement is essential if the land is to continue in productive agricultural use. The variations in problems encountered are many but a number of basic techniques should solve most of them:

When ditches are to be diverted, the new channel should be based on normal design requirements for the size and nature of catchment involved.

Where two or more carrier channels are to be amalgamated, the new carrier should be of adequate capacity for the larger catchment.

Where ditches are to be piped or culverts constructed, the discharge capacity should make allowance for the loss of overload capacity.

When ditches are diverted, the leaders of field drainage systems must be extended along a suitable route to reach the new channel.

All drains exposed by the new ditch cutting should be provided with protected outlets.

Underdrainage systems disrupted by major pipeline trenches should be provided with a new collector drain of adequate capacity to divert drainage water from the upslope side to a new outlet point.

For minor pipelines such as water pipes requiring a narrow trench only, field drains may be bridged across the track by using short lengths of firm, solid-walled piping, set in stable, undisturbed soil at each side of the trench.

Where leader and carrier drains must cross wider trenches, they should be supported by bridges of sufficient strength set into solid material on both sides of the trench.

Where leader and carrier drains must cross a trench but the pipeline is at the same level and no alternative route is available, it is necessary to construct a siphon system which must have a silt trap at each side of the pipe.

Where engineering works release confined groundwater, it is necessary to install suitable drains to intercept the flow and carry it to an outlet.

3.9 General design and supervision requirements

Successful land drainage requires accurate design, good workmanship, suitable choice of materials and adequate supervision. Drainage design must also be based on sound economic principles. It is important to recognise that some sites will present unsurmountable physical difficulties whilst for others, although drainage is technically possible, the cost of doing so may be prohibitive when assessed against the likely returns on the investment.

Even where design and choice of materials are satisfactory, the workmanship must be of a matching standard. Care is needed to ensure that design gradients are being achieved, and for this it is not enough to rely on sophisticated machine-mounted gradient control devices. The work must be checked. Most important of all, the conditions must be suitable for drainage traffic. Drainage machines and ancillary equipment are heavy and cause compaction. Operations in wet conditions cause smearing and compaction of the topsoil. Sinking and crabbing can cause poor gradient control and smearing of the trench sides and produce slurried soil which may block the pipe inlets. All of these difficulties are reduced or eliminated when the work is carried out in dry conditions.

Decisions on investments in land drainage should be based on three main factors. It is necessary, firstly, to establish, as far as possible, that drainage improvement to a significant extent is technically feasible; secondly, that it will not result in unacceptable damage to the countryside; thirdly, that the installation and running costs will be reasonable in relation to the likely extra income derived as a consequence of improved drainage. It may be necessary to seek ecological/countryside advice on environmental matters, and the likely returns will be assessed by the investor, but a field drainage adviser can be expected to assess feasibility and provide installation costs.

4 Field drainage in non-temperate climates

P.B. LEEDS-HARRISON and R.J. RICKSON

In many tropical climates the pattern of rainfall differs greatly from that in temperate regions. In particular, rainfall intensity in some areas is very much higher than in temperate climates, while in others the annual quantity and distribution of rain can be such that profitable agriculture is not possible without irrigation. These two features, high rainfall intensity and irrigation, can lead to drainage problems specific to these areas. This chapter examines drainage design for erosion control in areas of high rainfall intensity and for the control of waterlogging and salinity in irrigated arid and semiarid areas.

4.1 Drainage in irrigated areas

More than 200 million hectares of the world are irrigated, and in over 50% of this area rainfall on an annual basis is low and occurs in only a few weeks of the year. Such semiarid and arid climates rely almost entirely on irrigation water for agricultural production. Much of this water is derived from river systems or groundwater aquifers, and irrigation in these areas can turn arid lands into highly productive ones.

Irrigation systems impose dense networks of canals and water courses on the areas which transform the soil environment from a dry one to a much wetter one. Water in irrigation canals dominates the area to be irrigated, and inevitably seepage and percolation of water occur. Intercepting runoff from these areas with surface drains or controlling water tables by subsurface tube drains become important considerations in the design and layout of an irrigated area.

4.1.1 *The drainage problem*

It is a feature of all irrigation schemes that more water is added to the soil than is actually required to make up the deficit in the soil which results from evapotranspiration by crops. In addition to the excess water which drains through the root zone of the crop, water seeps from irrigation canals and water courses, and together these can lead to a problem of waterlogging.

In many older irrigation schemes, drainage for water table control was not included in the design, and in many instances the problem of waterlogging only becomes obvious many years after the commissioning of the scheme. For example, the water table in Bhantinda Mansa in India rose at a rate of $0.4\,m\,yr^{-1}$ after the scheme was introduced at the turn of the century and has now reached the point where yields have dropped considerably (Bos, 1984). The great irrigation systems of the Indus Valley are only now experiencing massive loss in yield as a result of waterlogged soils some 50–100 years after the schemes were first introduced; but the rate of rise of the water table has been estimated at $2.5\,m\,yr^{-1}$ in a more recent scheme in West Nubaria in Egypt. To understand how to deal with this emerging drainage problem it is first necessary to understand something of the efficiency of irrigation systems.

4.1.2 *Irrigation efficiency*

Irrigation practice is concerned with the replenishment of soil water which has been transpired by the crop or evaporated from the soil surface. Figure 4.1 shows the water balance situation in the field during the irrigation season. The water used by the crop comes from the root zone, so that just prior to irrigation there is a soil-moisture deficit. Irrigation water applied to the soil aims to make up this deficit and return the soil to near field-capacity condition.

Methods of applying water to the soil can be divided into three groups: above ground, below ground and surface. Of these, surface methods of

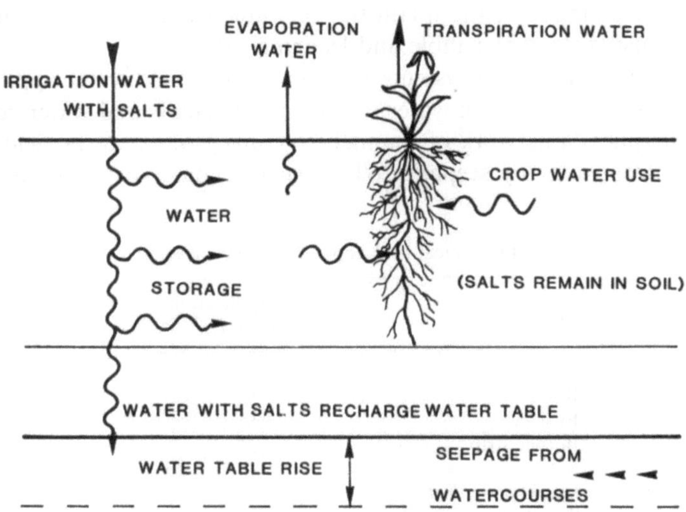

Figure 4.1 Water and salt balance during the irrigation season.

applying water are by far the most widely used from a worldwide perspective, and this is particularly so in developing countries. In highly developed agricultural systems, above-ground methods are more common, particularly where irrigation supplements rainfall.

All irrigation methods are inefficient in that more water is applied to the field than is stored in the root zone. Water is lost from the area being irrigated by evaporation from open-water surfaces, by seepage from canals and water courses, by drainage through the base of the root zone of the crop and by runoff. However, in terms of field application of water, some methods are more efficient than others. Field application efficiency, E_a, is defined as the ratio of the water stored in the root zone immediately after irrigation divided by the gross amount of water applied to the field and expressed as a percentage. Table 4.1 shows typical efficiencies of water application for different irrigation methods.

In arid situations where surface methods of irrigation are practised, much of the inefficiency of water application comes from overwatering, although such factors as the concentration of water in low spots in the field and the direct transmission of water through the root zone in soil cracks and fissures are important considerations. Overwatering arises from poor irrigation water management, and there is little doubt that improved management practice through water control and scheduling can greatly reduce the scale of the drainage problem.

It will be seen, however, that there may often be a need to ensure that there is a drainable surplus and that water passes through the root zone to maintain a suitably low salt concentration in the root zone. A knowledge of irrigation efficiency is essential in drainage design, as it is from this that estimates can be made of the quantities of water which drain through the root zone, raising the water table and leaching salts.

Inefficiencies in irrigation systems arise not only in field water application but also in the conveyance of water to the field in canals and water courses. Irrigation requires a network of channels to convey water to the field, all of which may lose water by seepage. Where such seepage losses occur, water

Table 4.1 Typical field application efficiencies.

Method	Field application efficiency E_a(%)
Surface methods	
Basin	50
Furrow	55
Border strip	55
Overhead methods	
Sprinkler	60–65
Trickle	up to 90

infiltrates downwards through the soil, causing a rise in the water table of the area. Conveyance efficiencies may be very low for poorly constructed earth bank canals but may be very high for lined canals. Where an earthen channel conducts water only on the day of irrigation and is dry in between irrigations, cracking of the banks of the channel may lead to extremely high losses.

Conveyance efficiency, E_c, is defined as the the ratio of water received at the field or block of fields to the water put into the conveyance system. Field canals and water courses have typical conveyance efficiencies of 70–80%, while lined canals have efficiencies of 80–95%.

4.1.3 *Irrigation intervals*

It is important that intervals between irrigations are known, as recharge to the water table by seepage through the root zone or from field water courses occurs predominantly at the time of water application, and the interval between irrigation is the time during which the water table must be allowed to fall.

Irrigation is usually practised on a rotational basis, supplying water either at regular fixed intervals or at an interval determined by the demand for water. The intervals between irrigations and the quantities of water required at each irrigation will thus depend on the nature of crop, the environmental demand for water, and the water-holding capacity of the soil. The scheduling of irrigation takes these factors and the efficiencies of the system into account. Methods of making estimates of water demand, irrigation quantities and intervals may be found in various texts (e.g. Doorenbos and Pruit, 1977).

4.1.4 *The salinity problem*

In many irrigated areas the problem of high salt levels in the root zone of the crop is associated with the drainage problem. Where the environmental demand for water is high and it is satisfied by irrigation water, there is a risk that the level of salinity will rise in the root zone of the crop. Figure 4.1 shows the situation which occurs in the soil during the irrigation season. Irrigation waters often contain dissolved salts which are not readily taken up by the plant but instead are left in the soil after water has been transpired. Hence irrigation at 100% efficiency inevitably leads to a rise in soil salinity levels, perhaps to a level at which crop production suffers. Many plants have some salt tolerance, and some can stand quite high levels of salt in the root zone without any detrimental effect. Doorenbos and Pruit (1977) list the expected yield of crops as a percentage of the maximum possible yield for increasing salinity levels in the root zone. This shows, for instance, that barley and cotton are tolerant of quite high levels of salinity whereas corn and legumes have a low tolerance.

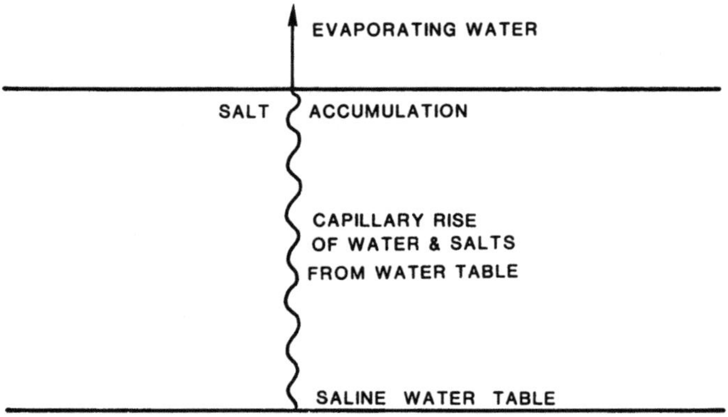

Figure 4.2 Capillary rise from a saline water table during a fallow period.

An additional salinity problem shown in Figure 4.2 can arise during a fallow season when there is no irrigation. Here the groundwater itself is high in soluble salts, so that during the fallow period, when the water table is close to the soil surface, capillary rise takes water and salts into the upper layers of the soil. Evaporating water leaves very high salt concentrations in the surface layers of the soil, which can often be seen as white crystalline deposits. Such deposits can be removed by leaching the salts with irrigation water and flushing them out by means of a drainage system.

In practice, the problem of capillary rise only occurs when the water table is kept high by incoming seepage from outside the fallow area. In this situation drainage to control the position of the water table is required. The depth, Z, to which the water table should be controlled can be estimated from the following equation:

$$Z = \frac{\ln(1 + k_0/E)}{C} \tag{4.1}$$

where k_0 is the saturated hydraulic conductivity of the soil, C is the exponent term in eqn 2.10 (which uses k for the k_0 here), and E is the evaporation rate from the soil surface. For a given soil the calculated value of Z from this equation depends on the chosen value of E; a value of $2\,\mathrm{mm\,d^{-1}}$ is usually

Table 4.2 Some values of k_0 and C for different soil types.

Soil type	$k_0\,(\mathrm{m\,d^{-1}})$	$C\,(\mathrm{m^{-1}})$
Sandy loam	1.8	18.0
Silty loam	0.85	4.00
Fine sand	1.1	2.00
Structured clay	0.5	10.0

considered sufficiently low to prevent excessive salinisation of the root zone. In general, as the size of the pores in the soil increases both k_0 and C become larger (Table 4.2). However, structure and aggregation in the soil have a large effect on the values, so it is not possible to give typical values of the exponent C on the basis of texture alone.

4.1.5 *Leaching requirement*

Where irrigation water is saline and there is a danger of salinity developing, excess irrigation water must pass through the root zone to maintain the required average salinity. The leaching requirement is calculated as that depth of water required for leaching and which must pass through the root zone. It is calculated as a fraction of the water needed to satisfy crop water demand less any effective rainfall. The leaching requirement, LR, may be estimated from the following equations:

$$\mathrm{LR} = \frac{\mathrm{EC_w}}{f(5\mathrm{EC_e} - \mathrm{EC_w})}(\mathrm{ET_c} - P_\mathrm{e}) \quad \text{for surface or sprinkler irrigation} \tag{4.2a}$$

or $$\mathrm{LR} = \frac{\mathrm{EC_w}}{2\mathrm{EC_{e\,max}}}(\mathrm{ET_c} - P_\mathrm{e}) \quad \text{for trickle irrigation} \tag{4.2b}$$

where $\mathrm{EC_w}$ is the electrical conductivity of the irrigation water, $\mathrm{EC_e}$ is the required electrical conductivity of the soil saturation extract for an acceptable level of yield, $\mathrm{EC_{e\,max}}$ is the maximum acceptable electrical condutivity of the soil, $\mathrm{ET_c}$ is the crop water evapotranspiration over the period considered, P_e is the effective rainfall over the period considered and f is the leaching efficiency. Where water leaches uniformly through the soil, as in a single-grained graded sand, efficiencies are high. Where structural cracks and large vertical pores exist, efficiencies can be low. Salt levels are expressed as electrical conductivities rather than concentrations, because electrical conductivity is considered to be linearly related to solution concentration and is relatively easy to measure.

4.1.6. *Estimation of drainage quantities and water table rise*

Drainage quantities to be dealt with by field drains are calculated as the excess irrigation water recharging the water table at each irrigation. This leads to the general statement:

$$\mathrm{DR} = r(\mathrm{IR} - \mathrm{SMD}) \tag{4.3}$$

where DR is the drainable surplus recharging the water table, IR is the irrigation water supplied to the area, SMD is the soil-moisture deficit at the end of the irrigation interval and r is the fraction of the excess irrigation water which recharges the water table; r often has a high value of between 0.9 and 1.0, however, some water losses may be intercepted by surface drainage, and in these cases r may be lower.

The excess water passing through the root zone (the deep percolation loss, DPL) is found from the field application efficiency. Here:

$$\mathrm{DPL} = r_1[(\mathrm{SMD}/E_a) - \mathrm{SMD}] \tag{4.4}$$

Losses in the field water courses, WL, which will occur at the same time as the field losses, are found by considering the water course conveyance efficiency:

$$\mathrm{WL} = r_2[(\mathrm{SMD}/E_a \times E_c) - \mathrm{SMD}/E_a] \tag{4.5}$$

These two losses, from the field and from the water course, can be considered to act together to recharge the water table on the day of irrigation.

The resulting rise in the water table at irrigation may be calculated from:

$$\mathrm{WTR} = \frac{\mathrm{WL} + \mathrm{DPL}}{p} \tag{4.6}$$

where p is the drainable porosity. However, it is usual to multiply this value by 1.5 (Dumm and Winger, 1964) to take into account the inability of many simple transient flow equations to describe adequately the early part of the water table recession. This provides an estimate of the maximum rise of the water table midway between drains.

Irrigations occur at defined intervals, and the water table rises rapidly at this time, declining slowly between irrigations as water is removed by the drainage system. Thus drains are placed at a depth which allows the water table to fluctuate and ensures that it does not enter the root zone of the crop. The minimum drain depth for the irrigation season is determined by the root zone depth, the zone needed for water table fluctuations and the capillary fringe. However drainage theory shows that the water table would take an infinitely long time to be drawn down to drain level midway between the drains. Consequently drains are placed somewhat lower than this minimum in the soil. The limit to which drains are placed below the minimum will depend on the nature of the drainage control required, the depth to which drain-laying machines can work, allowing for the need to grade the pipe to an outfall, and the costs associated with deeper working.

4.1.7 *Drain-spacing requirements*

The spacing to which drains should be placed can be estimated from drainage equations, knowing the quantities of water that have to be discharged within the interval between irrigations. Inputs to the water table are considered to recharge it instantaneously, resulting in the rise given in eqn 4.6. The average drain flow rate, q_{av}, will be:

$$q_{av} = (\mathrm{WL} + \mathrm{DPL})/T_1 \tag{4.7}$$

where T_1 is the irrigation interval.

This value, q_{av}, may be used in a steady-state equation such as that of Hooghoudt (1940), (see section 2.6), but it is often more satisfactory to use a transient-state drainage equation for the calculation of the spacing knowing that the water table must decline from a maximum immediately after irrigation to a minimum just before the next irrigation. Such an approach allows the fluctuation of the water table to be modelled over the whole irrigation season and the effect of varying drain spacing to be assessed. Such equations include that of Dumm (1954) or Youngs (1985) (see section 2.7).

For drainage design, Hooghoudt's equation is written as:

$$L^2 = 1/q(8kdh + 4kh^2) \tag{4.8}$$

where L is the required drain spacing to control the water table to a mid-drain water table height, h, under a steady state through flow q, k is the saturated hydraulic conductivity of the soil and d is called the equivalent depth. The equivalent depth is a function of drain spacing, the depth to the impermeable layer and the wetted perimeter of the drain (see Chapter 2).

Dumm's equation is written as:

$$L^2 = \pi^2(kd_{av}t/p)/(\ln 1.16\, h_0/h_t) \tag{4.9}$$

Here k is as above, p is the drainable porosity and t is the time required for the mid-drain water table to drop from height h_0 to h_t during the recession. D_{av} is the average depth of the saturated zone during the recession and is taken as being equal to $(d + h_{av}/2)$. Note that many drainage equations have been developed from soil-water physics (see Chapter 2).

In transient-state analysis it is usual only to consider the recession of the water table as it falls from its maximum height above the drain immediately after irrigation to just prior to the next irrigation. It is normal to consider the situation where the capillary fringe is at the base of the root zone, and this determines the maximum height of the water table at the start of the recession. As the rate of drawdown depends on how far apart the drains are spaced, appropriate drain spacings can be found to allow the water table to fall sufficiently before the next irrigation. Such calculations are made in the first instance for the most critical period during the irrigation season, which will be when the irrigation interval is at its shortest and/or quantities of water input are greatest. Having made a preliminary calculation for the required drain spacing and depth, it is useful to simulate the fluctuation of the water table throughout the irrigation season.

4.1.8 *Rainfall during the irrigation season*

When rainfall occurs during the irrigation season it may affect the quantities of water draining to the water table. The worst situation occurs when there is rainfall just after irrigation. At this time the water table is already at or just below the base of the root zone and the soil in the unsaturated zone is at field capacity, so the water table will inevitably rise into the root zone, and the drainage design should allow for its rapid removal. Crops vary in their tolerance to waterlogging, but in general it is recommended that where the root zone is completely saturated the drainage scheme should lower the water table to 0.3 m from the soil surface within 24 hours and achieve a completely aerated root zone within 3–5 days. Often this criterion is met by designs based on the removal of irrigation inputs only.

4.1.9 *Example of a drainage design calculation*

The starting point for the design is a knowledge of the soil properties, crop, climate, irrigation quantities, intervals and efficiencies. Table 4.3 lists the required data. In this example, the peak water application is 92 mm, with a corresponding irrigation interval of 14 days. The deep percolation loss in the field:

$$\text{DPL} = 0.94 \times [(92/0.65 - 92] = 47\,\text{mm}$$

(taking 0.94 as the fraction of the field losses which go to deep percolation).

The leaching requirement is calculated from eqn 4.2(a) as 22 mm for this

Table 4.3 Soil, crop and irrigation data for the critical crop and irrigation season.

Soil									
Soil texture									Sandy loam
Hydraulic conductivity									$1.6\,\text{m}\,\text{d}^{-1}$
Drainable porosity									$0.14\,\text{m}\,\text{m}^{-1}$
Assumed capillary fringe									0.09 m
Leaching efficiency									70%
Irrigation									
Field application efficiency									65%
Water course conveyance efficiency									85%
Irrigation water quality									$5\,\text{dS}\,\text{m}^{-1}$
Irrigation data for whole season:									
Irrigation no.	1	2	3	4	5	6	7	8	9
Deficit at irrigation (mm)	33	47	47	61	80	92	85	78	59
Irrigation interval (d)	30	20	20	17	17	14	14	17	40
Crop									
Root zone depth									1 m
Maximum permissible soil salinity									$7\,\text{dS}\,\text{m}^{-1}$

$1\,\text{dS}\,\text{m}^{-1}$ = 1 decisiemen per metre.

irrigation interval. Since the leaching requirement is much less than the deep percolation loss, no extra water needs to be added to the soil to maintain the required salt balance. If the leaching requirement had been close to or greater than the deep percolation loss in the field then extra leaching water would have been needed, increasing the amount to be dealt with by the drainage system.

The conveyance loss:

$$\mathrm{WL} = 0.95 \times [92/(0.65 \times 0.85)] - (92/0.65) = 24\,\mathrm{mm}$$

(taking the fraction of the conveyance loss contributing to water table rise as 0.95). (Note that conveyance losses do not contribute to leaching.)

Water recharging the water table at this irrigation $= 47 + 24\,\mathrm{mm} = 71\,\mathrm{mm}$ (the drainable surplus). Thus the average flow rate to the drains is $(71/14) = 5\,\mathrm{mm\,d^{-1}}$. Note that this is the value for the peak part of the irrigation season: average flow values for the whole season may be typically 1.5–$3\,\mathrm{mm\,d^{-1}}$.

Using eqn 4.6 and a factor of 1.5, the water table rise at this irrigation is:

$$\mathrm{WTR} = 1.5 \times (0.071/0.14) = 0.76\,\mathrm{m}$$

Hence the required minimum depth to the drain can be estimated as

$$0.76 + 0.09 + 1.0 = 1.85\,\mathrm{m}$$

In practice, the drains are laid perhaps 0.1–0.2 m lower than this. If there is a steady input from outside the area, an additional depth allowance must be added to account for the control of this recharge. In the example it will be assumed that the drains are placed at a depth of 2.0 m. This should be deep enough for the control of capillary rise during the fallow season if there is an inflow of water to the area keeping the water table at drain depth. For a sandy loam using the values in Table 4.2 and eqn 4.1 it is found that a depth of 0.4 m will control capillary rise to less than $2\,\mathrm{mm\,d^{-1}}$ and so the depth of 2 m for the irrigation season is quite satisfactory.

The assumption is that just prior to recharge the water table is at a depth of 1.85 m below the soil surface and rises to 1.09 m from the soil surface just after irrigation so the logarithmic average height of the water table above drain level midway between drains during recession is 0.46 m. (Note that the logarithmic mean is used as the fall of the water table follows an exponential decay. The arithmetic mean is 0.53 m, i.e. higher than the logarithmic mean, as would be expected.)

Using Hooghoudt's steady-state equation, taking $h = 0.46\,\mathrm{m}$ and $q = 5\,\mathrm{mm\,d^{-1}}$, and noting that the depth to the impermeable boundary is infinite or at least more than 0.25 times the drain spacing, it is found from an iterative procedure or from nomographs that the required spacing is 76 m.

Using the transient-state drainage equation of Dumm, the drain spacing required to lower the water table from 0.7 to 0.19 m above the drain within the 14-day irrigation interval is 55 m. A close agreement between these two approaches is often not found, and in general taking the transient approach is preferable, as it accounts for actual soil-water storage changes and ensures a rapid initial drawdown of the water table.

4.1.10 *Simulation of the whole irrigation season*

At the start of the irrigation season the water table may be at or below the level of the drains if there is no incoming seepage from outside the area. In the above example with drains placed at 2.0 m depth the fluctuations of the water table throughout the irrigation season can be simulated using a transient drainage equation. In Figure 4.3 such a simulation has been carried out for the above data using the irrigation data given in Table 4.3.

It can be seen that, with the spacing found from the initial calculation, the water table is easily contained below the root zone. Drain spacing can be increased, as shown, to 65 m without compromising root zone aeration or salinity. In addition, it can be seen that the water table is at a high level for only a short time and rapidly falls away from the root zone. An increase in spacing from 55 to 60 m (9%) can allow significant reductions in costs in large drainage schemes, although it may be of little importance in small schemes.

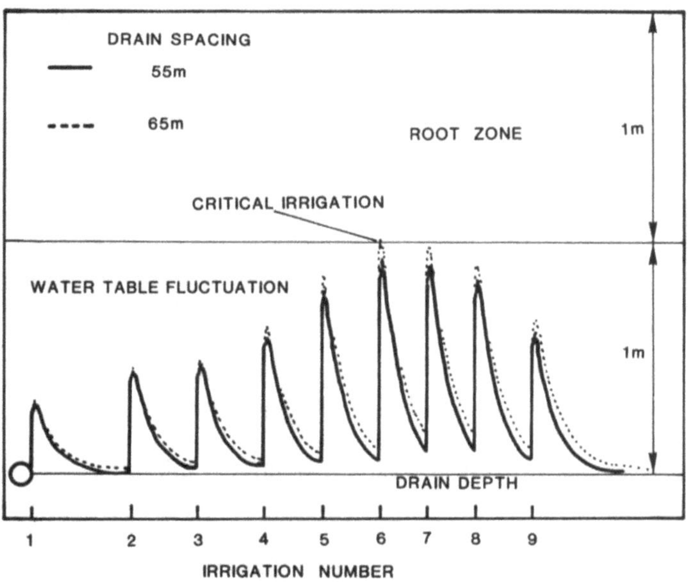

Figure 4.3 Simulation of water table fluctuations during the irrigation season for drain spacings of 55 m and 65 m.

4.1.11 *Rainfall immediately after irrigation*

If there is a rainfall event immediately after the irrigation water has been applied to the soil, then the added water input from the rainfall will directly recharge the water table. If the drainage design has aimed to allow the water table to rise to just below the root zone, then the water table will now rise into it, excluding air. Suppose drains are spaced at 60 m (as in the above example) and the fraction of the 1 in 5 year rainfall event which percolates into the soil is 50 mm. In this case, the additional rise in the water table is $1.5 \times (0.05/0.14) = 0.54$ m. Thus initially the water table will be 1.54 m above the drain at mid-drain position. The Dumm equation can be used to estimate the time that is required for the water table to drop to the base of the root zone, i.e. by 0.54 m.

From eqn 4.9:

$$t = (1/a)\ln(1.16H_0/H_t)$$

where $a = \pi^2 kD_{av}/pL^2$. For the soil data given and a spacing of 60 m, $a = 0.154$ and $t = 3.7$ days. This would probably be an acceptable period for reaeration of the root zone for all but the most sensitive crops. The rainfall event chosen for this analysis will depend on the rainfall return period and the value of the enterprise being drained. Typically a 1 in 5 year return period might be chosen for irrigated arable crops.

4.1.12 *Interception of seepage water from canals*

So far only those losses which raise the water table locally at each irrigation have been considered. In the case of seepage losses from canals, these may occur all year round, and this small but continuous input to the general area may be a major contributor to water table rise. The use of interceptor drains or ditches to prevent waterlogging is shown in Figure 4.4 (a and b). The amount of water that will be intercepted by such drains depends on the geometry of the system. Flownets are a useful way of estimating seepage to the drain, and on the basis of such analyses drain size can be estimated. However, note that the deeper the interceptor drain is placed the greater will be the loss from the canal. Generally the drain should be placed as far from the canal as is practical. While it is theoretically possible to intercept all of the seepage with a fully penetrating ditch drain, this is not possible when there is a deep aquifer below the drain. In some cases only a small percentage of the seepage can be collected in this way. Lining canals is expensive but can cut down on seepage loss dramatically, and in some situations silt deposits around the perimeter of the canal can greatly reduce losses. It is not uncommon to re-use seepage water intercepted in this way for irrigation either by placing the drain at a shallower grade than that of the canal so that the intercepted water may be reintroduced into the canal

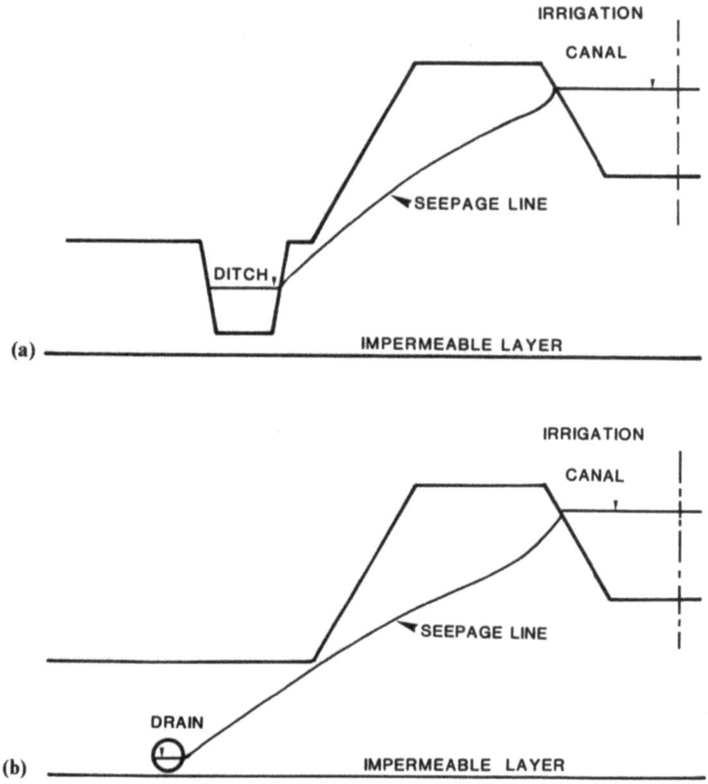

Figure 4.4 Control of seepage losses from an irrigation canal where there is a shallow depth to the impermeable layer; (a) by a ditch drain; (b) by a tube drain.

further downstream or by using the water directly in fields adjacent to the canal.

4.1.13 *Pipe drainage outfalls*

The depth to which drains are placed in irrigated areas is considerably deeper than that usually required in humid, temperate areas. This introduces a problem of lack of outfall in those cases where natural land gradients are low. For the above example, a lateral drain requires a depth of 2 m to control the water table. If the lateral is 500 m long and laid to a gradient of 0.1% (i.e. 1 mm in 1 m), then the depth of the lateral outfall will be 2.5 m. If this is fed to a collector, which in turn is laid to a suitable gradient, then the outfall may be 3 m or more below the soil surface. It is unlikely that surface drainage canals to which the water is to be discharged will have a level lower than this, so water has to be lifted by pumping. Such pumping systems would typically serve perhaps 500 ha (see Chapter 9).

4.1.14 *Drainage materials*

In general, the methods of installation of drains and the materials used for drainage do not differ from those used in humid, temperate areas. However, drainage machines, of either the excavating or non-excavating type, must be capable of working at greater depths. Lateral pipes for water table control are almost always of corrugated plastic, but collectors may be of clay or concrete.

The size of the drainage pipe chosen depends not only on the gradient to which the pipe is laid and the quantity of water it has to discharge but also on the design procedure used. Two methods are commonly used in drainage design, the dewatering or drainage approach and the transport approach (e.g. Cavelaars, 1973). In the drainage approach the drainage pipe is designed to run full over its entire length with a surcharge which results in a piezometric head over the pipe. In the transport approach the pipe is designed to be full only at the outlet and runs partially full with no surcharge over its length. A consequence of this is that pipes designed using the transport approach will be larger than those chosen using the drainage approach.

Where the drainage lateral provides water table control on an area which is irrigated all at one time, then the design flow rate must be based on the maximum flow expected. However, in some cases a lateral pipe serves areas in which subdivisions of the area are irrigated sequentially, and in this case the average discharge from the area is the appropriate flow rate to use for pipe sizing.

The use of an envelope material to surround the pipe to increase the hydraulic conductivity adjacent to the pipe and to provide some stability to the soil may also be required in those soils in which the soil has an extremely uniform grain size lying between 20 and 200 μm. Increased hydraulic conductivity of the drain surround reduces the hydraulic gradient near the drain and so helps to prevent soil movement and entry into the drain. Pipe envelopes may be graded sands, gravels or synthetic materials such as woven nylon sock or other geotextile material. The specification of drainage envelopes is often based on empirical relationships between the grading curve of the soil particles and that of the envelope material (see, for instance, Dieleman and Trafford, 1976).

4.1.15 *Surface runoff*

Surface runoff may occur as a result of either irrigation water or rainfall exceeding infiltration rates. In all irrigated areas there will be the need for surface drainage, and some provision at field level will nearly always be required. Without adequate control of runoff there may be an increased risk of soil erosion by water. Sustained agricultural production is not possible without attention to this erosion hazard.

4.2 Erosion

4.2.1 *Causes and effects of erosion*

Erosion is the removal of soil or rock by agents such as water, wind or gravity. Natural soil erosion presents no local problem as long as its rate is balanced by the rate of new soil formation; however, erosion can be accelerated by agriculture, urban and industrial development and recreation. Both natural and accelerated erosion can lead to irreversible loss of soil and siltation in rivers and reservoirs. Erosion by rainfall and runoff occurs through the detachment and transport of soil particles. Rainsplash is only effective in detaching soil; the transport capacity of rainsplash is very limited because of the short distances over which splashed particles can travel (Morgan, 1986). However, runoff is effective in both detaching and transporting particles. Erosion rates are greatly increased over and above those for rainsplash alone when runoff is generated. Sediment will be deposited when the energy of the erosive agent is insufficient to transport the soil particles any further. Once eroded, the sediment is highly vulnerable to further detachment and transport.

One common form of erosion is the uniform removal of soil by overland flow (sheet erosion) which can lead to undetectable soil-surface lowering. When runoff becomes concentrated into channels, such as rills or gullies, rates of soil loss increase dramatically. Rills are small, often discontinuous, eroded channels which are often obliterated by subsequent non-erosive rainfall, frost action or tillage operations. Gullies are permanent erosion features, with deeply incised channels and steep sides, indicating severe rates of soil loss. Flow within gullies is ephemeral and highly erratic, but it is capable of detaching and transporting vast quantities of sediment.

Gully development is very unpredictable. Often, channels are eroded in one rainfall event and then completely abandoned in the next storm, when a new gully system may develop. This results in constantly changing drainage networks. Development of the gully upslope through headcutting results in new catchment areas and watershed divides. Piping or tunnel erosion can be the first stage of gully formation, and may change the hydrology of an area. Piping is caused by concentrations of flow beneath the soil surface, often along the interface of soil horizons with different hydraulic conductivities. Evidence of such subsurface erosion must be a warning sign to the drainage engineer that artificial subsurface drainage may accelerate the development of pipes and tunnels.

Massive slope failure results from the downward and outward movement of large masses of slope-forming materials under gravity (Gray and Leiser, 1982). Mass movements have been classified according to the type and rate of movement, and by the processes involved (Varnes, 1958). Slope instability can be triggered by excessive rainfall and high infiltration rates, leading to an increase in mass or surcharge, higher pore water pressures and a reduction in cohesion and shear strength of the slope material. Surcharge may be difficult to drain away naturally because of the poor hydraulic conductivity of the material.

Rates of soil erosion vary throughout the world, as do the impact of erosion and the perception of erosion as a land management problem. The effects are seen both on site and off site. Sheet erosion is often only detected when highly erodible and infertile subsoil is exposed by erosion of the top soil. There will be an inevitable decline in vegetative productivity, aggravated by the declining depth of soil and consequent reduction in water-holding capacity of the eroded soil profile. Reduction in crop yield is often masked or compensated by the addition of inorganic fertilisers. Sheet erosion can therefore continue unchecked, often until it is too late to reverse the trend of land degradation.

Deeply incised gullies cannot be traversed by machinery, and the effective land area for production is reduced and dissected. For example, when overgrazing initiates erosion, eroding gullies will reduce the carrying capacity of the land, yet stock numbers are likely to stay constant, which results in further overgrazing and erosion.

Any loss of soil leads to preferential depletion of nutrients, fertilisers and organic matter at source. Erosion is highly selective in transporting these vital soil resources away. Even crops can be washed out or damaged by water and wind erosion.

These on-site effects of erosion have great impact on the land user in terms of the financial and environmental costs incurred. However, off-site consequences of erosion have serious impact on the whole environment, and hence the whole of society is affected. These include the deposition of sediments in rivers, lakes, reservoirs and canals. Serious sedimentation reduces the capacity of these water sources, and supplies for irrigation, hydroelectric power and domestic use can be seriously reduced. With the reduced water-holding capacity, flooding risks are increased after storm events. Water quality is reduced by high sediment concentrations, aggravated by the high concentrations of chemicals found in eroded sediments, which can act as pollutants.

4.2.2 *Need for drainage in erosion control*

Runoff energy for erosion is dependent on the volume and velocity of the flow. Both influence the kinetic energy of flow to detach and transport sediments. Meyer and Wischmeier (1969) showed that soil detachment varies with velocity squared and transport capacity with the fifth power of velocity. This implies that even a small reduction in the runoff velocity and volume can dramatically reduce the erosive power of the water flow.

Drainage techniques can be used to enhance infiltration into the soil, and hence reduce runoff velocities and volumes. This has been illustrated by Fausey and Schwab (1969), who reported that on undrained plots a hard crust formed which impeded infiltration, but this was not found on plots with a pipe drainage system. Drainage can also improve transmission of water down through the soil profile (Leyton and Yadav, 1960) so that runoff is less likely to generate on the soil surface. Chisci and Lodi (1974) found, on drained plots, annual reductions in runoff of 29% when compared with undrained plots.

Drainage can be manipulated to ensure soil moisture conditions which minimise erosion risk. Soils with high moisture contents are quick to generate surface runoff. Free-draining soils require higher rainfall intensities and longer storm durations before runoff is generated. Soil moisture content also affects soil erodibility and susceptibility to massive slope failure. There is a strong relationship between moisture content and soil shear strength. Wet soils have fewer cohesive bonds, because of the effect of water weakening the cementing agents within soil aggregates. Weak aggregates are highly susceptible to raindrop impact and the shearing forces of runoff. Drier soils are associated with higher shear strengths, and more resistance to erosive forces. Leyton and Yadav (1960) found more water-stable aggregates in pipe-drained clay soils than in soils with surface ditching.

However, dry, friable soils such as peats are highly susceptible to wind erosion. Moisture in the soil helps to increase the resistance of the soil to flowing air. Maintaining adequate moisture in the soil is essential for wind erosion control as well as for maintaining healthy vegetation, which can provide in-field shelter by reducing wind velocities close to the ground surface (Morgan, 1989). Controlled drainage with maintained water levels at a specified depth can reduce susceptibility to wind erosion (Schwab *et al.*, 1981).

Ponding on the soil surface, caused by poor drainage, can enhance erosion processes. Studies by Palmer (1964) have shown that ponded water of shallow depths (1.0–1.5 mm) increases rainsplash erosion, as a result of the turbulence in the ponded layer set up when impacting raindrops strike the ponded water. However, deeper water will cushion the effect of raindrop impact. Ponded water may also increase the risks of piping development and mass soil failure.

Indirectly, drainage aids soil erosion control by improving conditions for vegetation growth which can dramatically reduce erosion rates through the effects of the canopy, stems and roots (Rickson and Morgan, 1988). Healthy vegetation also has a vital role to play in slope stabilisation (Coppin and Richards, 1990). Adequate drainage has been shown to increase crop productivity (Chisci, 1976; Hundal *et al.*, 1976; Eriksson, 1979; De Crecy,

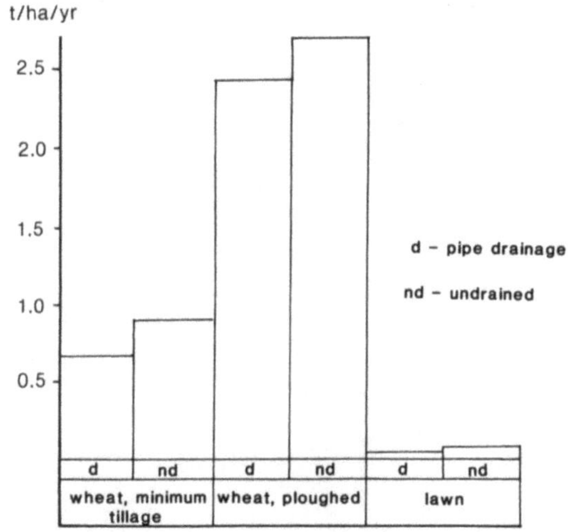

Figure 4.5 Annual soil losses as a function of pipe drainage, crops and tillage.

1982) as a result of increased soil temperatures and increased porosity and hence water-holding capacities (Leyton and Yadav, 1960). Waterlogging, however, caused by inadequate drainage rarely favours vegetative growth. Seed germination and plant establishment and growth are severely hindered in waterlogged soils.

Figure 4.5 illustrates the reduction in soil loss by pipe drainage (Chisci and Zanchi, 1981); runoff was also reduced. The effectiveness of pipe drainage in controlling soil erosion has been estimated (Chisci *et al.*, 1981) to give a value of 0.8 to the support practice factor (*P*) used in the universal soil loss equation (Wischmeier and Smith, 1978). Drainage also permits land consolidation and field enlargement without incurring erosion risks (Zanchi, 1989).

4.3 Drainage techniques for erosion control

4.3.1 *Introduction*

Engineering structures, especially surface drainage schemes, are often used to control runoff velocity, whilst tillage can be manipulated to reduce runoff volume by enhancing water movement through the soil profile.

A network of diversion ditches, waterways and terrace channels acts like hillside surface drainage lines to dispose of runoff without causing erosion (Figure 4.6). All these measures are designed to convey runoff generated by the 10-year return period storm, which can be predicted using empirical procedures such as the rational method (see sections 1.4.5 and 9.5), Cook's

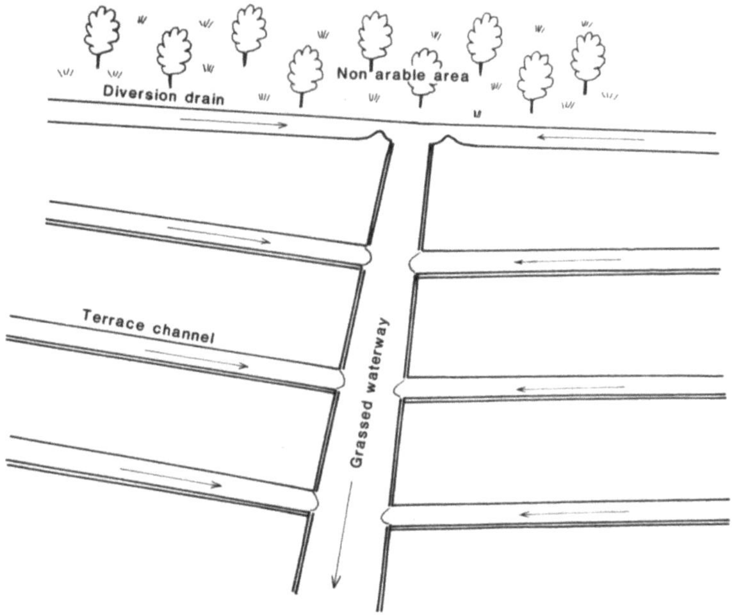

Figure 4.6 Terrace and waterway system.

method or the US soil conservation curve method when direct runoff data are not available (Hudson, 1981).

4.3.2 *Diversion drains*

Diversion drains are used to protect arable land from runoff generated upslope, or to divert runoff away from an area of active gully development. They can be designed using the Durbach method (Hudson, 1981) or following

Table 4.4 Maximum safe runoff velocities based on cover expected after two seasons (m s^{-1}).

Material	Bare	Medium grass cover	Very good grass cover
Very light silty sand	0.3	0.75	1.5
Light loose sand	0.5	0.9	1.5
Coarse sand	0.75	1.25	1.7
Sandy soil	0.75	1.5	2.0
Firm clay loam	1.0	1.7	2.3
Stiff clay or gravelly soil	1.5	1.8	2.5
Coarse gravels	1.5	1.8	*
Shale, hard pan, soft rock, etc.	1.8	2.1	*
Hard cemented conglomerates	2.5	—	—

*Unlikely to form very good grass cover.

Table 4.5 Depth of cut channel (m).

		Velocity of flow ($m\,s^{-1}$)						
Slope (%)	S*	0.25	0.50	0.75	1.0	1.5	2.0	2.5
1.00	100					0.3	0.45	0.60
0.66	150	Minimum value			0.20	0.4	0.60	0.85
0.50	200	0.20			0.25	0.5	0.75	0.90
0.40	250			0.20	0.30	0.6	0.90	
0.33	300			0.25	0.35	0.65	1.00	
0.25	400			0.30	0.45	0.85		
0.20	500			0.35	0.50	1.00		
0.17	600		0.20	0.40	0.60			

*1 in *S* is the channel gradient, and 0.20 is the minimum value of excavation.

Table 4.6 Values of *F* (= discharge per unit width of channel, $m^3\,s^{-1}$).

Depth of cut channel (m)	S 100	150	200	250	300	400	500	600
0.2	0.35	0.25	0.20	0.20	0.20	0.15	0.15	0.15
0.3	0.60	0.45	0.40	0.35	0.30	0.25	0.25	0.25
0.4	0.90	0.75	0.65	0.60	0.55	0.45	0.40	0.35
0.5	1.30	1.15	0.95	0.85	0.80	0.65	0.60	0.55
0.6	1.80	1.55	1.30	1.20	1.10	0.95	0.80	0.75
0.7	2.25	2.00	1.70	1.50	1.35	1.20	1.05	1.00
0.8	2.80	2.45	2.15	1.90	1.70	1.50	1.30	1.25
0.9	3.40	3.00	2.65	2.35	2.10	1.80	1.60	1.50
1.0	4.05	3.60	3.15	2.75	2.50	2.15	1.90	1.85

Values of *F* shown above are limited to a maximum velocity of $2.5\,m\,s^{-1}$ (assuming a Manning's *n* value of 0.035).

the procedures used in grassed waterway design (see next section). Both approaches are based on the concept of maximum safe runoff velocity in the ditch.

The Durbach method involves selection of a maximum safe runoff velocity (Table 4.4) and suitable ditch gradient (usually taken as 0.4%). These values are used to obtain the maximum depth of cut channel (Table 4.5). The depth and gradient of the channel are then used to obtain an *F* value or the discharge in $m^3\,s^{-1}$ per metre width of channel (Table 4.6). Dividing the *F* value by the predicted maximum flow ($m^3\,s^{-1}$) gives the required width of channel.

Example

Design a diversion drain to carry 2.0 $m^3\,s^{-1}$ on a gradient of 1:250 over a sandy soil.

(1) Select maximum permissible velocity (Table 4.4) = $1.5\,m\,s^{-1}$.
(2) Using $S = 1{:}250$ and $V = 1.5\,m\,s^{-1}$, read depth of cut channel from Table 4.5 = 0.60 m.

(3) Using $S = 250$ and $D = 0.60\,\mathrm{m}$, read F value from Table 4.6 = $1.2\,\mathrm{m^3\,s^{-1}}$ per m width.
(4) Width = $Q/F = 2/1.2 = 1.67\,\mathrm{m}$.

The effective depth of the channel is twice the design depth, as the soil excavated to construct the channel is used to form a bank on the downhill side.

4.3.3 *Waterways*

Waterways have to drain high quantities and rates of runoff from terrace channel networks which divert surface runoff across the hillside to points where it would not naturally concentrate. Waterways are often located in natural depressions, so that few cut-and-fill operations are needed to ensure effective drainage of the slope. Waterways are designed to convey the water quickly but safely downslope, often down the fall line, without causing scour or siltation.

The salient properties of designed waterways needed for effective surface drainage are (a) waterway shape; (b) type of vegetation; and (c) channel capacity. Most designed waterways are parabolic in shape, because this approximates a natural channel shape; other shapes (triangular or trapezoidal) tend to become parabolic as a result of localised scour and deposition within the channel. Whether the waterway has to be constructed, or simply located in a natural depression, will depend on the design specifications calculated (see later) and the form of the natural depression.

Vegetation in the waterway in crucial as it helps to dissipate and protect against the erosive forces of the flow (Hewlett *et al.*, 1987). Thus, vegetated waterways can withstand higher velocities of flow, without scour, than would be permissible in unvegetated channels. The maximum non-eroding velocity within vegetated waterways depends on the depth of flow, the type of vegetation, planting density, percentage cover, condition of the sward and resilience to water flows and periodic waterlogging (Ree, 1949).

Waterway design is also based on the concept of maximum flow velocities and open-channel hydraulics. The Manning equation for flow velocity is applied to specify the dimensions (width and depth) of a parabolic channel, capable of conveying runoff from the 10-year return period storm. The design procedure requires the input parameters of discharge (Q); slope (S)—here it is the natural slope angle, rather than an imposed gradient as for diversion drains and terrace channels; maximum permissible velocity (v), which is dependent on vegetation and soil type; and Manning's n value (n), representing roughness imparted to the flow by the vegetation and soil. These values are then substituted into the Manning equation to obtain the hydraulic radius of the channel:

$$r = \left(\frac{vn}{S^{0.5}}\right)^{1.5}$$

The cross-sectional area required is calculated from the discharge and maximum permissible velocity values:

$$A = \frac{Q}{V}$$

The design channel depth for a parabolic section can be approximated by:

$$d = 1.5r$$

and top width can be calculated by:

$$w = \frac{A}{0.67d}$$

Example

Design a parabolic grassed waterway to convey a peak flow of $7\,m^3\,s^{-1}$ on a 3% slope, over an erodible sandy soil with short grass.

(1) Select maximum permissible velocity (Table 4.4) = $1.5\,m\,s^{-1}$.
(2) Select Manning's n value (Table 4.7) = 0.045.
(3) Substitute into Manning's equation:

$$r = \left(\frac{1.5 \times 0.045}{0.03^{0.5}}\right)^{1.5} = 0.243\,m$$

Table 4.7 Manning's roughness coefficient (n).

	n
(a) *Channels free from vegetation*	
Uniform cross-section, regular alignment free from pebbles and vegetation, in fine sedimentary soils	0.016
Uniform cross-section, regular alignment free from pebbles and vegetation, in stiff clay soils or hardpan	0.018
Uniform cross-section, regular alignment, few pebbles, little vegetation, in clay loam	0.020
Small variations in cross-section, fairly regular alignment, few stones, thin grass at edges, in sandy and clay soils, also newly cleaned, ploughed and harrowed channels	0.0225
Irregular alignment, ripples on bottom, in gravelly soil or shale with jagged banks or vegetation	0.025
Irregular section and alignment, scattered rocks and loose gravel on bottom, or considerable weeds on sloping banks, or in gravelly material up to 150 mm diameter	0.030
Eroded irregular channels, channels blasted in rock	0.030
(b) *Vegetated channels*	
Short grass (50–150 mm)	0.030–0.060
Medium grass (150–250 mm)	0.030–0.085
Long grass (250–600 mm)	0.040–0.150
(c) *Natural stream channels*	
Clean and straight	0.025–0.030
Winding with pools and shoals	0.033–0.040
Very weedy, winding and overgrown	0.075–0.150

(4) Calculate required cross-sectional area:

$$A = \frac{Q}{V} = \frac{7}{1.5} = 4.67\,\text{m}^2$$

(5) Calculate design depth:

$$d = 1.5r = 1.5 \times 0.243 = 0.365\,\text{m}$$

(6) Calculate design top width:

$$w = \frac{A}{0.67d} = \frac{4.67}{0.67 \times 0.365} = 19.12\,\text{m}$$

(7) Check capacity of the channel is adequate to convey the flow:

$$\begin{aligned} Q &= 0.67\,wdv \\ &= 0.67 \times 19.12 \times 0.365 \times 1.5 \\ &= 7.013\,\text{m}^3\,\text{s}^{-1} \end{aligned}$$

(8) Add 20% freeboard to the final design depth

$$\begin{aligned} d &= 0.365 \times 1.2 = 0.44\,\text{m} \\ w &= 19.12\,\text{m} \end{aligned}$$

Waterways are usually designed in sections to avoid overdesign and excessive land take at the top of the catchment. The procedure shown above has to be repeated for each section, accounting for changes in discharge (Q) and slope gradient downslope. Ideally the sections should gently increase in width and depth downslope, but this is not automatic when using the Manning design procedure. Thus some trial and error adjustments have to made to avoid the channel becoming narrower or shallower downslope, which will inevitably cause severe channel scouring. Checks should also be made to ensure maximum permissible velocity is never exceeded.

Flow in waterways should only be intermittent, but in some waterways on gentle slopes, the ground may remain wet for some time. This will increase the likelihood of subsequent erosion and seriously impair the growth and vigour of vegetation and its ability to reduce flow velocity. Hence, it may be necessary to instal subsurface pipe drains to ensure adequate and rapid drainage of the waterway. These should be placed within the waterway, slightly to one side of the lowest point, so that should the waterway erode the pipe will not be damaged or exposed. Installation of the pipes will increase the cost of the soil conservation scheme considerably.

Grassed waterways are usually constructed one or two seasons before the installation of the terrace channel network. This allows the vegetative lining to reach its required design characteristics. Before the vegetation matures, the waterway will be susceptible to erosion, and should be protected from runoff scour. One technique is the application of geotextiles, which can also aid vegetation establishment (Rickson, 1990).

4.3.4 *Pipe outlets*

An alternative drainage technique to vegetated waterways is a pipe outlet scheme. Terrace channels are graded toward the natural depression which is filled in to straighten the terraces. At this point, the riser of the pipe (Figure 4.7) will drain any accumulated runoff, at a rate determined by the size and position of the orifice plate. Slow drainage rates will lead to temporary, localised waterlogging, with sediment deposited at this point. This helps to level the terrace channel and reduce the off-site impact of erosion. However, it must be noted that sedimentation can cause blocking of the pipe inlet, thus incurring costs in clearing out the sediment. Frequent waterlogging can adversely affect crop yields adjacent to the riser pipe. The installation and maintenance costs of this technique may prove prohibitive.

4.3.5 *Terrace channels*

The salient design features of terrace channels for effective drainage are (a) the spacing of the channels; (b) their gradient; (c) their length; and (d) their cross-sectional area or capacity.

Terrace channels are spaced at a regular interval known as the horizontal interval, HI, which can be determined theoretically or empirically. The theoretical formula used is based on Manning's equation and estimates the critical slope length over which surface runoff can flow before it becomes erosive:

$$\mathrm{HI} = \frac{v^{5/2} n^{3/2}}{(R - i)\sin\frac{3}{4}\theta \cos\theta}$$

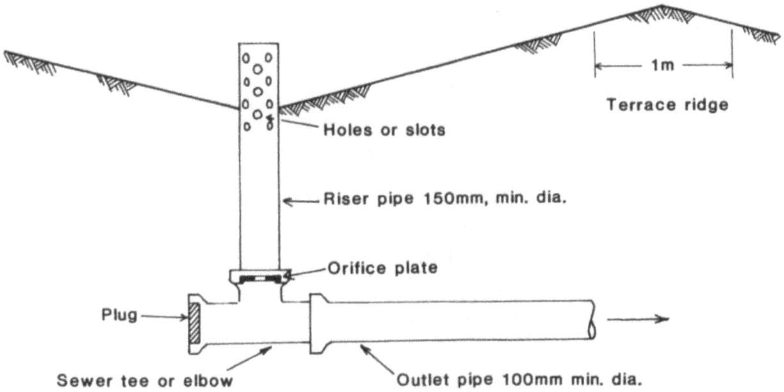

Figure 4.7 Pipe inlet.

where v = maximum safe runoff velocity (varies with soil type—see Table 4.4; values of between 0.46 and 0.61 m s^{-1} are given by ASAE [1972]), n = Manning's roughness parameter (often taken as 0.20 for bare soil in terrace channel design), R = rainfall intensity, i = infiltration capacity and θ = slope angle.

Example

Calculate the spacing of terrace channels on a 7° bare soil slope with moderate infiltration rate and under tropical rainfall conditions. Let $R = 100$ mm h^{-1} for 10 minutes (= 0.0167 m depth of water); $i = 20$ mm h^{-1} (= 0.003 m equivalent depth); $v = 0.60$ m s^{-1}; $n = 0.2$; $\theta = 7°$.

$$\mathrm{HI} = \frac{0.6^{5/2} \times 0.2^{3/2}}{(0.0167 - 0.003) \times \sin\frac{3}{4}7^\circ \cos 7^\circ}$$

$$= 8.91 \text{ m}$$

Empirical formulae for terrace spacing are easier to use and are based on readily available data. They have been derived for many countries worldwide. They assume that:

$$\mathrm{HI} = \frac{\mathrm{VI} \times 100}{S}$$

where VI = vertical interval, or height difference between two successive terrace channels, and S = slope (%). This is calculated from empirical formulae (Morgan, 1986). Some examples are given in Table 4.8.

Example

Use the Zimbabwe formula (Table 4.8) to calculate the spacing of terrace channels on a 7° slope

Table 4.8 Examples of empirical formulae for terrace channel spacing.

Origin	Formula
United States Soil Conservation Service	$\mathrm{VI\,(ft)} = aS + b$
where a varies from 0.3 in the south to 0.6 in the north, and b is 1 or 2 depending on the soil erodibility.	
Zimbabwe	$\mathrm{VI\,(ft)} = \dfrac{S + f}{2}$
where f varies from 3 to 6 according to the soil erodibility.	
Kenya	$\mathrm{VI\,(m)} = \dfrac{0.3(S + 2)}{4}$

on highly erodible soil. For $\theta = 7°$, $S = 12\%$. For highly erodible soil, $f = 3$.

$$VI = \frac{S+f}{2} = \frac{12+3}{2} \text{ ft} = 7.5 \text{ ft} = 2.29 \text{ m}$$

$$HI = \frac{VI \times 100}{S} = \frac{2.29 \times 100}{12} \text{ m} = 19 \text{ m}$$

To enable drainage, terrace channels must be placed at a grade off the contour which is neither so steep that flow erodes the channel nor so gentle that the channel silts up through deposition. The gradient can be uniform along the length of the channel (often 0.4%), or variable to cope with the different runoff velocities and volumes along the channel. Gentle gradients (0.1%) are used in the upper reaches of the channel, with steeper gradients (0.4%) at the outlet end (Hudson, 1981). This effectively increases the capacity of the channel to cope with the greater runoff volume at this point, but the increased capacity comes about through an increase in the flow velocity, which may cause scour if the maximum permissible velocity is exceeded.

Even at a safe gradient, long terrace channels will accumulate high runoff volumes and velocities, thereby increasing erosion risks along the length of the channel. Recommended maximum terrace channel lengths are given as 250 m for sandy soils and 400 m for clay soils in Africa and 500 m for all soils in the United States. These limits can be extended to 400, 450 and 600 m respectively in special circumstances, providing the horizontal interval of the terraces is reduced (Hudson, 1981).

The capacity of each channel must accommodate the runoff generated from the interterrace area above (Figure 4.6). The channel dimensions can be based on the modified Manning equation used in grassed waterway design or by designing a balanced cut-and-fill cross-section (Figure 4.8), whereby the front slope width (W_f) is taken as equal to the construction machinery width, and the depth of flow (d) determined from the runoff rate for a 10-year return period storm (Schwab *et al.*, 1981).

Terrace channels are designed to convey runoff at a grade across the slope at safe velocities. The runoff is then discharged into designed waterways which act as the main drainage line of a mechanical soil erosion control scheme.

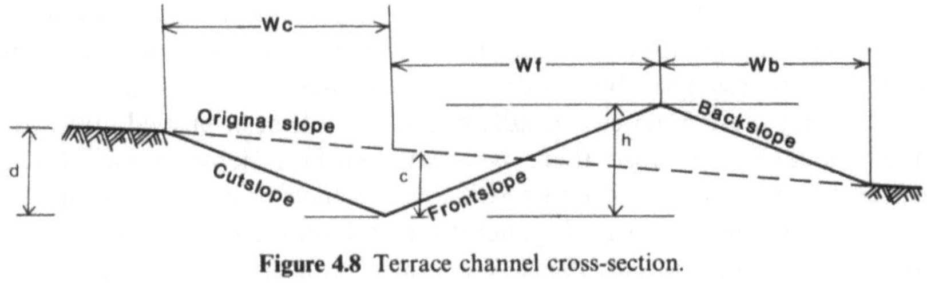

Figure 4.8 Terrace channel cross-section.

4.3.6 *Maintenance*

As with all engineering structures it is essential that water courses are maintained regularly. Deposited sediment must be removed after every storm event or channel capacities will be reduced; vegetation must be mown to the design height and protected from grazing livestock in order to keep its design properties; and care must be taken with machinery so that the channel dimensions are not ploughed out with subsequent tillage operations.

4.3.7 *Slope stabilisation*

Drainage systems such as French drains, trenches, vertical wells and horizontal drains can release the build up of the excessive surcharge and pore-water pressures within slopes prone to mass movement. These techniques have been used widely as both a preventive and curative method of slope stabilisation (Zaruba and Mencl, 1969; Royster, 1979).

4.4 Soil management techniques for erosion control

The principle of soil management for erosion control is to maintain a fertile seed bed whilst retaining maximum resistance to erosion. Soils can be managed so that runoff volume and velocity are reduced, thereby controlling soil erosion rates.

Primary and secondary cultivations can increase soil drainage by encouraging infiltration in the short term. Compacted layers are broken up and bulk densities tend to be lower, so that infiltration rate and capacity are higher after tillage. However, tractor wheelings can lead to localised compaction (Pidgeon and Soane, 1978) and reduced infiltration rates, as evidenced by severe water erosion in tramlines (Tatham, 1989). Whilst loose, uncompacted soil has good drainage characteristics, it is also susceptible to rainsplash erosion, with detached soil particles deposited to form an impermeable crust with very low hydraulic conductivity. Conventional tillage practices can also lead to smearing on wet, heavy soils which will impede water movement through the soil. Surface ponding and runoff may result, thus increasing the erosion hazard.

Conservation tillage techniques such as strip or zone tillage, minimum tillage or zero tillage (Sprague and Triplett, 1986) are useful in controlling erosion but are less desirable for drainage purposes. Runoff volumes can be reduced under these practices, usually not as a result of improved infiltration and drainage but because there is greater surface depressional storage. Reduced tillage can lead to dense soil layers which have lower infiltration rates. This can increase runoff generation and seriously affect crop yields (Triplett and Van Doren, 1977). Generally, conservation tillage is not recommended for poorly drained soils, such as the highly plastic, sticky calcareous black clay soils of the tropics and subtropics (i.e. vertisols).

For these soils, special soil management techniques have been developed, such as the broad bed and furrow technique at ICRISAT (Krantz, 1981; Pathak *et al.*, 1985). This surface drainage system comprises broad beds of approximately 100 cm width, set on a grade of 0.4–0.8%, separated by furrows of 50 cm width. Two to four crop rows are set out on each bed, depending on the size of machinery used. Runoff accumulated in the furrows is conveyed to a grass waterway. This technique is particularly effective on the heavy, black clay or cotton soils, in areas with rainfall usually over 750 mm per annum. It has been applied on vertisols in India and Ethiopia, on alfisols in Brazil (Lal, 1985) and on light soils in Zimbabwe and Kenya (Hudson, 1987).

Traditional small open drains are used in the teff growing regions of Ethiopia. The purpose of these closely spaced drains is not so much for erosion control but to prevent the washing out of the fine teff seeds after planting. Channel terraces are used in combination with these drains to control soil erosion.

Temporary waterlogging at crucial times can be solved through soil management. In Portugal, winter cereal planting is impeded by very wet soil conditions. A system of 'pnudivales' is used; these are small channels constructed by mouldboard plough and a mounted ridger after seed bed preparation, but before drilling. The drains are 3–4 m wide and 0.25 m deep, on a gradient of 0.6–0.8%. Subsequent cultivations of the cereal are carried out in straight lines, ignoring the lie of these drains.

An alternative soil management approach is the use of hydrophilic soil conditioners which encourage water movement down through the soil profile, and hence reduce potentially erosive runoff (De Vleeschauer *et al.*, 1979). These products can be made from natural substances (such as seaweed extract) or synthetic materials (such as polyacrylamide). These conditioners can improve soil aggregation, hydraulic conductivity and porosity, so can be applied to leach out salts from saline soils. Soil conditioners are expensive and have a limited effective lifetime (usually sufficient to protect slopes from erosion prior to vegetation establishment and growth). They are mostly used in civil engineering projects (road and railway cuttings and embankments) or for the protection of high value crops.

5 Urban drainage

F.H.M. VAN DE VEN, A.J.M. NELEN and G.D. GELDOF

5.1 Urban hydrological cycle

The drainage system in urban areas serves a large number of functions. The most important are:

Prevention of flooding.
Discharge of polluted wastewater in a sanitary acceptable way.
Maintaining a minimum bearing capacity of the soil.
Guaranteeing accessibility within the area.
Providing reasonable hydrological conditions for urban aquatic and terrestrial ecosystems;
Creating an aesthetically acceptable environment.

Large social and economic interests are involved. As a result, the drainage system in urban areas has to meet strict standards. A system of open drains is generally inadequate for proper drainage and a sewer system is installed to drain the surface runoff and the wastewater flow in a controlled way. In cases where the groundwater level is too high this may also be controlled by a subsurface drainage system. Moreover, it is considered unacceptable from an environmental point of view to discharge polluted wastewater directly into a receiving water and as its treatment is centralised the drainage system serves as a collection system for the treatment plant. This in combination with the land use features of the urban environment means that the drainage of urban areas is complex, artificial and expensive.

Typical pathways for water in the urban environment are shown in Figure 5.1. For an impression of the amounts of water involved, two examples of water balances are shown in Figure 5.2: the first for a small housing area in Lelystad (The Netherlands), with 41% paved area and measurements over a long period, and the second for the city of Lund (Sweden), with 37% paved area and measurements over a 1-year period. Both cities are located in a temperate, maritime climate.

As may be seen from Figure 5.2, both precipitation and the public water supply system are large sources of water. Most of the input is discharged through the sewage treatment plant. Evapotranspiration, together with the discharge of the subsurface drainage system (Lelystad) and the inflow of

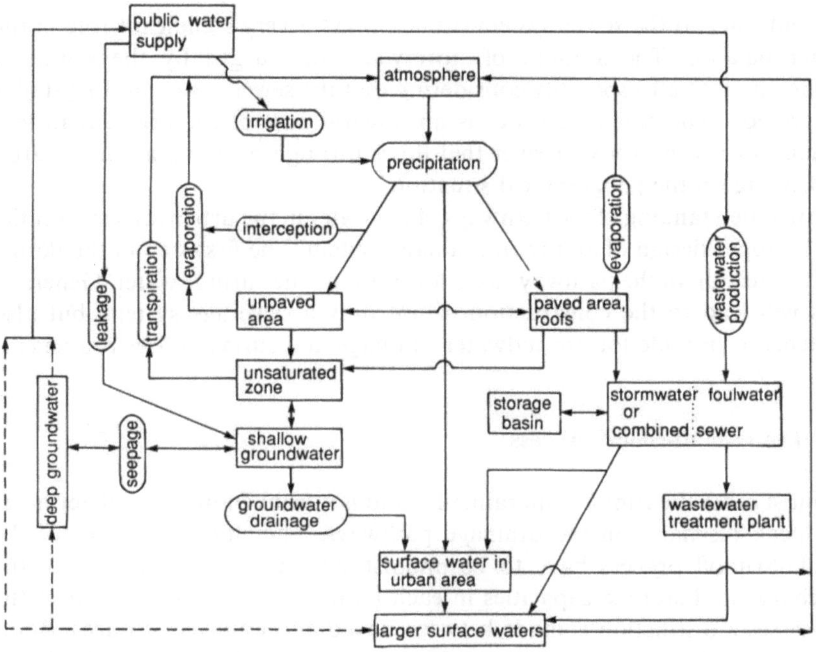

Figure 5.1 The urban hydrological system (Van de Ven, 1988).

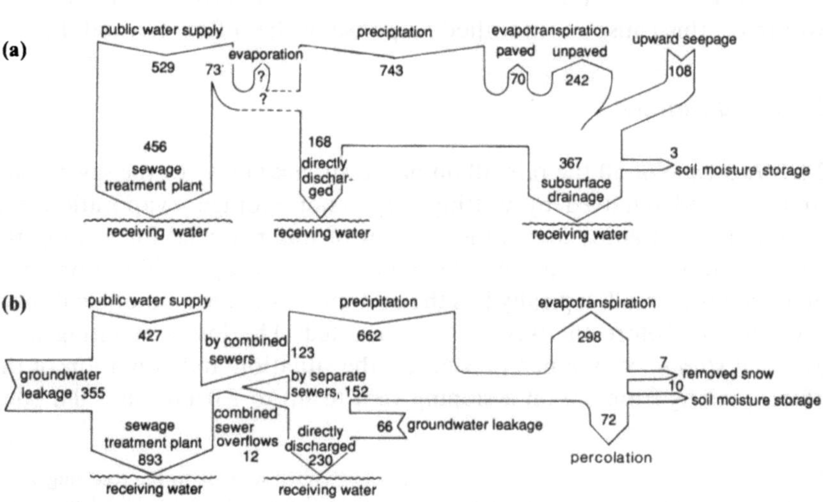

Figure 5.2 Annual water budgets of housing areas in (a) Lelystad, The Netherlands, and (b) Lund, Sweden. Amounts in mm (Hogland and Niemczynowicz, 1980; Oldenkamp, 1988).

groundwater to the sewer system (Lund), plays a very significant role in the water balance. The amount of stormwater discharged by the sewers is surprisingly small, especially considering that the sewer system in Lelystad is separated*. The receiving water is an integral part of the urban plan (e.g. canals), or it is a brook or river that flows through or along an urban area, depending on the geographical situation.

An understanding of the pathways of the water in the urban area is essential for a proper design of an urban drainage system. The first step in the design is the selection of the pathways used for draining the surplus water. Generally this will lead to the construction of not only a sewerage system, but also systems to provide for groundwater drainage and surface water drainage.

5.2 The rainfall-runoff process

In most cases the runoff from rainfall—and not from snowmelt—determines the peak discharge in the drainage pathways. Therefore the basics of the rainfall-runoff process have to be understood for a correct design of the discharge and storage capacities in each pathway. For a description of the processes a distinction is made between paved and unpaved surfaces. Roofs and any kind of pavement are considered to be paved area, while bare and green areas are considered as unpaved. The runoff process from both areas can be divided into two subprocesses. The first is the group of loss processes. These cause a reduction in the amount of rainfall that flows into the drainage system. The second is the transformation of the rainfall to sewer inflow. Because it takes time for the water to flow over the ground surface to the sewer inlet, this causes a smoothed response of the inflow to rainfall.

5.2.1 *Paved surfaces*

5.2.1.1 *Losses.* Not all the rainfall on paved surfaces flows to the sewer; part is retained and removed by wetting, depression storage, evaporation and infiltration. The *wetting loss* is the amount of water needed for wetting the surface material, and can only be removed by evaporation. For most materials this is small; typically less than 0.5 mm. For some materials it takes a few minutes before the wetting is completed. The losses resulting from *depression storage* very much depend on the situation and condition of the surface, ranging from 0.0 on a sloping roof to up to 5.0 mm on a flat roof.

*In the *separated sewer system* the stormwater is discharged directly to the receiving water by storm drains, while the wastewater is discharged to the sewage treatment plant. In the *combined sewer system*, stormwater and wastewater are collected in one system with limited capacity and transported to the treatment plant; the surplus is discharged as combined sewer overflow.

In most cases the losses resulting from wetting and depression storage are integrated into the so called *initial loss.* Falk and Niemczynowicz (1979) reported initial loss values for 13 small basins with slopes from 1 to 4% ranging from 0.1 to 1.1 mm. For 19 basins in Sweden, the Netherlands and the United Kingdom, Kidd (1978) reported values ranging from 0.1 to 1.5 mm and gives the relation:

$$L_i = 0.77S^{-0.49} \qquad r = -0.85 \tag{5.1}$$

where L_i is the initial loss, S is the catchment slope and r is the regression correlation coefficient. Approximately the same relationship is used in the Wallingford procedure for sewer design. The *evaporation loss* of paved surfaces is hard to assess. Only a very limited number of studies are available, e.g. Grimmond and Oke (1986) and Van de Ven (1989a). The heat flux in the surface material strongly influences the evaporation process. A hot pavement can evaporate some 1.0 mm during the first hour of a rainstorm. But the pavement is not always warm. As a reasonable approximation for design purposes, evaporation of water from paved surfaces is said to be negligible during a storm event, but for the water balance of urban areas it is certainly not negligible, as can be seen in Figure 5.2. *Infiltration* has only recently been recognised as a loss process of significant importance on brick, tile and other permeable pavements. Van den Berg (1978) and Jensen *et al.* (1985) reported that in four different basins some 15–30% of the rainfall on a brick-paved area infiltrated. Measurements by Bebelaar and Bakker (1981) and Van Dam and Schotkamp (1983) on different types of pavement showed infiltration capacities of 9–34 mm h^{-1} on different forms of brick and tile pavement (medians of the observations). All these pavements rested on a sandy, permeable substratum. The observed capacities strongly depended on the condition of the pavement. Old, dirty pavement is far less permeable than new.

The infiltration process can be modelled by the well-known Horton equation:

$$I_{\mathrm{cum}} = at + b[1 - \exp(-ct)] \tag{5.2}$$

where I_{cum} is the infiltrated amount, t is time, and a, b and c are model parameters; a is the final infiltration rate attained after a long period of infiltration. Van de Ven (1989a) gives the following values for the Horton parameters for the experiments of Van Dam and Schotkamp (1983):

	a (mm h^{-1})	b (mm)	c (h^{-1})
Bricks	5.2	15	0.56
Concrete bricks	7.2	16	0.88
Tiles	5.4	16	0.57

The actual infiltration capacity of a pavement depends on the antecedent wetting condition. If the terrain is wet at the beginning of a storm, reductions of the available infiltration capacity can reach up to 50% or more. But even then infiltration remains an important loss.

5.2.1.2 *Transformation.* The surplus water that remains on the surface flows to the sewer inlets. This takes some time. This retardation is illustrated by the unit hydrographs (see Figure 5.3 and Chapter 1) of the sewer inflow in two flat experimental basins with a drainage area per gullypot of approximately 100–200 m^2. It takes more than 10 minutes before the largest part of the unit input reaches the inlet point. This leads to a significant reduction of short-lasting rainfall peak intensities. The transformation can be modelled with a Nash model:

$$\begin{cases} h(t) = \dfrac{1}{k}\dfrac{1}{\Gamma(n)}\left(\dfrac{t}{k}\right)^{n-1} \exp(-t/k) & t \geqslant 0 \quad (5.3a) \\ h(t) = 0 & t < 0 \quad (5.3b) \end{cases}$$

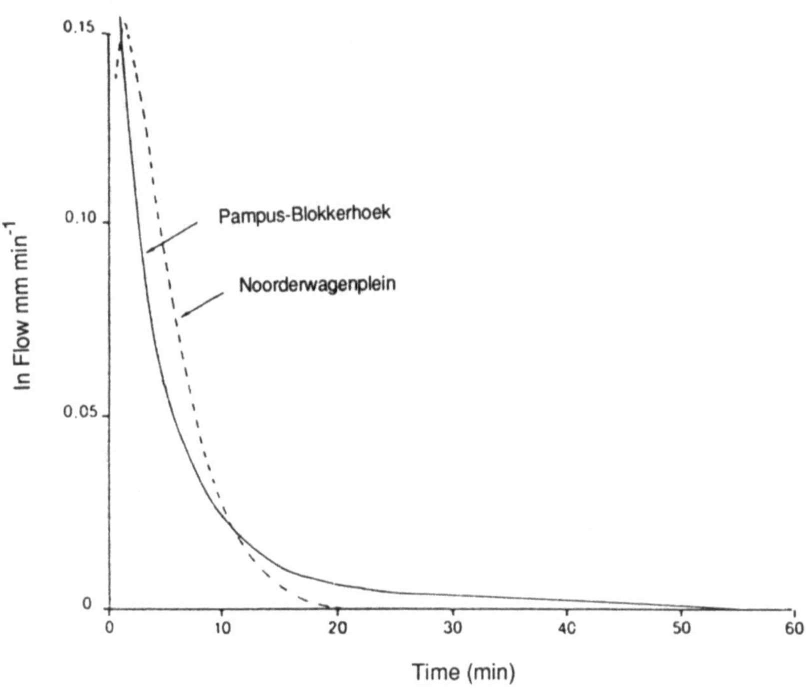

Figure 5.3 Unit hydrographs for the inflow in two experimental basins in Lelystad, The Netherlands (after Van de Ven, 1985).

where $\Gamma(n)$ is the gamma function, which is defined as:

$$\Gamma(n) = (n-1)! \qquad (n = 1, 2, 3, \ldots) \qquad (5.3c)$$

$$\Gamma(n) = \int_0^\infty x^{n-1} \exp(-x)\,\mathrm{d}x \qquad (n > 0) \qquad (5.3d)$$

where $h(t)$ is the unit hydrograph and n and k are the parameters. For flat areas, Van de Ven (1989a) recommends $n = 0.7$ and $k = 400$ (s), while Kidd (1978) recommends $k = 180$ (s) and

$$n = 1.188 S^{-0.344} L^{0.15} \qquad r = 0.71 \qquad (5.4)$$

where S is the catchment slope and L is the length of the overland flow (m).

Another way of modelling the transformation is by the (slightly) non-linear reservoir model:

$$\mathrm{d}B/\mathrm{d}t = p_{\mathrm{n}} - q \qquad (5.5a)$$

$$B = Kq^{\mathrm{b}} \qquad (5.5b)$$

where B is the reservoir content, p_{n} is the net rainfall after subtraction of all the losses, q is the reservoir discharge (sewer inflow) and K and b are the model parameters. According to Van de Ven (1989b) $K = 5.1$ ($\mathrm{mm}^{-0.07}\mathrm{min}^{1.07}$) and $b = 1.07$ for flat areas. Note that the value of b differs significantly from the value 0.666, derived from the Chezy equation, which is often applied.

An efficient and simple model for the transformation is a linear reservoir ($b = 1.00$). For flat areas $K = 280$(s) approximately, while Kidd (1978) gives as estimation

$$K = 1.43 S^{-0.40} L^{0.22} I^{-0.4} \qquad r = 0.77 \qquad (5.6)$$

where I is the average rainfall intensity over the most intense 10 minutes of the storm (mm min^{-1}).

More complex rainfall inflow models containing a larger number of model parameters seem attractive for achieving a better model performance. However, because of the high field variability, these parameters are so variable in time and place that the model performance is at best only as good as that of the above-mentioned models.

In many designs the rainfall-runoff process was neglected in the past because of lack of knowledge. However, this process has a tremendous effect on both the volume and the rate of the discharge. Neglect leads to serious overdesign of the system.

5.2.2 *Unpaved surfaces*

5.2.2.1 *Losses.* Depending on climate and other factors, the assumption can be made that the unpaved surface does not contribute to the discharge of the sewers. Of course this is only true in the case where the potential losses exceed the rainfall depth of a storm. In all other cases overland runoff from the unpaved surface is drained either via the paved surface and the sewer or directly by surface water drains. The infiltrated water that is not used for evapotranspiration recharges the groundwater and is drained by surface or subsurface drains.

The *initial losses* are in general larger than on paved surfaces. Although very dependent on the type of surface, values of 2–4 mm are not exceptional for flat areas; for sloping surfaces 0.0–2 mm seems reasonable. Measurements to confirm these figures are not available. The *evapotranspiration loss* is slightly increased because of the oasis effect that is introduced by the unpaved surface (Grimmond and Oke, 1986). It is however impossible to quantify this effect for a specific situation. Therefore the oasis effect is generally neglected. The *infiltration* capacity not only depends on soil type and antecedent wetness, but also on the function of the terrain. Figure 5.4 illustrates the variability of the final infiltration rate—parameter a in the Horton equation (eqn 5.2)—as a function of the land use on a loamy soil. This variability leads to the conclusion that runoff may occur from one part of the unpaved surface, while the other parts remain almost dry. Based on the median of numerous observations, the subsequent values for the Horton parameters for infiltration in sandy, humus-rich soil (Van de Ven, 1989a) are as follows:

	a (mm h^{-1})	b (mm)	c (h^{-1})
Grass, lawn	100	7.5	8
Bush	170	14	7.5
Bare soil	135	14	9

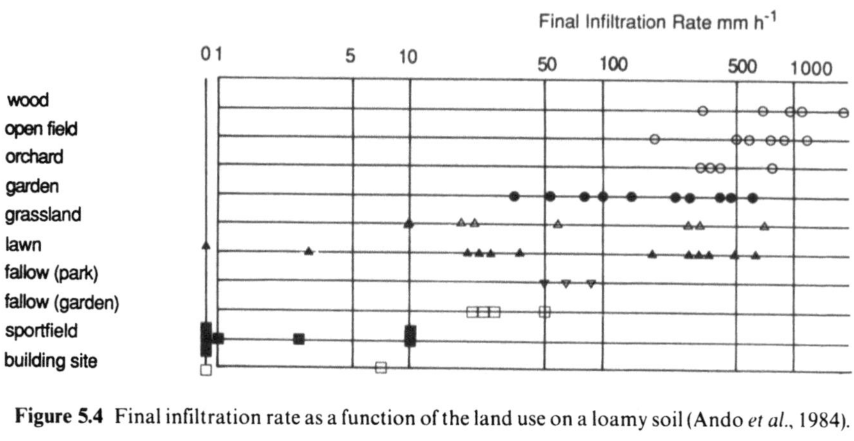

Figure 5.4 Final infiltration rate as a function of the land use on a loamy soil (Ando *et al.*, 1984).

This infiltration process is strongly influenced by the antecedent wetness of the catchment. In the case where the catchment is wet, a reduction of the calculated infiltration capacity of up to 50% is applied. The total loss is estimated by adding the initial loss, the evapotranspiration and the infiltration loss.

5.2.2.2 *Transformation.* In cases where a substantial contribution from the unpaved area to the surface drainage system (including sewers) is expected, the runoff can be calculated from the net rainfall using a unit hydrograph, as is shown in Chapter 1. If the soil can be considered impervious, the transformation formulae of the previous section (5.2.1) can be applied. In many cases the runoff from unpaved areas is only moderate, if not negligible. Snowmelt runoff over a frozen soil is, if relevant, considered in the design as a fixed load; in Sweden a load of $0.5–1.0\,m^3\,s^{-1}\,km^{-2}$ is used.

In very extreme storm events the runoff from unpaved areas can be significant, even if it is not under normal design conditions. If this runoff is not taken into account during the design process, tremendous damage may result: damage that could have been avoided by relatively simple and cheap means. In general, ponding of the surplus water on the surface is an effective way to avoid problems with erosion and downstream flooding.

5.3 Design methods

5.3.1 *Groundwater*

5.3.1.1 *Introduction.* Apart from the preservation of wooden foundation piles in cities such as Amsterdam and Rotterdam, urban groundwater serves no real purpose. As long as the water level is neither too high nor too low, nothing needs to be done with the groundwater. However, if the groundwater level is a problem, measures have to be taken to deal with it. This is extremely difficult because of the many conflicting elements which are present in urban areas, and a systematic solution is nearly impossible.

There are, however, several tools available which can assist the engineer in designing optimal measures. Several will be highlighted in this section. Attention will be given to two situations:

(a) Temporary measures to lower the water table.
(b) A high water level.

5.3.1.2 *Darcy's law.* Solving of groundwater problems is synonymous with changing the level of the groundwater. In urban areas this almost always concerns the phreatic level in the aquifer (the groundwater table). Darcy's law can be used as the basis for the necessary calculations. As has been previously discussed in Chapter 2, Darcy's law describes the relationship between the groundwater flow density and the water level gradient. In its most common form Darcy's law is as follows:

$$q_x = -k \frac{\mathrm{d}h}{\mathrm{d}x} \tag{5.7}$$

where q_x is the flow density or specific discharge (m s^{-1}), k is the permeability (m s^{-1}) and dh/dx is the water level gradient (dimensionless).

5.3.1.3 *Computer models.* With Darcy's law as a base, numerous computer programs have been developed to describe the effects on the water levels of any proposed remedial measures. More than 400 programs are registered at TNO-DGV in Delft. All of these programs have their specific advantages and disadvantages.

It is possible to classify the computer models as:

(a) Analytical models.
(b) Finite difference models.
(c) Finite element models.

The analytical method uses Darcy's law and continuity equations to determine relationships which can be used to calculate one continuous surface of water levels. In many cases simplifications are made. By introducing image wells, it is possible to model complex situations. The analytical relationships are, in many cases, manageable without the use of a computer. In section 5.3.1.4 a simple example of an analytical equation is given. Further examples are given in Chapters 10 and 11.

The use of finite difference and finite element methods is inextricably connected to the use of computers. By discretising a problem area and dividing it into elements, and within these elements creating linear relationships, very complex situations can be analysed (see Figure 5.5).

In section 5.3.1.5 an example of a model based on the finite difference method will be discussed. In addition to differences in the calculation method, the models also differ in:

The range, i.e. local or regional.
The number of layers that is taken into consideration.
Steady or unsteady flow.
With or without unsaturated zone.

New models are still being brought onto the market. The following developments have been observed:

(a) Many models which until now could only be run on large mainframe computers are now available for the personal computer. The programs have in many cases also become more user-friendly (the pre- and post-processing).

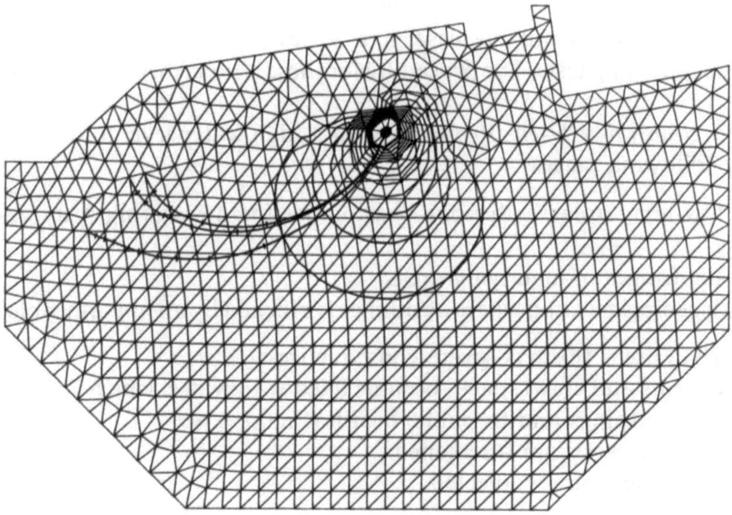

Figure 5.5 Example of output using the finite element method (Micro-Fem).

(b) Many models now have quality parameters. With these models it is possible to predict precisely the spread of pollution or calculate fresh and salt water behaviour.

(c) More co-ordination with other disciplines, for example water management (integral water management).

5.3.1.4 *Lowering of the water table.* In urban areas it is sometimes necessary to lower the groundwater level in connection with building projects. In these cases the level of the water table is lowered by means of rows of wells. By withdrawing groundwater from the building site and pumping it into the ground a short distance from the site (return drainage to prevent damage at a short distance from the building site), the shape of the groundwater level surface can be adapted to the needs of the building project. As is discussed in detail in Chapter 11, many techniques are available for dewatering sites. However, if a well is used, its effect can be predicted by the equation:

$$s = \frac{q}{2\pi kD} \ln\left(\frac{r}{R}\right) \tag{5.8}$$

where s is the lowering of the water level (m), q is the discharge of the well ($m^3 s^{-1}$), k is permeability ($m s^{-1}$), D is the thickness of the aquifer (m), r is the distance from the well (m) and R is the diameter of the area of influence of the well (m).

The problem in practice is often to make a good estimation of the permeability and the thickness of an aquifer (the combined kD value, the transmissivity of the aquifer). In some cases adequate groundwater data are available. If this is not the case, it is necessary to drill test wells and to conduct pumping tests. The procedure for these is described in Chapter 10.

5.3.1.5 *High water levels.* Problems with a high water level frequently occur in the following places:

In low-lying areas with poor possibilities for dewatering (clay and peat areas).

At the fringes of high-lying areas.

On a geological fault, where an aquifer is blocked by an impermeable layer.

For urban areas this has severe consequences:

Basements and crawl spaces become filled with water, which is detrimental both to furnishings and to public health (Figure 5.6).

Cables and wires are threatened.

'Green zones' can be affected.

To prevent or solve the problems, dewatering measures are required. With the help of well drainage, horizontal pipe drainage or open water drains, the groundwater level surface can be controlled.

To estimate accurately the effectiveness of the measures, it is necessary to conduct a model study. In the study the following two water balances should be evaluated:

$$\Delta B_{onv} = (N - E - Q_{opp} - P + C)\,\Delta t \tag{5.9}$$

$$\Delta B_{verz} = (P - C - Q_{ont} - I + K)\,\Delta t \tag{5.10}$$

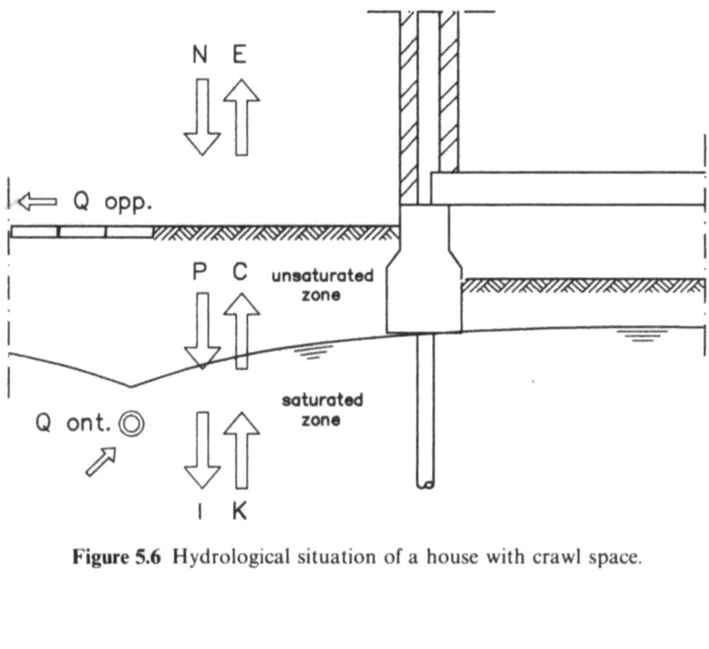

Figure 5.6 Hydrological situation of a house with crawl space.

where N is the precipitation ($m^3 s^{-1}$), E is the evapotranspiration ($m^3 s^{-1}$), Q_{opp} is the surface drainage ($m^3 s^{-1}$), (see section 5.3.2), P is the percolation ($m^3 s^{-1}$), C is the capillary rise ($m^3 s^{-1}$), Q_{ont} is the water drainage ($m^3 s^{-1}$), I is the infiltration to deeper groundwater ($m^3 s^{-1}$), K is the seepage ($m^3 s^{-1}$), ΔB_{onv} is the change in groundwater storage in the unsaturated zone (m^3) and ΔB_{verz} is the change in groundwater storage in the saturated zone (m^3).

HYSTED is a computer model which calculates the water balances mentioned above and which is specially designed to evaluate the measures to control and prevent high water levels in urban areas. It is a computer program based on the finite differences method which conducts quasistationary calculations. In HYSTED, an urban area is discretised by dividing it into nodal areas. Within each area (for example 10 × 10 m) the two water balances mentioned would be set up as a function of time.

In the saturated zone the flow exchange between two areas (see Figure 5.7) is calculated as follows:

$$q_{12} = \frac{2}{l^2} \frac{T_1 T_2}{T_1 + T_2} (h_1 - h_2) \tag{5.11}$$

where q_{12} is the specific discharge from section 1 to section 2 ($m s^{-1}$), l is the length of the nodal area (m), T_1 is the transmissivity (kD value) of nodal area 1 ($m^2 s^{-1}$), T_2 is the transmissivity of nodal area 2 ($m^2 s^{-1}$), h_1 is the groundwater level in nodal area 1 (m) and h_2 is the groundwater level in nodal area 2 (m).

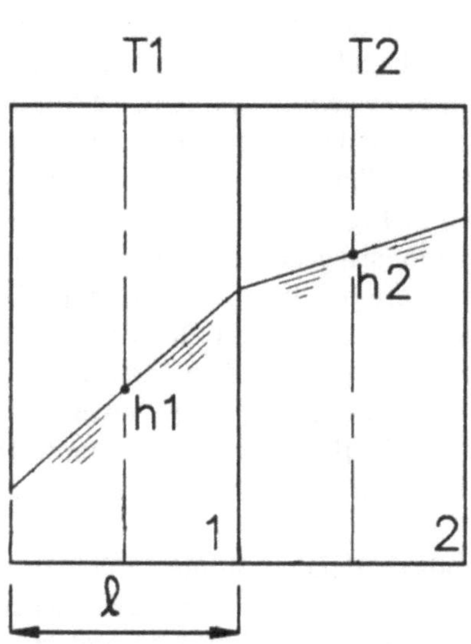

Figure 5.7 Cross-section of a saturated zone.

The work scheme is as follows:

(a) Water level observations are taken in test or observation wells (over at least one winter period).
(b) The model is calibrated using actual meteorological statistics and other data.
(c) The model is used to divide the observations into two parts:
    (1) The explicable part (that part which agrees with the computed values of the model).
    (2) The inexplicable part, the noise. If the noise component is too large, additional investigations are necessary.
(d) Measures (for example, drainage) are evaluated to see if high-groundwater problems can be alleviated.

5.3.2 *Storm sewers*

As described in section 5.2, a part of the precipitation is drained via a storm sewer system. Although different design philosophies are applied in different countries, they show one common feature: storm sewers are expensive, and it is generally desirable to minimise this cost while maintaining a low frequency of urban surface flooding causing disruption to services and property damage. A risk-based design, based on the probability of occurrence of a state variable (such as flow, discharge, water level) greater than the design magnitude during a specified period of time, is not yet fully developed for sewer pipe design. Until now, the optimisation of sewer systems has been expressed by the choice of the design return period. It is noted that in designing storm/combined sewers not only the design discharge is relevant, but also the quantity and quality characteristics of sewer outflows. In general, the governing factor in sewer system design is to be found in the effects on the receiving waters. This section deals with the water quantity aspects; water quality control is handled in Chapter 6. Typical components of an urban drainage model are shown in Figure 5.8.

In order to provide hydrological criteria for the design of drainage systems, rainfall-runoff calculations are of great importance. One of the main requirements is obviously an accurate figure for precipitation. Rainfall data should be collected and further processed in such a way that they can be used for further calculations. Rainfall data themselves are of no value; what matters in drainage design is the amount of runoff that results from precipitation. Finally, using hydraulics, the appropriate size of the conduit has to be chosen.

Flood estimation methods that may be applied to the design of stormwater drainage systems can be divided into two broad categories: those which produce only an estimate of the peak flow rate and more comprehensive approaches that also provide the shape of the runoff hydrograph. The

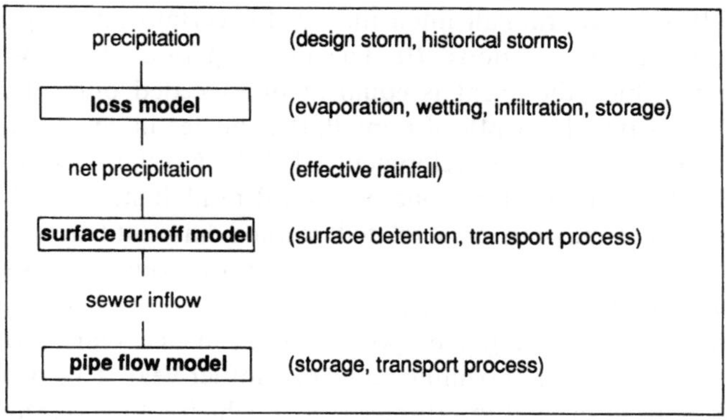

Figure 5.8 Scheme of an urban drainage model.

principal example of the former approach is the rational method. Representatives of the latter are the unit hydrograph and flood routing. The basic idea of flood routing is to predict runoff as a function of time and place $Q = f(x, t)$. Flood routing may further be classified in two major categories: simple hydrological routing and more complex hydraulic routing. Hydrological routing involves the balancing of inflow, outflow and volume of storage through the use of the continuity equation and a storage–discharge relation. Hydraulic routing differs from hydrological routing in that both the equation of continuity and the momentum equation are solved simultaneously.

In the first part of this section some standards methods for storm sewer design will be presented. These are all methods that allow calculation by hand or by pocket calculator. In the last decade, many computer packages have been developed for designing and analysing urban drainage systems, and in the second part of the section three well-known packages are briefly described.

5.3.2.1 *Precipitation.* Two different kinds of rainfall data can be used for the design of storm sewers (Arnell, 1982):

(1) Design storms estimated from intensity–duration–frequency (I–D–F) relationships or from historical rainfall data. A design storm can be defined as a rainfall which is developed for a certain design return period, and the discharge value which is calculated by means of the storm is said to obtain the same return period as the storm.
(2) Historical storms or time series generated by statistical methods are run through a runoff model, and the statistical analysis is applied to the simulated flow values to determine the flow value coupled with the design return period.

In an *I–D–F* curve, rainfall intensities (*I*) for certain return periods are plotted against given durations (*D*). The return period of an event is the period during which the event is equalled or exceeded only once on the average. The greater the depth of rainfall, the shorter in general the length of time it continues. The development of *I–D–F* relationships requires statistical analysis of data from one or several rainfall stations. A Gumbel analysis of annual maxima or a related method has until now been used frequently for assessing the return period of certain events. A disadvantage of annual maximum series is that only the maxima of each year are taken into account, whereas it might be possible that, in one year, two or more measurements exceed the maximum value of another year. This problem can be avoided by using partial duration series, in which all measurements that exceed a certain value are counted. Sevruk and Geiger (1981) indicated that the annual maximum method is most suited for estimates of events with large return periods (of the order of 10–1000 years). Yevjevich (1984) showed that the applicability of both methods depends on the distribution of the measured values. If in partial duration series a threshold is chosen, so that on average two or three values per year are counted, the method will give in general more reliable predictions of extreme values than the traditional annual maximum methods. For a description of *I–D–F* analysis, refer to, for example, Arnell (1982), Geiger *et al.* (1987) and Van de Ven (1989b).

It should be noted that *I–D–F* curves are evaluated for use in connection with the rational method and its derivatives, which are discussed below, and give no information on the temporal variation of the rainfall. Design storms have the advantage of being easy and inexpensive to use. The use of historical storms gives in general more accurate results and takes into account non-linear effects in the runoff process that influence the flow statistics. However, this method requires that a large number of storms are run through a model in order to facilitate a statistical assessment of the flow, which may make the method more expensive and time-consuming.

5.3.2.2 *Losses and surface runoff.* In storm sewer design, input flows are difficult to predict with a great deal of confidence. It is stressed, however, that dimensioning sewers and storage facilities on standards that are derived directly from precipitation data will lead to a significant over-dimensioning: the rainfall-runoff process is not to be neglected in the design process (Van de Ven, 1989b). Possible loss models and surface runoff models have been discussed in section 5.2.

5.3.2.3 *Flow in pipes.* The rate of change of discharge in a drainage system is usually sufficiently slow to treat the flow as steady when calculating pipe sizes (kinematic wave approximation). Several flow formulae are available to determine flow and the size of pipe required. They have in common the fact that they relate capacity, hydraulic gradients, coefficients of friction and pipe size. Some basic equations for the flow in pipes are:

Manning–Strickler:

$$v = k_{\mathrm{m}} R^{2/3} I^{1/2} \tag{5.12}$$

de Chezy:

$$v = C R^{1/2} I^{1/2} \tag{5.13}$$

Colebrook–White:

$$\frac{1}{\sqrt{\lambda}} = -2\log\left(\frac{1}{0.4\,\mathrm{Re}\sqrt{\lambda}} + \frac{k}{3.7D}\right) \tag{5.14}$$

where v is the mean flow velocity ($\mathrm{m\,s^{-1}}$), I is the gradient, i.e. friction loss per unit length, R is hydraulic radius = area/wetted perimeter (m) (for circular pipes counts $R = \frac{1}{4}\pi D^2/\pi D = \frac{1}{4}D$), D is the pipe diameter (m), k_{m} is the roughness coefficient of Manning ($\mathrm{m^{1/3}\,s^{-1}}$), C is the roughness coefficient of de Chezy ($\mathrm{m^{1/2}\,s^{-1}}$), λ is the dimensionless friction coefficient, k is the roughness coefficient (m) and Re is the Reynolds number for full-bore flow [$= vD/\nu$; where ν = kinematic velocity ($\mathrm{m^2\,s^{-1}}$)]. (Note: The Colebrook–White equation may be considered as the most up-to-date one, as it describes turbulent as well as laminar flow.)

The friction loss in a circular conduit can be calculated using the Darcy–Weisbach formula, which is:

$$z = \lambda \frac{L}{D}\frac{v^2}{2g} \tag{5.15}$$

where z is the friction loss (m), L is the length of the conduit (m) and g is the gravitational acceleration ($\mathrm{m\,s^{-2}}$).

5.3.2.4 *The rational method.* Several methods have been employed by engineers to determine the sizing requirements for storm sewers. The most popular is the rational method. In American literature, the method was first mentioned in 1889 by Kuichling for a determination of peak runoff for sewer design in New York. However the principles were expounded much earlier by the Irishman Mulvaney (1851). In the UK, the method is often referred to as the Lloyd–Davies method owing to the implication ascribed to a paper of 1906 (Chow, 1964). The rational formula is:

$$Q = CiA \tag{5.16}$$

where Q is the design peak discharge ($\mathrm{m^3\,s^{-1}}$), C is a dimensionless runoff coefficient, i is the constant (net) rainfall intensity ($\mathrm{m\,s^{-1}}$), lasting for a critical period of time t_{c}, t_{c} is the time of concentration (s) and A is the size of the drainage area ($\mathrm{m^2}$).

In Figure 5.9, the basis of the rational method is set out. The method

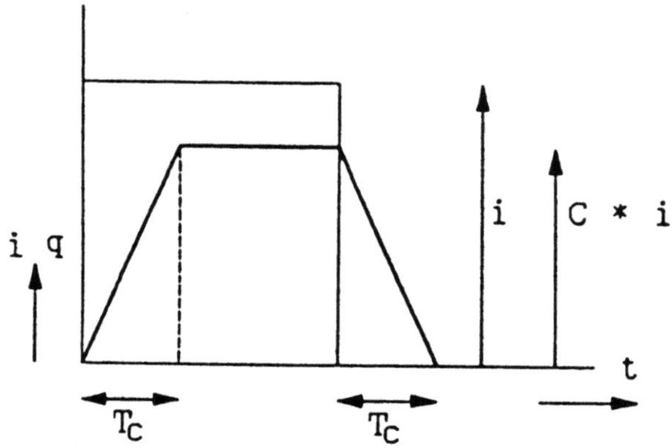

Figure 5.9 The rational method, basic principles.

assumes that the peak discharge occurs at a time t_c (time of concentration) after the beginning of the rain storm when the entire basin starts contributing to the runoff. The parameters t_c and C are assumed to be constant. The time of concentration is usually taken as the time for water to flow from the most remote part of the drainage area to reach the point being considered and is computed assuming that flow velocities are constant.

The calculation procedure to determine the pipe size involves the following steps:

(1) Determine the area contributing to the pipe under consideration.
(2) Choose an adequate pipe diameter, d_i.
(3) Calculate the flow velocity, v_i, assuming full bore velocity, using, for example, Manning's equation (eqn 5.12) or the formula of Colebrook–White (eqn 5.14). Establish the gradient from the contours. Minimum values depend on the required minimum flushing velocity.
(4) Calculate the time of concentration, t_c, which equals:

$$t_c = t_e + t_v \tag{5.17}$$

where t_c is the time of entry (of the order of 2–10 minutes), t_v is the travel time in the sewers up to the point of consideration and for pipe section N counts:

$$t_v = \sum_{i=1}^{N} \frac{L_i}{v_i}$$

where L_i is the length of each pipe.
(5) Use t_c to obtain the design rainfall intensity i from an I–D–F relationship for a selected return period for which surcharge may occur.
(6) Compute the design discharge Q using the rational formula (eqn 5.16). The runoff coefficient C_i for each subcatchment is either taken to be

equal to the fraction of the area that is impervious or is obtained from a table or formula.

(7) Compute the discharge capacity of the pipe: $Q_i = \frac{1}{4}\pi d_i^2 v_i$.

(8) If $Q_i < Q$, the procedure should be repeated from step 2 with a larger diameter.

The main objections to the use of the rational method may be summarised as follows:

The runoff coefficient is a constant.

No variation in the rate of rainfall with time.

No storage effects (backwater) in the sewer system.

No variation in the rate of increase in contributing area.

Antecedent conditions, the storm sequence, non-uniform rainfall, etc., are not taken into account.

5.3.2.5 *The time–area method.* The inability of the rational method to deal with catchment areas in which the rate of increase in contributing area is variable led to the introduction of design methods based upon the use of the time–area diagram. The principle of the time–area method is shown in Figure 5.10. During time, the area contributing to the discharge increases. The same applies to the situation as given in Figure 5.11. First, the contributing area increases for the time of concentration T_1. Somewhat later, the second catchment will start contributing. Hence the area will increase between T_3 and $T_2 + T_3$. At that moment the area contributing is at its maximum.

Using time–area diagrams, the rational method may provide quite useful results, even when dealing with variable contributing areas. It is noted that more sophisticated, so-called tangent, methods have been derived from the time–area method. However, these methods show problems in their estimation of peak runoff rates and have now largely been abandoned.

5.3.2.6 *Typical storm methods.* These methods differ from the time–area method only in that the variation of rainfall intensity with time (i.e. the

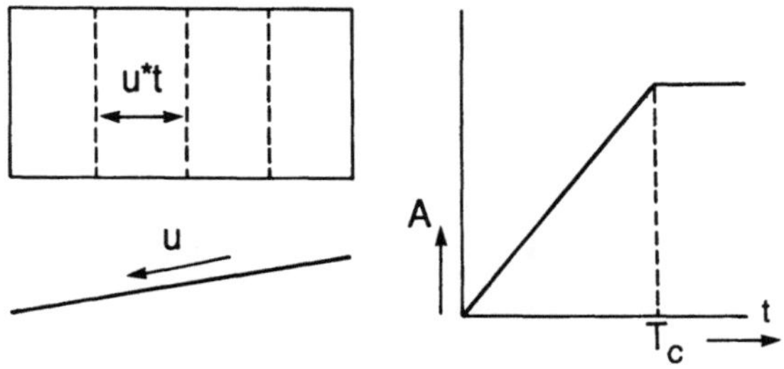

Figure 5.10 The time–area method, basic principles.

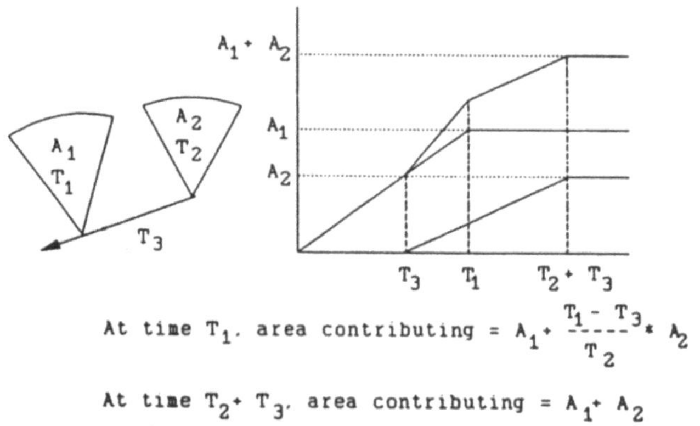

Figure 5.11 The time–area method, two catchments.

storm profile) is included. This approach generally assumes an arbitrary shape of storm profile, constructed from the *I–D–F* relationship for a given frequency of occurrence.

Arnell (1982) investigated the results of several design storms: the *average I–D–F design storm*, which is simply the constant intensity obtained from the *I–D–F* curve, gave underestimated peak flow values. The same applies for the *Illinois State Water Survey* (*ISWS*) *design storm*, which consists of the rain volume obtained from the *I–D–F* curve and with a certain time distribution. As both methods gave underestimates and consist of more or less a constant intensity only, they are not recommended for use. The *Chicago design storm*, which is determined from the mathematical expression of the *I–D–F* curve and whose most important characteristic is that the maximum average intensities for all durations follow an *I–D–F* curve, is also not recommended. The use of the *Sifalda design storm*, which compounds the

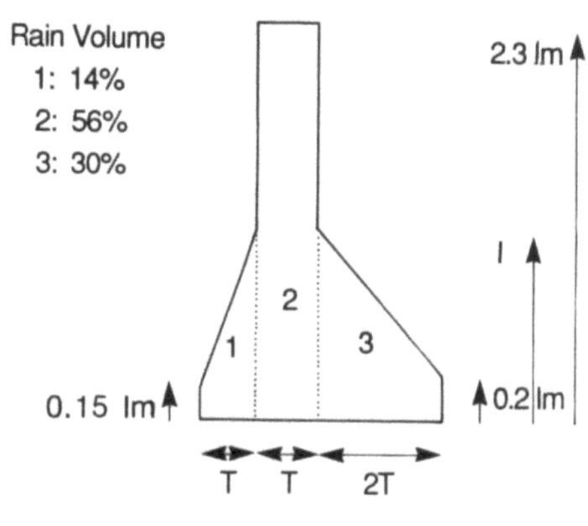

Figure 5.12 Design storm suggested by Sifalda (Arnell, 1982).

I–D–F design storm with precipitation added before and after, giving the Sifalda storm a total volume similar to the total volumes of the historical rainfalls (Figure 5.12), gave the best results when using design storms.

The development of the typical storm methods in the UK culminated in what is now referred to as the Transport and Road Research Laboratory (TRRL) hydrograph method (Watkins, 1962). Nowadays, the *Flood Studies Report* (*FSR*) *design storm*, which has a total volume obtained from the I–D–F curve and with a time distribution equal to the average distribution for the historical storms centred around the most intense parts, has been recommended in the UK for practical use (NERC, 1975).

5.3.2.7 *The unit hydrograph.* The methods discussed above are mainly directed towards the estimation of peak flow. For certain problems, such as design criteria for pipes and structures, this may be sufficient. However, for many purposes it is essential to know the distribution of the runoff volume in time, in order to assess peak discharge, time lag and runoff duration. The time–area method forms the first attempt in estimating the whole runoff hydrograph. A more sophisticated approximation is the unit hydrograph, which may be defined as the hydrograph of direct runoff, resulting from a unit depth of effective rainfall generated uniformly over the catchment area at a constant rate during a specified period of time. The method is outlined in Chapter 1.

5.3.2.8 *Hydrological routing.* Flood-routing methods are used to predict the temporal and spatial variations of flood waves through the system. The rate of change of storage (S) can be written as the balance between inflow (I) and outflow (O) (the continuity equation):

$$\mathrm{d}S/\mathrm{d}t = I - O \tag{5.18}$$

Considering a lumped storage approach, this equation can be generalised to a finite-difference equation for two points in time. An easy method of performing hydrological routing is reservoir routing, in which the storage is only related to outflow. Examples of such relations are the linear reservoir, the non-linear reservoir and the Nash model, as described in section 5.2. Reservoir routing may be applied to, for example, flood prediction, reservoir design and urban drainage.

If one considers water surface profiles at various times during a flood wave, e.g. in rivers or channels, a storage–discharge relationship as a function of both inflow and outflow is required. This is accomplished in the Muskingum method, which is described by, for example, Bedient and Huber (1988). The method assumes uniform, steady flow and is based on the linear relationship:

$$S = K[xI + (1 - x)O] \tag{5.19}$$

where K is the travel time constant for the reach and x is a weighting factor, which varies from 0 to 0.5. For a linear reservoir, $x=0$. For a detailed description and determination of the Muskingum coefficients, see, for example, Bedient and Huber (1988) and Shaw (1988).

Lumped hydrological models are in general capable of describing the flow retention in sewer networks; however, they fail in simulating backwater and surcharge effects.

5.3.2.9 *Hydraulic routing*. Hydraulic routing is more complex and accurate than hydrological routing and is based on the solution of the continuity equation and the momentum equation for unsteady flow in open conduits. Three different levels of hydraulic descriptions can be distinguished, incorporating different terms of the equation of Saint Venant:

Continuity equation:

$$\frac{\partial Q}{\partial x}+\frac{\partial A}{\partial t}=0 \tag{5.20}$$

Momentum equation:

$$\frac{\partial Q}{\partial t}+\frac{\partial}{\partial x}\left(\beta\frac{Q^2}{A}\right)+gA\frac{\partial h}{\partial x}+gAI_{\mathrm{f}}=gAI_{\mathrm{o}} \tag{5.21}$$

- $gAI_{\mathrm{f}}=gAI_{\mathrm{o}}$: Kinematic wave approximation
- $gA\frac{\partial h}{\partial x}+gAI_{\mathrm{f}}=gAI_{\mathrm{o}}$: Diffusion (non-inertia) approximation
- all terms: Full dynamic wave approximation (Saint Venant equations)

where Q is the flow rate ($m^3\ s^{-1}$), A is the cross-sectional area (m^2), h is the flow depth (m), g is the gravitational acceleration ($m\ s^{-2}$), x is the longitudinal axis (m), t is time (s), β is the velocity distribution coefficient ($-$):

$$\beta=\frac{A}{Q^2A}\int u^2\mathrm{d}A;\ \text{where } u \text{ is the flow velocity (m s}^{-1})$$

I_{o} is the bottom slope ($-$) and I_{f} is the friction slope ($-$).

Since no closed-form solution for these differential equations exists, various numerical methods have been developed for the computer. When computing the runoff in conduits, the governing equations may often be simplified to a one-dimensional continuity equation and a uniform flow relationship (kinematic wave), meaning that only the frictional and the gravitational forces are considered. This implies that backwater and surcharge phenomena cannot be computed with the kinematic wave approach. The diffusive wave approximation also takes the pressure gradient forces into account. In many cases the model makes a fairly good computation of surcharge phenomena. In the dynamic wave version all terms of the Saint Venant equations are included. The main difference between the diffusive wave and the dynamic wave versions is that the latter is better at computing sudden changes in the runoff, e.g. the effect of a rapidly rising water level. Further consideration is given to the methods of solution of the Saint Venant equations in Chapter 7.

5.3.2.10 *Computer models.* In the last decade, many computer packages have become available for runoff calculations and urban drainage design. A distinction can be made between design methods and simulation methods. The former are used in designing new systems and are based on one or more of the standard methods described above. Since computer runs are fast, it is possible to calculate various options within a short time. Simulation models are used for analysing the performance of existing systems or as a checking procedure on the hydraulic performance of new systems. Some models are capable of handling water quality features. In general much attention is being paid to the development of suitable numerical techniques to calculate pollutant transport; however, up until now, these efforts have not yet resulted in accurate models. This topic is discussed in more detail in Chapter 6.

Proper use of computer programs requires good preparation and fundamental knowledge of the phenomena under consideration. Even if totally misused, most programs will provide attractive figures and graphs, but in fact these may only represent nonsense. First of all a model should be used that fits the specific problem. Furthermore a data check and calibration should be included whenever setting up a model. A manual calculation should be made with one of the previously described standard methods and the results compared with the model results, using the same data set. This will lead the user through a major part of the program and the gross blunders will normally be found.

The Wallingford procedure (WASSP). The Wallingford procedure for the design and analysis of urban storm drainage, often referred to as WASSP (Wallingford Storm Sewer Package), was developed in the 70s and 80s in the UK by, amongst others, Hydraulic Research Limited and the Institute of Hydrology, both at Wallingford. The Wallingford procedure includes several models:

WASSP, MicroWASSP: the original UK implementation of the Wallingford procedure for urban storm drainage, incorporating a hierarchy of methods: the Wallingford modified rational method, the Wallingford hydrograph method, the Wallingford optimisation method, the Wallingford simulation method, a data-checking program and a resource cost program. For more detailed information refer to NWC (1981). This paper includes flowcharts showing how to use WASSP and how to choose the appropriate method.

WALLRUS, the international version of MicroWASSP.

MicroRAT, the spreadsheet implementation of the modified rational method with storage pond design.

SPIDA, the simulation model for looped networks.
MOSQITO, the water quality submodel.
NEMOSYS, the graphics-based network modelling system.
GURVIL, the graphics presentation program.

Further information may be obtained from Wallingford Software Ltd (UK). The programmer's manual is only supplied with the programs.

The storm water management model (*SWMM*). The US Environmental Protection Agency Storm Water Management Model, or SWMM, is a computer-based model for simulation of the quantity and quality of runoff in urban areas, with extensions to non-urban areas as well. The first version of SWMM was developed in the early 70s for mainframe computers; version 4 was released in 1988 and can be run on microcomputers. The model consists of four computational 'blocks': the runoff block, the transport block, the extended transport block (EXTRAN) and the storage/treatment block. In addition six 'service blocks' are available for amongst others statistics, presenting graphs and rain input and to link the different routines. Generally speaking, water quality modelling is difficult. This holds for SWMM as well. Furthermore, the deterministic approach as used in SWMM is difficult to calibrate. Thus most users stick to water quantity modelling only. The model, including source files, is delivered all over the world, but the majority of the users can be found in the USA and Canada. The EXTRAN block, which performs the hydraulic routing, is also available as a separate version. The University of Technology in Hanover (West Germany) developed a menu-driven user's interface and made some small modifications of the numerical solution methods as applied in EXTRAN. This model is called HYSTEM–EXTRAN.

The SWMM is fully described by Huber and Dickinson (1988). The EXTRAN block is further dealt with by Roesner *et al.* (1988). More information may be obtained from the University of Florida, Department of Environmental Engineering Sciences.

MOUSE. The Danish MOUSE package (*mo*delling of *u*rban *se*wer systems) was developed in the 80s by the Danish Hydraulic Institute, Emolet, I. Kruger and PH-Consult especially for application on microcomputers. MOUSE is a menu-driven program and consists of several computational modules for simulation of surface runoff, pipe flow and pollution loads, together with a number of auxiliary modules for data input and presentation of results. The model input is handled by a catchment database containing an inventory of the geometric, hydrological and hydraulic features of the catchment, and a rain database, which consists of measured and/or synthesised time series and the *I–D–F* formula. The runoff module includes a time–area method and a kinematic wave routing of hydrographs. The pipe flow module is built up in such a way that it is possible to choose the appropriate hydraulic description (kinematic, diffusive or dynamic wave) for the same set of catchment data. The pollution module, SAMBA, is used for analysis of pollution loads in connection with combined sewer overflows (CSO) and inlets to treatment plants. A relatively simple routine, based on the time–area diagram and assuming ideal mixing of rainwater and foul water, is used to allow for long-term simulations in order to facilitate statistical assessment of pollution discharges. As previously stated, water quality modelling is difficult and, because of its simplicity, SAMBA may lead to inaccurate results with regard to estimates of pollution loads. Several investigations have shown that, especially in flat areas, processes such as settlement and resuspension of settled material are important sources of CSO pollution and therefore not to be neglected. Upgrades of SAMBA may be expected within the near future.

MOUSE is available in several languages, and the majority of its users can be found in Europe. More detailed information may be obtained at the Mouse Service Center, Gentofte (Denmark), and the Danish Hydraulic Institute (see Mouse, 1989).

5.3.3 *Surface water*

The drainage process in urban areas is different from that in rural areas. Because of the paved surfaces in urban areas, precipitation is drained immediately and the losses are minimal in comparison with those in rural areas. Urban surface drainage has two functions: the removal of drainage water and the temporary storage of drainage water. In designing the system one should take into account the storage required and the discharge capacity of the drains.

The design of the system of open waterways and ponds depends to a great extent on the local circumstances. An important characteristic is the slope of the terrain. Different designs are applied to areas with steep slopes than to those with low gradients. Often, and certainly in a country as flat as The Netherlands for example, it is not possible to drain the precipitation directly. In this case the water must be temporarily stored.

If rainfall can be drained immediately, the waterways and the structural works in the area will be designed based on the drainage capacity. In general, this is determined using the Chezy or Manning–Strickler formula (see eqn. 5.12, section 5.3.2.3). To calculate temporal effect a hydrodynamic model, based on the Saint Venant equation, is generally used (see eqn. 5.20, section 5.3.2.9).

If it is not possible to drain the rainfall directly, the waterways must be designed based on the required storage capacity. The surface area of open water is then of major importance and the drainage capacity of minor importance. In this situation only the continuity equations are solved (see eqn. 5.20, section 5.3.2.9).

In general, the following criteria must be considered in the design of open waterways in urban areas:

Sufficient land reclamation.
The maximum water level rise for a given rainstorm with a given recurrence time.
Ease of maintenance.
Ease of cleaning (to control water quality).
Minimum ground use.
Minimum number of structural control works.

5.3.4 *Surface drainage from roads*

One of the main problems in urban areas is the removal of water from road surfaces. This is essential, since excess surface water can lead to the loss of adhesion between vehicle tyres and the road surface and also to a spray hazard for all road users, including pedestrians. As in the case of storm sewers, design of facilities to deal with surface water is dependent on a hydrological assessment of the amount of water to be disposed of and a hydraulic assessment of the way in which the water moves towards and ultimately in the channels, pipes, etc., carrying it away from the area. Frequently surface water is discharged into a sewer system, either combined or separate, and this aspect of the design has already been considered in section 5.3.2. What has yet to be considered is the way in which the water is collected from the road surface. There are essentially two collection systems, one in which water is allowed to flow over the edge of the road pavement into an open drain or ditch, and the other in which water flows in a channel formed by a raised kerb, verge or other boundary and discharges into gullies or outlets placed at regular intervals. In temperate climates and in large conurbations the latter system is more usual.

In order that water may flow off the road pavement, a transverse gradient is required, and then to allow the water to flow towards an outlet a longitudinal gradient is required. When the road is kerbed the result is to produce a triangular channel sloping towards the outlet. Problems arise when for traffic engineering reasons shallow gradients are required, leading to loss of hydraulic efficiency. One solution is to produce 'false channel profiles' by creating artificial gradients in the kerbside channels by raising and lowering these in relation to the overall longitudinal gradient. For drainage design purposes roads are classified according to their longitudinal gradients, the categories being longitudinal gradients greater than 0.5% and less than 0.2% with a transition zone between 0.5 and 0.2%. Detailed design procedures are given by Russam (1969) and Whiffin and Young (1973). These are summarised as follows.

5.3.4.1 *Longitudinal gradients greater than 0.5%*. Consider rain of intensity I mm h^{-1} falling on a section of road surface B m wide, with transverse gradient C (expressed as a fraction), longitudinal gradient S (as a fraction) and draining into a triangular kerbside channel. In order to limit the width, W(m), of flow in the channel, outlets or gullies have to be placed at regular intervals of J m. Russam (1969) showed that the outlet spacing may be obtained from:-

$$J = 0.315 \frac{K}{nBI} W^{8/3} C^{5/3} S^{1/2} \qquad (5.22)$$

where K is a constant equal to 1 when metre units are used throughout, and n is Manning's roughness coefficient, often taken as 0.01 for road surfaces.

Introducing a gulley or outlet efficiency factor, E%, usually of the order of 90% for gullies set into the road surface, then

$$J = 0.315 \frac{K}{nBI} W^{8/3} C^{5/3} S^{1/2} \frac{E}{100} \qquad (5.23)$$

Design rainfall intensities can be predicted using the procedures outlined in Chapter 1 and section 5.3.2.

5.3.4.2 *Longitudinal gradients less than 0.2%*. Roads with gradients of less than 0.2% are referred to as level or near-level roads. Typical examples are motorways. Inspection of eqns 5.22 and 5.23 shows that, for gradients of zero or near zero, outlet spacings of zero are predicted. This is clearly not the case in practice. Hence a different form of prediction equation is required. Whiffin and Young (1973) give suitable equations, one in which it is envisaged that the water spills into a trapezoidal channel set at the edge of an unkerbed hard shoulder and the other in which, as in the previous case, a triangular channel forms at the edge of a kerbed hard shoulder.

For the trapezoidal channel:

$$J = \frac{0.235(s + 0.5GH)^{12/13} H^{16/13}}{(IB)^{10/13}} \qquad (5.24)$$

where s is the bottom width of the channel (mm), G is the sum of the cotangents of the angles of the channel sides and H is the depth of the channel (mm).

For the triangular channel:

$$J = 545\left[\frac{W}{IB}\right]^{3/4} C^{23/16}\left[1 + \frac{kW^{7/4}S^{\omega}}{(IB)^{7/8}}\right] \tag{5.25}$$

where k is a coefficient related to C such that

$C = 0.01$	0.015	0.02	0.025	0.03	0.04	0.05
$k = 190$	265	326	380	416	448	448

and ω is an index related to C such that

$$\omega = 2.32 - 0.13C$$

C and S are expressed as percentages.

As in the case of equation 5.23, outlet efficiency can be included by the addition of the multiplier $E/100$ to eqns 5.19 and 5.20.

As before, rainfall intensities can be predicted using the procedures given in Chapter 1 and section 5.3.2.

5.3.4.3 *Transition zone, longitudinal gradients between 0.5 and 0.2%.* For longitudinal gradients between 0.5 and 0.2%, the outlet spacing should be calculated by both eqns 5.22 and 5.25 and the greater value accepted as the required spacing.

5.4 Runoff control

Various methods of runoff control are considered in the modern, innovative design of urban drainage. Runoff control comprises measures taken to reduce the volume of surface runoff entering the sewer system and measures involving control by storage and treatment of the collected flow. The former group is referred to as source control; the latter represents collection or off-line control. Real-time control is a way of providing maximum use of the storage and discharge facilities.

5.4.1 *Source control*

The most cost-effective methods for reduction of runoff in urban areas are source controls. Several measures can be considered, all based on the principle of increasing rainwater infiltration and hence reducing runoff. Porous pavements, soak-away pits, seepage trenches, etc. are basically groundwater recharge facilities which are dispersed throughout the catchment and therefore difficult to control and maintain. Although such source controls may be very effective in reducing runoff volumes and peaks, the protection of groundwater quality must restrict their application to less polluted stormwater originating from rooftops, backyards and residential streets. Another possibility is to discharge flows into a cistern which may be used to store water, for example for garden watering.

Centralised groundwater recharge facilities allow good operational control and maintenance. Sometimes detention ponds or sedimentation basins are used in conjuction with infiltration basins so that suspended solids will settle before the water is released into the basin. Design of recharge–storage facilities should account for the fact that lateral drainage through the basin is generally several times more rapid than vertical percolation. For this reason a control drain should be installed to infiltrate water into the soil by means of trenches or vertical wells. The use of infiltration basins is particularly popular in areas where groundwater recharge is required, such as coastal areas, where urbanisation may lead to saltwater intrusion, or in other areas where groundwater depletion would cause problems. Without proper maintenance, open-surface storage-infiltration facilities accumulate pollutants and become a community nuisance. On the other hand, well-landscaped and well-maintained basins can be used as a recreation area, which then requires plants, trees and facilities capable of withstanding temporary inundation. Basin sides should be gently sloped to give a park-like appearance.

5.4.2 *Storage facilities*

Retention and detention are the most frequently employed methods of runoff control and can be used to achieve virtually any degree of runoff control, provided that the costs of such facilities are not prohibitive. The basic principle is to provide sufficient storage in the drainage system to keep the water in the system until there is sufficient discharge capacity to lead it away (e.g. to the treatment plant). By using a system of storage facilities it is possible to reduce peak flows drastically and to use existing systems to convey runoff from new urban developments. Storage facilities can be constructed as in-line or off-line reservoirs.

Off-line reservoirs can be defined as reservoirs that are only activated if a preset level of flow or stage is exceeded. The advantage of off-line reservoirs is that pollutant removal by sedimentation can take place in the reservoirs. The removal efficiency depends strongly on the hydraulic design and local conditions. Investigations in The Netherlands showed a 40–60% reduction in chemical oxygen demand (Hove and Wensveen, 1986). Although off-line reservoirs are relatively expensive to construct and need routine maintenance since sediments have to be frequently removed, they are probably the best technique for improving the performance of combined sewer systems. This is because they are effective for both flood protection and reduction of pollutant outflow to receiving waters.

In-line reservoirs can be defined as reservoirs that are permanently activated, since they are a part of the conduit. In-line reservoirs can be constructed as basins or just by using pipes with large diameters in sections of the system. The advantage of in-line reservoirs is that they are generally cheaper to construct and, when properly designed, they do not need so much maintenance. Sedimentation cannot occur undisturbed since they are permanently activated. For flood protection they are as effective as off-line reservoirs.

In areas with adequate open space, the most cost-effective solution is to use open-surface reservoirs. In densely developed areas, for safety reasons and because of space limitations, storage facilities are often built underground. Underground storage facilities obviously require more resources for their design, construction and maintenance. Such facilities include in-line and off-line reservoirs with regulated outlets. It is good practice to subdivide larger storage facilities into a number of cells. The entire storage capacity is used only for the largest storms. Runoff from more frequent storms is stored in a limited number of cells in order to reduce maintenance. The facility might be designed so that runoff during 'normal' conditions is stored in the underground part and additional volumes from extreme events are retained in an open reservoir.

5.4.3 *Real-time control*

The conventional design of urban drainage systems is based on the concept of a design storm. Proper design of the urban drainage system does not imply that the system performs optimally under all conditions. Important aspects are:

The discrepancy between planned and real performance of the urban drainage system as a result of the schematisation and assumptions made in the design.

Variations of the loading of the system in time and place; the design storm will never occur as a physical event.

Sewer construction and maintenance work may modify the system's capacity.

The tuning of storage–discharge capacities of various subcatchments.

The relation between urban discharges and the treatment plant capacity/efficiency.

Temporal effects on receiving waters and local differences in sensitivity of the receiving water bodies.

It is normally assumed that no intervention is required in the operation of a drainage system since it has been well designed. However, because of the above-mentioned aspects, the system will never perform 'optimally' and during most storms the storage and discharge capacity of the system will not be utilised to capacity. It may be concluded that most conventionally designed systems contain an unutilised potential for reducing flooding problems and pollution from combined sewer overflows. Furthermore it has become clear that the total drainage system—the sewer system and the treatment plant—has to be designed and operated as an entity. Only by using an integrated approach can an optimum be found in relation to the pollution load on receiving waters, which is generally the main governing factor in designing urban drainage systems.

An urban drainage system is operated in real time if process data currently monitored in the system are used to operate flow regulators during the actual process (Schilling *et al.*, 1987). In the context of real-time control (RTC), the meaning of 'system' is the controllable part of the drainage system. The general objective of RTC is to use the capacity of all facilities of the urban drainage system as well as possible under all operational situations. RTC means continuous monitoring and controlling of the flow process. In principle, the control of a process can be schematised to a simple control loop (Figure 5.13). This control loop requires a sensor to measure the process, a regulator to adjust the process and a controller to process the measurements and to activate the regulator. Data have to be transmitted between the elements.

Several hierarchised levels of control can be distinguished, i.e. local control, unit process control and global control, with the last-mentioned being the top level. Depending on the requirements of the specific drainage system, the control can be decentralised or fully centralised, or some mixed arrangement can be applied. Distributed systems are most common in practice. These allow for local automatic control of the regulators and for central

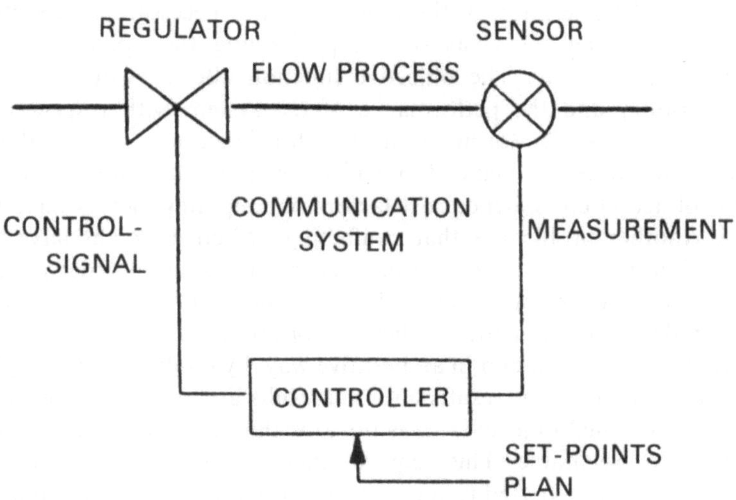

Figure 5.13 A simple control loop.

modification of the local control. Communication is usually realised by a telemetry network using public telephone lines. Global control can be executed manually (supervisory mode) or automatically (central automatic mode). For safety reasons it should allow for all kinds of interference, such as malfunctioning of hardware, communication system failure or on-site manual operation.

The technology of RTC systems, including their hardware, is becoming well known, and their use is rapidly increasing. The key problem for the drainage engineer when applying these systems to urban drainage systems is the formulation of the control strategy, which can be defined as the time sequence of all regulator setpoints. In automatic RTC systems, the control strategy is often referred to as the set of rules to specify such a time sequence. In urban drainage systems the optimum setpoints vary with each flow pattern. Hence, a flexible method has to be used to react to whatever loading may occur.

The main features of the problem determining the control strategy are:

The operational objectives.
The physical constraints.
The system loading.
The solution technique.

In order to determine the way the urban drainage system should react under different conditions, the operational tasks of the system have to be specified. Mostly these are to avoid flooding and environmental problems while keeping the costs of operation and maintenance low. It is often useful to rank the objectives according to their priority. In order to make rational and consistent decisions on the operation of the regulators it is necessary to specify the ideal operation and the costs of not performing the operational tasks (the objective function). The objective function allows evaluation of the control strategy and the performance of the system with respect to the specified objectives. The formulation of such a function is usually difficult, as several objectives are included, of which some are impossible to quantify in terms of actual costs, hence cost factors or weighting factors have to be applied. Another problem is that conflicting objectives might have to be included. For example, storing stormwater in the system in order to reduce combined sewer overflow might lead to a higher risk of flooding. In such cases a trade-off between the conflicting objectives has to be defined. The best strategy is mostly found in an iterative way: by modifying the weighting factors and evaluating the results until the results are in accordance with the required operational objectives. It is obvious that a control strategy has to be physically executable. This requires that the state variables (storage, discharge, etc.) are restricted to their physical bounds (static constraints) and that the physical laws of water motion in a drainage system, i.e. continuity and energy balances, have to be obeyed (dynamic constraints). In general, the determination of the control strategy requires the use of a model, as described in section 5.3.2.

The physcial capacities are generally known with sufficient accuracy. The loading of the system (storm inflows, pollutant discharges) is more difficult to determine in real time. Information on the input of the drainage system can be gained by:

Flow and water level measurements in upstream parts of the system, which allow reaction within the travel time of the flow.

Rain measurements, in connection with rainfall-runoff models, which extend the reaction time by the travel time for water to flow over the surface to the sewer inlet.

Rain forecasts (e.g. by radar images) would allow gain of additional time, depending on the forecast horizon.

Several techniques are available to generate a suitable control strategy. Heuristic methods are based on the experience of the operators. In finding the appropriate strategy they might use an interactive decision support system (e.g. a flow simulator). The techniques which may be used for automatic control can be divided into three categories:

Control scenarios or decision matrices, which are based on rules of the 'if..then..else..' type.

Mathematical optimisation techniques, which are based on the minimisation of an objective function subject to a set of static and dynamic constraints. Well-known optimisation routines are linear programming, quadratic programming and dynamic programming. The mathematics behind these techniques are described in various handbooks on optimisation, e.g. Kirk (1970), Lasdon (1970) and Bryson and Yu-Chi Ho (1975).

Expert systems, which are based on known information about the system, its operational state and precisely described reasoning processes to produce a control strategy. The control decisions are, simply stated, not found through a model of the physical system but through a model of the expert, i.e. the operator.

Heuristic control is applied in most cases. A few examples can be found of control systems using control scenarios. Practical applications of automatic control, based on optimisation and/or expert systems, do not yet exist, but several feasibility studies are being carried out.

The first comprehensive approaches to RTC in urban drainage were initiated in the United States in the 70s, but most RTC applications in the US, Europe and Japan started in the 80s, after the introduction of the microprocessor. The increasing complexity of urban water management and the increasing possibilities of measuring equipment stimulated many water managers to install computerised monitoring systems. As yet, the reasons for installing such systems are mostly acquiring data (e.g. for maintenance planning), monitoring the state of operation and giving an alarm in case of technical trouble. Until now, the real-time control of the regulators (pumps, gates, weirs, etc.), based on the actual state of the drainage system, has only been used in a few cases. Although several research projects have shown the potential of RTC, it is still not widely accepted in urban drainage. The main obstacles to the use of this technique are to be found in administrative borders within the urban drainage system, funding arrangements and inflexible regulations and standards that are in favour or even prescribe static solutions to urban drainage problems. Nevertheless, it can be expected that, because of the change in attitude towards environmental protection and the need to minimise costs, RTC will be a common feature in urban drainage systems in the near future.

6 Pollution control

M.P. OSBORNE and J.A. PAYNE

6.1 Introduction

Pollution of rivers by drainage systems can occur as a result of discharges from combined sewer overflows, surface water outfalls, pumping station overflows and sewage treatment works. In the UK and Europe, most sewage pollution incidents are caused by combined sewer overflows (Figure 6.1).

Drainage discharges have a measurable adverse effect on river quality, and these effects need to be minimised. This can be achieved by source control to prevent pollutants entering the system, or by better design and management of drainage systems, treatment works and outfalls. This requires relevant legislation, so that decisions can be taken within a sensible framework which allows water quality objectives to be met, and appropriate tools, including water quality models which can predict pollutant levels in sewerage systems and receiving waters, thus allowing the engineer to assess the water quality effects of proposed new systems, the benefits of rehabilitation of existing systems and the relative merits of management alternatives. Predictive tools are already widely used in the hydraulic design of drainage systems to prevent flooding, and in rivers to design flood defences. Water quality models are not as widely used but have been applied in the US and are increasingly being developed for use in Europe and the rest of the world.

The following sections describe the sources, nature and effects of pollutants in drainage discharges; the relevant legislation; structural and non-structural controls; general approaches to water quality modelling; and sewerage and river water quality models.

6.2 Nature and sources of pollutants

6.2.1 *Mechanisms of pollution*

Drainage discharges which affect water quality can be categorised into four groups:

(1) Those which contain oxygen-demanding substances, either organic, such as faecal matter, or inorganic. Heated discharges, such as cooling waters, reduce the concentration of dissolved oxygen.

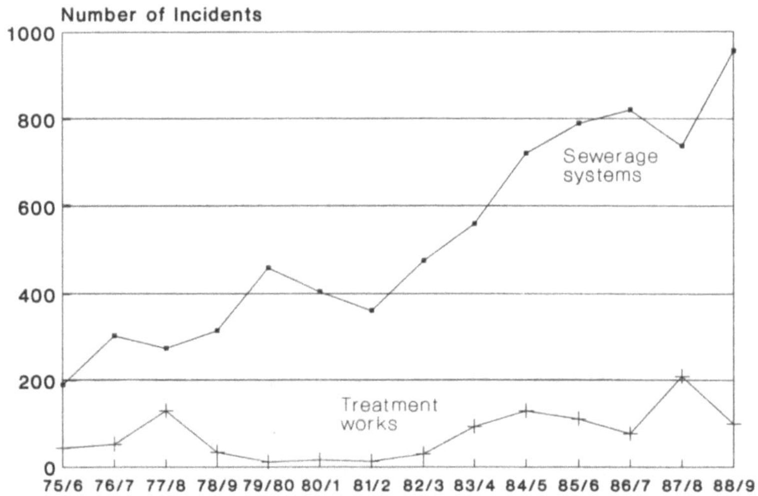

Figure 6.1 Types of sewage pollution incidents (NRA Severn–Trent Region).

(2) Those which contain substances which physically hinder reoxygenation at the water surface, such as oils.
(3) Discharges containing toxic compounds, including ammonia, pesticides and some industrial effluents.
(4) Discharges high in suspended solids, which inhibit biological activity by excluding light from the water or by coating the bed.

Discharges containing oxygen-demanding substances are assessed by measuring the amount of oxygen required for their stabilisation, using biochemical oxygen demand (BOD) and chemical oxygen demand (COD) tests. BOD measures the potential of the pollutants present in the effluent to sustain bacteria which consume oxygen. The test attempts to represent the conditions likely to occur in a river as a result of the natural purification capacity of the water. COD measures the oxygen demand in the presence of a strong oxidising agent, and is a measure of the total amount of oxygen required to stabilise the waste.

6.2.2 *Domestic sewage*

In addition to human faecal waste, domestic sewage contains detergents, other household chemicals and waste from food preparation. The volume of domestic sewage produced is similar to the volume of water supplied to an area, and in the UK this is approximately 220 litres per person per day.

In the UK and Europe, most older communities have combined sewer systems, in which domestic sewage and surface runoff are conveyed in the

Table 6.1 Typical quality of domestic sewage.

	Raw*	Treated†	Overflow
Suspended solids (mg l^{-1})	426	5	200
BOD (mg l^{-1} O_2)	367	10	300
Ammonia (mg l^{-1} N)	39	7	30

*Tebbutt (1971).
†Severn-Trent Water (1988).

same pipe. During dry weather the sewage is treated before discharge to a watercourse, but during wet weather the volume of domestic sewage plus runoff can exceed the capacity of the sewers and the treatment works, and the mixture spills into rivers via combined sewer overflows. Overflows are generally designed to limit the maximum flow in the sewer to between six and 12 times the dry weather flow, so that they operate only infrequently. In practice, many poorly designed or overloaded combined systems spill domestic sewage at times of low flow. Combined sewer overflows are one of the major causes of river pollution in the UK.

Since 1950, the practice in the UK has been to sewer new developments with separate foul and surface weter sewers. Domestic sewage is conveyed in a separate pipe directly to a sewage works, where it receives treatment before discharge to a watercourse. Surface runoff is collected in a second pipe and generally discharged without treatment. Separate systems prevent the overflow of domestic sewage to rivers, but are more expensive to construct because of the need to provide two sets of sewers.

Domestic sewage therefore enters rivers in three forms:

(a) As effluent from treatment works.
(b) Diluted with runoff in wet weather from overflows.
(c) Undiluted from old or poorly designed systems.

Discharges of all three types can be controlled by better design and management of sewerage systems. Examples of the quality of these discharges are given in Table 6.1.

6.2.3 *Surface runoff*

Runoff from urban surfaces contains pollutants derived from atmospheric deposition, street refuse, traffic emissions, urban erosion, and road de-icing salts. Industrial site runoff can contain oils and toxic chemicals, and runoff from agricultural land can contain pesticides and fertilisers.

Measured runoff quality is extremely variable and is influenced by many factors. Table 6.2 gives typical ranges for pollutant concentrations in runoff from different sources.

Table 6.2 Pollutant concentrations in urban runoff.

	Highway runoff	Residential areas	Commercial areas	Industrial areas
Suspended solids (mg l^{-1})	28–1178	112–1104	230–1894	34–374
BOD (mg l^{-1} O_2)	12–32	7–56	5–17	8–12
COD (mg l^{-1} O_2)	128–171	37–120	74–160	40–70
Ammonia (mg l^{-1} N)	0.02–2.1	0.3–3.3	0.03–5.1	0.2–1.1
Lead	0.15–2.9	0.09–0.44	0.1–0.4	0.6–1.2

From Hall and Ellis (1985).

6.2.4 *Industrial and agricultural discharges and spillages*

Many industrial effluents are discharged, with consent, directly to sewers, where they can be treated with domestic sewage. At times of high flow, these effluents are spilled over combined sewer overflows. Industrial wastages can also enter rivers via sewerage systems following accidental spillage or deliberate illegal discharge.

Industrial effluent quality varies with the nature of the discharger's business and the degree of treatment provided prior to discharge. Highly polluting effluents include food-processing wastes, which are rich in organic matter and exert a high oxygen demand, and metal-finishing effluents, which contain toxic metals and cyanides. In some cases, discharge of spilled wastes to rivers may be preferable to attempting to treat them at a sewage treatment works, where they can cause disruption of the biological treatment process, thus adding domestic sewage to the works effluent.

Pollution from agricultural activities is increasing in developed countries, and the environmental impact is often more severe than in cases of sewage or industrial pollution. Milk pollution, for example, can be 700 times more harmful than raw sewage. Agricultural wastes can enter drainage systems as a result of poor farming practice, accidental spillage and discharges to sewers. The most common sources of pollutants are silage liquor, pesticides, farm slurry and agricultural chemicals.

6.2.5 *In-pipe deposits*

Deposits of sediments in sewers originate from domestic sewage, urban and rural runoff and industrial and agricultural wastes. Although not a primary source of pollutants, deposits provide a reservoir of pollutants in sewers which can be eroded during high flows and spilled into rivers via combined sewer overflows. The erosion of deposits from combined systems by rising flows is probably one of the prime causes of a first foul flush in which peak pollutant concentrations occur before the peak discharge (Figure 6.2). This can produce gross pollution even in modest storms. Sediment deposits can also

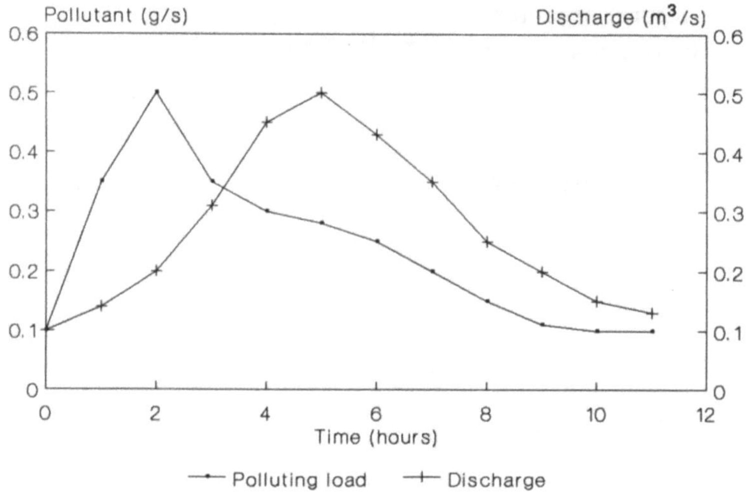

Figure 6.2 First foul flush in combined sewers.

affect the hydraulic capacity of sewers, thus causing premature overflow to rivers from combined systems.

In warm climates, hydrogen sulphide can be generated in sewers during anaerobic decay of organic matter. Research suggests that this takes place in sediment deposits, particularly in biofilms on pipe walls. Hydrogen sulphide is highly toxic and causes immediate fish kills if discharged to rivers, even at very low concentrations. Hydrogen sulphide can also combine with water in the sewer atmosphere to produce corrosive acids which attack the sewer fabric.

The problems of sediment in sewers can be reduced in new systems by designing them to be self-cleansing and by maintaining a minimum flow velocity often taken as 0.9–0.75 $m\,s^{-1}$ for small to large sewers (White, 1987). This requires provision of a sufficient gradient, or pumping, so that sediment does not have an opportunity to settle out. Some sediment accumulation is, however, inevitable and must be designed for.

6.3 Effects on receiving waters

Most domestic, industrial and agricultural effluents are eventually discharged, with or without treatment, into the sea or into freshwater lakes or rivers. Increased public awareness of environmental problems in most countries has led to legal controls on these discharges. The reduction of the effect of these discharges has therefore become of major importance.

All freshwater lakes and rivers can assimilate some wastes, which are stabilised by natural self-purification processes (Figure 6.3). Problems arise

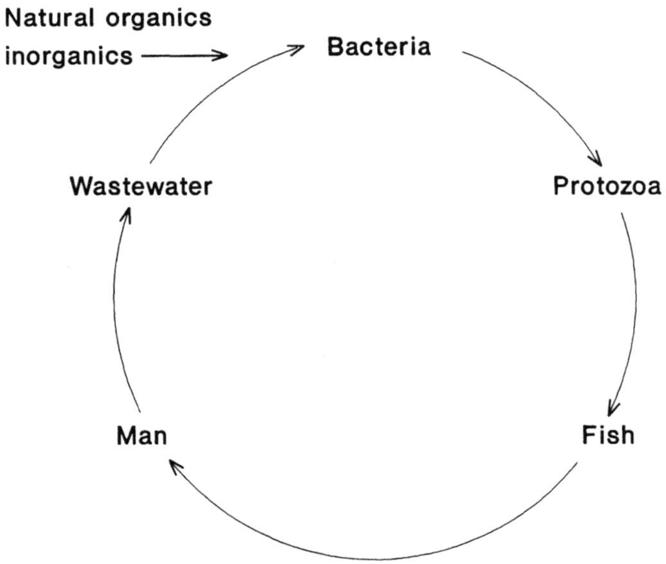

Figure 6.3 The natural self-purification cycle (after Tebbutt, 1987).

when pollutant loadings exceed the self-purification capacity of the receiving water, thus harming aquatic life and restricting the use of the water for supply and recreational purposes. The assimilative capacity for many toxic substances is very low. Water polluted by drainage discharges can create nuisances such as unpleasant odours, and can cause a direct hazard to health, particularly in tropical regions where water-borne diseases such as cholera and typhoid are prevalent.

Discharges are either continuous, such as those from sewage treatment works, or intermittent, such as those from combined sewer overflows and surface water outfalls. A high quality is probably required for continuous discharges as they exert a constant demand on the purification capabilities of the receiving water. Far less is known about the long-term effects of intermittent discharges, which are of variable quality, duration and frequency. The aim of good drainage design, in pollution terms, is to balance the effects of continuous and intermittent discharges against the assimilation capacity of the water, so as to optimise the quality of the receiving water.

6.3.1 *Sewage treatment works effluent*

The effects of domestic sewage pollution on river water quality are well documented elsewhere and will only be described briefly. The objective of sewage treatment is to reduce the pollution load to an acceptable level so that damage to the receiving water is minimal. The management of treatment works discharges must be considered in conjunction with other drainage discharges in the catchment, and with the assimilative capacity and environmental quality objectives of the receiving water.

The most serious effect of sewage effluent discharge is to reduce dissolved oxygen levels in the receiving water. Low dissolved oxygen concentrations injure or kill fish and other aquatic organisms, and hinder the natural self-purification process, thus eventually leading to severe pollution problems. Other important effects include nutrient accumulation, which is a problem in still and slow-flowing water, where it can result in prolific algal growths. The quality of treatment works effluent is usually assessed in terms of biochemical oxygen demand (BOD) and ammonia concentration. Ammonia also exerts an oxygen demand during purification as well as being toxic to aquatic organisms.

6.3.2 *Combined sewer overflows*

Discharges from combined sewer overflows can lower dissolved oxygen concentrations in the receiving water, have immediate toxic effects on aquatic life and cause aesthetic nuisance. They can also have a delayed, chronic effect, caused by high suspended solids loads, which settle in the receiving water where they can exert a bottom oxygen demand and act as a reservoir of toxic chemicals capable of being resuspended under high-flow conditions.

The effects of combined sewer discharges are difficult to quantify and regulate because of their intermittent nature. Their immediate impact can only be measured during a spill event, and their chronic effects are often difficult to isolate from other pollution inputs. Standards and performance criteria specifically for intermittent discharges are therefore needed to allow for these problems.

6.3.3 *Surface water discharges*

The effects of separate surface water discharges on water quality have recently received considerable attention, particularly in the US, where they have been the subject of a major national research programme. Although not as environmentally significant as combined sewer discharges, surface water discharges are likely to increase in comparative importance as a result of the reduction of pollution loads from combined sewers.

Runoff discharges to rivers can have physical, chemical and biological impacts, and again their intermittent nature makes them difficult to assess. However these discharges do have a measurable effect on the biological quality of the receiving water which can impair the use of a watercourse downstream of the outfall, particularly where water quality was initially high. Catchment land use is an important factor in determining the impact, with the most severe effects resulting from drainage of highway and industrial areas.

The problems of regulating surface water discharges are similar to those listed for combined sewer overflows. The current consensus of opinion in the UK, US and Europe is that surface water discharges should be controlled by a system of consents in conjunction with discharges from treatment works and combined sewer overflows.

6.4 Water quality standards and legislation

The legislation controlling water quality and drainage discharges varies significantly according to perceived priorities in the UK, the rest of Europe, the US and developing countries. This section outlines current practice in the US and Europe, where procedures are most highly developed, and explains the need for legislation appropriate to sewerage discharges.

6.4.1 *Legislation and practice in the UK and Europe*

Current practice in the UK is to discharge wastes to sewers and rivers by a system of consents. Under the Water Act of 1989, responsibility for the control of water pollution in territorial, coastal, inland and groundwaters has passed to the National Rivers Authority (NRA). The general approach is to determine objectives for the use of water from various sources, followed by an associated standard of quality for each objective. This is generally known as the environmental quality objective/environmental quality standard (EQO/EQS) approach. Thus waters designated for potable supply will have to meet more stringent quality standards than waters designated for industrial use, and this will be reflected in the strictness of discharge consents. The 1989 act has also provided a legal mechanism for the UK to implement EC directives on water quality (e.g. EEC, 1975, 1976).

Similar EQO/EQS practices are used in other European countries. At the moment, EC legislation has had little direct effect on drainage discharge standards because of the nature of directives, which generally address receiving water quality rather than discharge quality. Further EC directives are proposed, which will produce more uniform, possibly stricter, discharge criteria for member states. An exception to this is the recent directive requiring treatment of sewage before marine discharge.

Opinion differs on the approach which should be taken to setting and monitoring discharge consents. The procedures used for setting consents in the UK vary regionally. Some consider discharges in isolation, and others take account of the interaction of multiple discharges using catchment-based consent-setting models. The complexity of the procedures applied varies from simple mass balance techniques to mathematical models.

Some European countries, notably Denmark, already have some standards for intermittent pollution which include consideration of the time for which the discharge affects the water. It is necessary to use computational models to ensure that water quality objectives set in this form can be met. Bacteriological standards to protect against health risks are set out in EC directives for water to be used for water supply, and for bathing waters. These are being applied throughout Europe.

6.4.2 *Legislation and practice in the US*

The United States has had a programme to reduce the pollution from combined sewer overflows since 1967. In many states this problem has been overcome, although often at large expense by separating previously combined sewerage systems. Combined sewer overflows do still cause problems, but much of the official concern has moved to pollution from separate storm sewers, and to pollution from toxic substances.

The 1972 Clean Water Act introduced the requirement for discharge permits for industrial and foul sewage. The discharge consents were mostly based on the use of accepted process technology or on maximum levels of a range of pollutants. These controls were gradually extended to include large separate storm sewers with the final regulations introduced in 1988. The regulations require that stormwater discharges have a permit, and that to obtain this permit details of the quantity and quality of discharge must be provided. The constraints under which the discharges can continue can then be set in several ways. The first is by requiring an accepted technology, for example requiring primary sedimentation and high-rate biological filtration. The second is by setting maximum concentrations of specified pollutants. The third is by specifying a permitted environmental impact. The administrative burdens of this system are enormous, and there is still confusion over how to set permissible limits for intermittent discharges. An important part of the regulations is a requirement for the discharger to monitor and sample the discharge and to report the results of this to the Environmental Protection Agency. The discharger can be prosecuted for failure to comply based on this self-submitted evidence.

Disinfection of treated effluent and of storm overflow discharges is very common in the US. The 1972 Clean Water Act laid down limits on bacteria concentrations. This led to the universal use of disinfection, generally with chlorine. Since 1976 there has been a move away from this because of the polluting effects of residual chlorine. The requirements vary from state to state but generally require disinfection during the summer season. If chlorine is used then subsequent dechlorination is often required to reduce the residual chlorine level.

6.4.3 *Water quality standards in other countries*

Other countries either follow a similar approach to water quality standards to those defined above, or have no well-defined standards. The World Health

Organisation sets international standards for drinking water but has not set standards for effluent discharges.

6.5 Control of discharge quality

The pollution from drainage systems can be reduced by preventing pollutants from entering the drainage system or by reducing the pollutants discharged from the system by structural or non-structural means.

6.5.1 *Source control*

Domestic foul drainage is one of the fundamental purposes of urban drainage and it is not practical to control this source other than to discourage the discharge of pollutants such as motor oil.

Reducing the quantity of stormwater runoff by surface detention storage or infiltration areas will reduce the pollutant load. Care should be taken with infiltration that the polluted runoff cannot affect aquifers which are used for water supply. The pollutant load of the stormwater may be reduced by road sweeping. Research has generally indicated that road sweeping is effective at removing coarse particles, not the very fine particles which are the most polluting. Surface water generally enters the drainage system through gully pots or catchpits. These are effective at trapping coarse particles which would cause hydraulic obstruction and can also trap oil. However the breakdown of the sediment retained in gullies can provide a reservoir of polluted water to be washed out at the start of a storm to exacerbate the first foul flush. To be of any benefit gullies need to be cleaned regularly.

Industrial pollutants should be controlled at source by pretreatment before discharge into the sewerage system. Allowing them to be discharged into the system can not only cause pollution by the operation of overflows, but can also affect the operation of sewage treatment works.

6.5.2 *System separation*

Much of the pollution caused by drainage systems is the result of the operation of overflows on combined sewerage systems. One solution to this problem is to provide separate sewers for the foul flows and the relatively clean storm runoff. This is the preferred method of many countries, although the arguments in favour of separate systems are not conclusive because of problems of incorrect connections to the two systems. In the US it is now required to provide some form of treatment for storm runoff, so defeating the initial cost savings. Incorrect connections of storm water drains to the foul system also cause problems. The extra flow in the foul system then requires the provision of overflows. Keeping systems separate requires a continuous campaign of locating and removing incorrect connections.

6.5.3 *Storm overflows*

Any improvements to a combined system which reduce the volume of storm overflow discharges will reduce the pollutant discharge. However, improved design of overflow structures can provide even greater benefits. This will usually require the provision of a structure incorporating storage. There are two ways in which this can be used (Figure 6.4).

The first method is to *separate* pollutants from the flow by sedimentation in a stilling pond. This does not affect dissolved pollutants or those attached to fine sediment which is not easily settled. The overflow will generally be placed at the downstream end of the stilling pond so as to maximise use of the storage in the system upstream, so reducing the volume of storage which must be constructed. The overflow discharge therefore passes through the stored polluted water. The designs by Sharpe and Kirkbride (1959) have been widely used. A promising form of separation structure is the vortex or hydrodynamic separator, which can require less volume by forcing the flow to follow a spiral path through the separator.

The second method is to *detain* the flow during the period when it is most polluted, and discharge later flows. If the first foul flush is retained in the sewer, the subsequent flow can be spilled as it is cleaner. Unlike the separation structure the overflow will be at the upstream end of the storage. The overflow discharge does not pass through the stored polluted water and so the storage can be designed to encourage turbulent conditions to scour out sediment deposits. This is achieved by providing a drop from the incoming pipe to the floor level of the tank.

6.5.4 *Non-structural measures*

Sediment deposits which are washed out of combined sewers in storm conditions are a major source of pollution. These deposits are of two types. The first is consolidated deposits of mixed inorganic and organic material which are eroded only in large storms. This material will also cause an

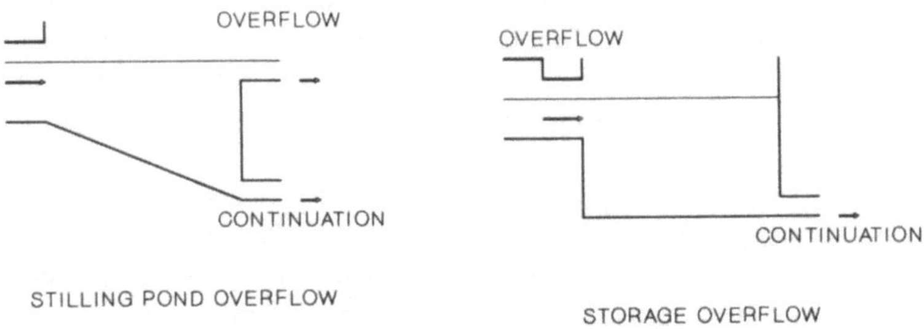

Figure 6.4 Operation of overflow structures.

obstruction to the flow. It can be removed by sewer cleaning using high-pressure water jetting or ploughing.

The second type of deposit contains more organic material and is unconsolidated. It is deposited during periods of dry-weather flow and eroded at the start of storm flows to form the first foul flush of pollutants. These deposits can be removed by flushing the sewers, either regularly using an automatic siphon or only when rain is forecast.

Control of the flows in the sewerage system in real time based on rainfall and flow measurements can make the best use of system capacity and storage. The first effect is to reduce the volume of overflow, but by controlling the detention of the first foul flush it can also reduce pollutant loads while still allowing overflow.

Chemical dosing with coagulants, usually aluminium sulphate, can improve the separation efficiency of stilling pond or hydrodynamic separator overflows. This technique has also been used in the US for separate stormwater discharged to detention ponds, where the small amount of sediment produced is not removed from the pond.

6.6 Modelling approaches

A model is a representation of a real system which can be used to investigate the operation of the system under a variety of existing or planned conditions. There are several choices which have to be taken to decide on the type of model to be used.

6.6.1 *Deterministic or stochastic models*

There are two modelling techniques which can be used to represent the behaviour of a system. These are:

Stochastic models.
Deterministic models.

A stochastic, or 'black box', model predicts the output from a system (flow, pollutants) caused by a certain input (rainfall) without describing why that input produces that output. Stochastic models are simple and quick, but need a large amount of data for calibration. They may not be able to represent the changes in output caused by changes to the system, such as the construction of new capital works.

A deterministic model represents the physical processes occurring in the system to determine the output from the system. Deterministic models are more complex and slower but need less calibration. They are able to represent the changes in output caused by changes to the system.

In practice, all drainage models are partly stochastic because of lack of knowledge of the processes taking place, and also because some of the processes are random. For example, the polluting load washed off a catchment surface could change drastically if a dog knocked over a dustbin. Some water quality models are completely stochastic.

Stochastic water quality models are justified on the grounds of their simplicity and because the processes involved are dominated by random components so that determinism will not improve the accuracy. Deterministic models are justified on the grounds that they are able to model the effects of changes or improvements to a system. This is particularly important for urban drainage systems where major capital works may be carried out. It is less important for receiving waters, although the processes in these can be changed by changing the discharges to them.

6.6.2 *Dynamic or steady-state models*

Most drainage processes are dynamic, that is they vary with time, as they are driven by rainfall. It is therefore usually necessary to use a dynamic model to study the change in conditions during a storm. For urban drainage systems the conditions change very rapidly, and a calculation timestep much shorter than 1 minute would normally be used. For sewage treatment and river models conditions change more slowly, and timesteps of several minutes or 1 hour can be used. It may even be possible to use a steady-state model in certain conditions.

6.6.3 *Design or simulation models*

Models can be used either to design a system to meet certain defined conditions (a design model) or to show the conditions which will occur in a defined system (a simulation model). For complex systems such as drainage water quality models, it is usual to use a simulation model. The model is not able to design improvements to the system; this is done iteratively by the user by analysing the system, incorporating proposed changes and seeing the effect which they have. The proposals can then be modified until the desired effect is achieved.

6.6.4 *Use of models*

Before starting to model water quality it is necessary to model the hydraulics of the flow (see Chapter 7). The type of hydraulic model will depend on the type of system being modelled. The hydraulic and water quality models do not have to be of the same type. For example, a river model for intermittent pollutant discharge could use a steady-state deterministic model of the hydraulics with a dynamic stochastic model of the water quality. There is a strong interaction between different parts of the drainage system requiring a range of models. For example, reducing the pollution load to rivers from overflows will necessarily result in an increased load on the treatment works, and therefore a possible reduction in effluent quality. It is therefore necessary to model three parts of the system: the sewerage system, to predict the overflow discharge and the flow to treatment; the treatment works, to assess its response to varying inflow rates; and the receiving water to assess its response to different patterns of overflow and treatment works discharge. These will generally be modelled separately and then linked together.

6.6.5 *Types of results*

The results of a water quality model can be expressed in several ways.

(1) As a total polluting load discharged for a given storm, or, by analysing a series of storms, the likely polluting load discharged in a year. The loads can be divided by the storm durations to give average concentrations.
(2) As the variation in pollutant concentration with time during a storm, a 'pollutograph'.
(3) A statistical treatment of the pollutograph results of a series of storms to provide the concentrations which are exceeded for defined percentages of the time. These are used for comparison with environmental standards, which are frequently expressed in this form.

6.7 Urban drainage water quality models

6.7.1 *Sewerage quality models*

There are two types of water quality process occurring in sewerage systems. The first is the transport of pollutants through the system by the flow. The pollutants are largely unchanged during this transport. The second process is the slow build-up and biochemical degradation of pollutants on the catchment surface, in gully pots or catchpits, and in sediment deposits in the sewers. The pollutant load for any storm therefore depends on the antecedent dry weather period as well as on the characteristics of the storm. The storms which cause overflow from combined sewerage systems, or significant discharge from separate systems, are much smaller than those analysed for the hydraulic design of systems for the prevention of flooding. The models will therefore be used with small recorded rainstorms rather than the large synthetic storms used for hydraulic design.

The pollutants to be considered in a sewerage model may include the following:

Sediment, possibly several different sizes and densities.
Oxygen demand (either as BOD or COD).

Ammonia.
Hydrogen sulphide.
Toxic pollutants, for example metals, pesticides, phenols, etc.

The pollutants can exist in both the dissolved phase and attached to the sediment particles. More complex models will treat each of these phases separately, as their behaviour is very different. The pollutants can be assumed not to decay during their transport through the system in storm conditions.

6.7.2 *Stochastic sewerage quality models*

Stochastic models are useful for identifying the scale of the problem caused by pollutants discharged from an urban drainage system, or for identifying the types of storms under which these problems will occur. However, as described in section 6.6, they have only limited ability to consider the effects of changes to the system. A stochastic model can include the length of the antecedent dry weather period as one of the parameters used to predict the pollutant load. It then requires calibration data from storms with different antecedent conditions.

6.7.3 *Deterministic sewerage quality models*

Deterministic models are required to consider the effects of changes in the system. They would use a dynamic solution for the pollutant transport during the storm event. The same solution could be used during the inter-event dry period to give a continuous simulation model. However, as the dynamic model would use a short timestep, typically much less than 1 minute, the computational effort involved in continuous simulation would be very large. A steady-state model or a stochastic model could therefore be used instead for the dry weather periods between events.

The sources of pollutants described in section 6.2 must be included, in particular the inflow of foul sewage, the pollutants stored in pipe sediments and pollutant washoff from the catchment surface. The foul flow will be based on measured inflows. The surface washoff model will be a partly deterministic model which calculates the eroding force of the raindrop impact and the flow across the catchment surface, but then is calibrated to relate this to the amount of sediment and dissolved pollutant washed off the surface.

The pollutants must then be transported through the sewerage system. The dominant process here is advection, where the pollutants travel at the same speed as the flow. The advection equation can be written as:

$$\frac{\delta c}{\delta t} = -U\frac{\delta c}{\delta x} \tag{6.1}$$

where x is the distance downstream, t is time, c is the concentration of pollutant and U is velocity of flow.

The equation can be solved by one of several explicit or implicit finite difference methods (see Chapter 7). Because of the importance of pollutants attached to sediment, especially in first foul flush, it is important to include a model of sediment erosion, transport and deposition. For fine organic sediment, a simple limiting shear stress model can be used, so that the sediment is transported when the critical shear stress is exceeded by the flow. For coarse sediment a model which considers the transport capacity of the flow, such as the Ackers and White (1973) equation, should be used.

6.7.4 *Sewage treatment works models*

For combined sewerage systems there is an interaction between the operation of the sewerage system and the sewage treatment works. Treatment works frequently include storm tanks to handle flows in excess of that which can be treated. The flows into the storm tanks can change very quickly with time, and it is therefore easier to include these as part of the model of the sewerage system.

The remaining flow to the treatment works is also affected by storm flows, although this may only be important in long storms. A dynamic model of a full treatment works would be an advantage to allow for this situation, and attempts are being made to develop such models.

6.8 River water quality models

The problems of modelling the effects of polluting discharges on rivers are different from those of modelling their transport through an urban drainage system. The main differences stem from the slower rate of change in conditions and the longer time scales and distances that need to be considered.

Flow velocities in rivers are generally lower than in urban systems, and there is more stratification of flows both vertically and horizontally. Because of this, dispersion, where the pollutants are spread throughout the flow along the length of the river, is as important as their advection at the velocity of the flow. Introducing dispersion into the transport equation gives:

$$\frac{\delta c}{\delta t} = -U\frac{\delta c}{\delta x} + D\frac{\delta^2 c}{\delta x^2} \tag{6.2}$$

where D is the dispersion coefficient.

The dispersion is not simply a process of molecular diffusion but is also the result of turbulent mixing as a result of large-scale eddies and pollutants being left in dead zones of slowly moving water at bends and between obstructions. The effect is therefore dependent on the course of the river, and also on the river level and flow velocity. It is therefore difficult to predict the appropriate value of dispersion coefficient to include in the model, and some calibration data are generally required. These are best obtained by measuring the dilution of a slug of salt solution introduced into the flow. The advection–dispersion equation can be solved by similar techniques to those for the advection equation.

The details of sediment transport are also different from urban drainage systems. Because of the slower flow velocity, much of the sediment discharged from storm overflows will be deposited close to the overflow. This sediment will be polluted, and its subsequent behaviour if eroded by future storm flows is important. Coarse sediment is of less concern: partly because it is generally less polluting than the fine organic sediment but also because most of this sediment should be retained in the sewerage system.

The largest difference between water quality models for urban drainage and for rivers is that it is necessary to model the self-purification ability of the river in reducing the pollutant concentration. If this was ignored then a simple mixing and dilution model would allow the concentration of pollutants to be calculated at any point downstream of the polluting discharge. Such models are in use, and for some toxic substances which are not broken down this may be sufficient. However, even these substances will be absorbed into the sediments and the plant and animal life along the river. A dilution and fate model is therefore needed to include these processes. As described in section 6.3, the most common effect of pollutants from sewerage systems is in reducing the oxygen levels in the river by requiring oxygen for purification. This is balanced by the reaeration of the water from the atmosphere, through the water surface and at weirs and other structures which cause turbulent flow. This leads to the typical 'oxygen sag curves' (Figure 6.5). The rate of uptake of oxygen by the pollutants is dependent on the source of the pollutants, and the rate of reaeration is dependent on the characteristics of

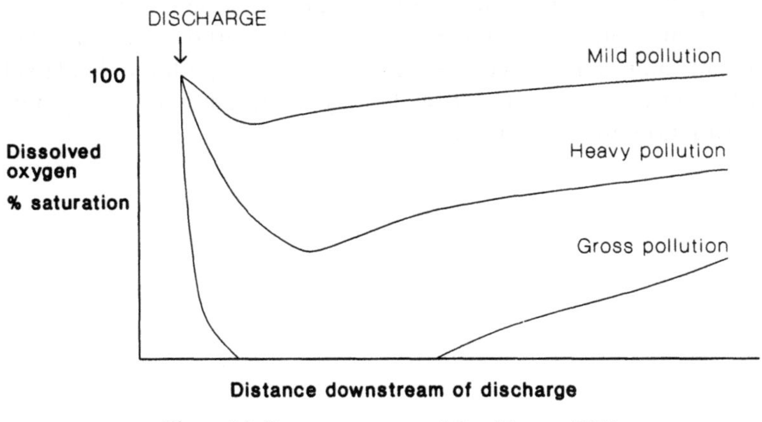

Figure 6.5 Oxygen sag curves (after Mason, 1981).

the river and the flow velocity. It is therefore necessary to calibrate these factors for different situations.

The advection–dispersion equation is then modified with a decay term to represent the reduction of BOD oxidation:

$$\frac{\delta c}{\delta t} = -U\frac{\delta c}{\delta x} + D\frac{\delta^2 c}{\delta x^2} - Kc \tag{6.3}$$

where K is the BOD rate coefficient.

A similar equation can then be applied to the concentration of dissolved oxygen (DO) by including a term for the reaeration from the atmosphere:

$$\frac{\delta c}{\delta t} = -U\frac{\delta c}{\delta x} + D\frac{\delta^2 c}{\delta x^2} - Kc + R(c_s - c) \tag{6.4}$$

where c_s is the saturated DO concentration and R is the reaeration coefficient.

The two equations need to be solved together to determine the oxygen sag curve. The reaeration coefficient depends on the velocity and depth of flow, and on the presence of weirs and other sources of turbulence.

The processes of oxygen demand are made considerably more complex by the effect of photosynthesis in plants and algae in the river. These will produce oxygen by photosynthesis during daylight, and will utilise oxygen for respiration during the night. Both the photosynthesis and respiration are temperature-dependent and seasonal. They are also dependent on the characteristics of the river, and on the background level of pollutants and nutrients, particularly nitrogen and phosphorus. The discharges from sewage treatment works and storm overflows contain a significant nutrient load, and this alone may be sufficient to cause low oxygen levels. The change in oxygen levels between day and night can be of the same order as the oxygen sag caused by pollutant discharges. For continuous discharges the worst case is given at night during summer when the respiration will be greatest, and when the pollutants will be more concentrated because of low flows in the river. For intermittent discharges from storm overflows the situation is considerably more complex because of the variation in pollutant load likely to be discharged at different times of the day. Procedures for analysing this type of situation are still being determined.

7 River systems

J. ELLIS

7.1 Introduction

Drainage systems for both urban and rural catchments often discharge into rivers or into lakes or reservoirs within river systems, and drainage in these catchments may be controlled by the conditions in the rivers; conversely, the rivers must themselves be designed and maintained to accept all the waters emptied into them both safely and economically. Thus, in drainage, river flows are important both directly and indirectly.

River flows are predominantly determined by the natural events of rainfall and snowmelt. The passage of these flows through networks of river channels poses the engineer with the problems of determining the resultant flow rates and water levels. In some instances where the variations of flow with time are relatively gradual, approximate steady-flow analysis techniques may offer a simple means of estimating water surface conditions. However, in general, time-dependent variations of flow conditions require to be studied in more detail in order to predict the movement of a flood wave through a network of river channels. The need to consider acceleration gradients becomes increasingly important with floods which rise swiftly or where man-made controls such as gates are used to regulate discharges. In such cases the potential for important accelerations cannot be overlooked. The problems of tracing the movement and related changes in the form and height of a wave are central to the work of the engineer engaged in studying river systems. The engineer must possess the ability to predict the effect on flood propagation of any changes, both natural and man-made, which may occur to the river channel.

7.2 Computer applications

The emergence of the modern digital computer has opened a new chapter in the history of hydraulics. A new and powerful means has been made available by which traditional problems may be solved. It has also revealed the existence of both new and previously overlooked hydraulics problems. A new discipline of computational hydraulics has emerged. Among the first of the hydraulics problems to attract the attention of both scientists and engineers using computer techniques was a range of unsteady or time-varying flow problems including flood routing.

7.3 Choice of numerical models

Since the introduction of these computational methods a range of numerical techniques has been tried and tested, and at the present time certain methods have become relatively well established. In carrying out any study of river systems there is considerable choice of method. It is possible to employ simpler methods in some circumstances and to provide a range of models which are each applicable to a limited range of circumstances. Examples of simpler methods are to be found in the kinematic or hydrological routing methods (Chow, 1950, pp. 604–613). One of the most popular of these is the Muskingum technique. The alternative to this range of restricted application models is to retain a model which has the capability of handling a wide range of flow conditions and river network configurations.

7.4 Essential attributes of a useable river model

In selecting or developing a worthwhile numerical model for flood routing purposes, the following are some of the essential qualities which the model should possess:

Ability to simulate, with little numerical distortion of the flood, a wide range of flow conditions in irregular or natural channels.

Ability to allow schematisation of a diversity of both straightforward and more complicated channel conditions, for example networks of branching channels, constrictions such as bridge crossings, weirs and other potential control sections and overbank flows.

Ability to provide accurate results using a computationally stable convergent numerical scheme.

Computational efficiency.

7.5 Equations of one-dimensional unsteady open-channel flow

The dynamic and continuity equations describing unsteady flow with a free surface in the nearly horizontal plane can be written in a number of forms. With reference to Figure 7.1 the continuity equation can be written as:

$$B\frac{\partial h}{\partial t}+\frac{\partial Q}{\partial x}-q=0 \tag{7.1}$$

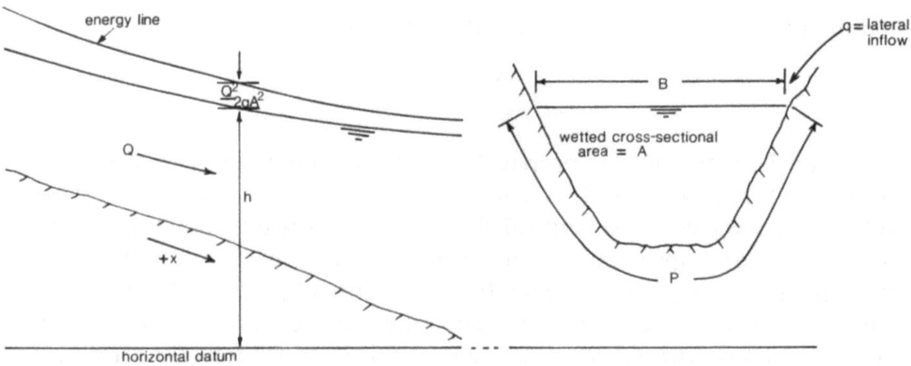

Figure 7.1 Definition sketch for derivation of equations of one-dimensional unsteady open-channel flow.

$$\frac{\partial Q}{\partial t}+\frac{Q}{A}\frac{\partial Q}{\partial x}+Q\frac{\partial(Q/A)}{\partial x}+gA\frac{\partial h}{\partial x}+\frac{k^{1/3}}{8.41^2A^2R^{4/3}}Q|Q|=0 \qquad (7.2)$$

where A is the wetted cross-sectional area at a channel section, B is the top width of wetted channel section, g is the gravitational acceleration, h is the water surface level at a section, k is the equivalent roughness height, P is the wetted perimeter of cross-section, Q is the discharge at a cross-section, q is the lateral inflow, t is time, x is the distance along channel axis and $R = A/P$ is the hydraulic radius of wetted cross-section.

7.6 Characteristic equations of one-dimensional unsteady open-channel flow

Before considering numerical methods it is instructive to examine the characteristic or ordinary differential equations which can be obtained from the partial differential equations 7.1 and 7.2 above. The characteristic equations may be obtained by means of several mathematical techniques, and the reader is referred to works by Abbott (1966) and Henderson (1966) for details of the derivation of the characteristic equations. These ordinary differential equations may be written as;

$$v \pm 2c = {}^{+}_{-}I \qquad (7.3)$$

where v is the mean velocity at a cross-section, $c = \sqrt{(gy)}$ is the celerity at a cross-section, $y = A/B$ is the mean depth at a cross-section and ${}^{+}_{-}I$ is 'quasi-invariant', that is its value changes gradually under the influence of friction or gradient.

Equation 7.3 applies along the paths defined by:

$$\frac{dx}{dt} = v \pm c \tag{7.4}$$

Equation 7.4 represents the propagation paths of infinitesimal wavelets. The wave front can be viewed as composed of an infinite number of these infinitesimal waves. In subcritical flow ($v/c < 1.0$) waves can travel both downstream and upstream, but in supercritical flow ($v/c > 1.0$) both sets of wave paths are swept downstream. In the majority of practical flood routing cases flow will generally lie in the subcritical range, except locally below control sections, where there may be a relatively short stretch of supercritical flow. Solutions for unknown velocity and depth of flow can be found where characteristics travelling in opposing directions cross (Figure 7.2). From an initial set of representative wave paths a set of intersection points can be obtained tracing the movement of waves in the channel. Typically this process will result in an irregular set of paths with solutions for the dependent variables of velocity and water depth at each intersection point. While this 'characteristic grid' method has been recognised as a benchmark against which other techniques may be measured when the full dynamic equation 7.2 is required (Wylie, 1980), for most practical purposes this approach becomes very unwieldy, particularly where irregular branched channels and other internal features are to be modelled. The vast majority of computational

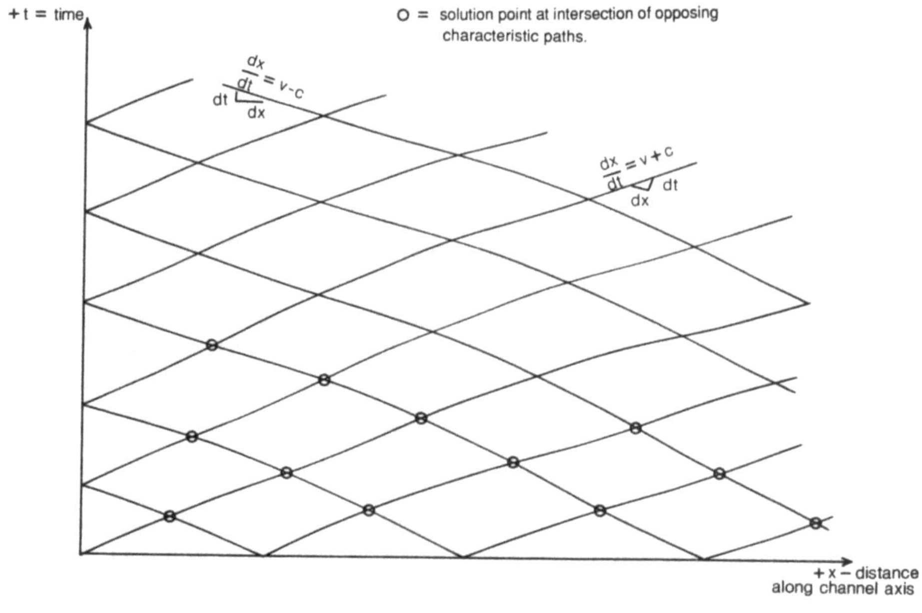

Figure 7.2 Characteristic mesh in the x–t plane resulting from selection of an initial set of paths.

schemes for flood routing are based on eqns 7.1 and 7.2 rather than on the characteristic eqns 7.3 and 7.4.

7.7 Boundary conditions for computations

Irrespective of the precise nature of the computational scheme adopted for simulation of flow conditions within a river network, it is necessary to input boundary conditions to the computer model. Commonly, at upstream or inflow boundaries of the system, values of changing flow rate, i.e. the inflow hydrograph, are specified with time over the flood event. Likewise, at tributary streams hydrographs will be required. Also, where drainage flows are entering the system along its length, values of inflow per unit length of channel axis, q of eqn 7.1, are required as a function of time. It should be noted that lateral inflow or outflow may arise from flow entering or leaving flood plains, and this topic will be discussed later in the chapter. At downstream limits of the system the boundary condition may take several different forms. Where a unique relationship exists between flow rate and water level, a rating curve may be employed at the downstream limit of a channel. An extreme form of this type of boundary occurs at entry to a very large reservoir whose water level does not rise significantly over the duration of a flood event. In this case a single value of water level applies for all downstream flow values. On the other hand, if, for example, the downstream boundary of a stream is sited upstream of a confluence with another river and yet lies within the region influenced by backwater effects from the confluence with this second river, then the boundary condition at the downstream limit of the model will no longer be uniquely determined by the model flow at this boundary but will also be a function of changing flow conditions within the second river. In cases such as this, or where the river enters a tidal estuary, the boundary condition may take the form of a time-dependent set of water level values which include the effects of a number of influences from downstream.

7.8 Factors influencing the computational mesh

Practical computational schemes for both steady and unsteady water surface profile computations employ a set of fixed sections, which are sited throughout the river system, and at which solutions for flow rate and water level are evaluated. From a practical viewpoint it is necessary to represent in the numerical model all important channel features and cross-sectional shapes. The siting of computational cross-sections will therefore be governed by the location of weirs, bridge constrictions, confluences and other features which require to be represented. The computational scheme should thus allow complete freedom in locating these cross-sections and should not be unduly dictated by the requirement to satisfy any numerical stability or other consideration.

In developed countries, particularly in urban areas which were centres of activity during the industrial revolution and subsequently, there are large numbers of bridge crossings, weirs and other man-made geometrical changes of river channels which require to be modelled. These are often in close proximity to one another. The longitudinal density of the representative cross-sections used to model such systems can thus become high in comparison with more rural areas, where the need for close spacing of sections is not so great.

Flood waves, by contrast, tend in the main to be relatively long, with a period of rise and fall extending over many hours or days. Exceptions to this do occur, particularly where gates are operated to regulate river discharges. In the interests of computational efficiency it is desirable to employ a timestep or increment in flood routing computations which reflects the rate at which flow conditions change within the model. Thus time increments of many minutes or longer are relatively commonplace. Depending on the relative magnitudes of cross-sectional spacing, Δx, and timestep, Δt, several different types of computational schemes may be identified. The characteristic paths represented by eqn 7.4 are helpful in this regard (Figure 7.3).

In Figure 7.3(a and b) are depicted cases in which the quotient $\Delta x/\Delta t > v \pm c$ and the solutions at the intersection point, A, of the opposing characteristic paths are determined by conditions within the adjacent reaches of channel. In the case of the scheme illustrated in Figure 7.3(a), conditions over the channel length BC are used to establish conditions at point A, whereas in Figure 7.3(b) conditions along the earlier segments, BD and CE, are employed in solving for conditions at A. Wylie (1980) has proposed the scheme represented by Figure 7.3(b) as a means of avoiding inaccuracies in the characteristic method. Both of these schemes are *explicit* in that the solution at point A is uniquely determined by previously known conditions at an earlier time or times and is not dependent on the concurrent solutions at adjacent points. As the time increment is increased and $\Delta x/\Delta t < v \pm c$, explicit schemes may still be employed. The characteristic paths (Figure 7.3c) extend beyond the adjacent channel reaches and intersect the previous solution line on further-removed reaches. This approach was proposed by Vardy (1976); it involves the use of known conditions along channel reaches further removed from the solution point and has some appeal in certain areas of application in flood routing computations. When a large time increment is used such that $\Delta x/\Delta t < v \pm c$, the more usual approach is to allow the characteristic paths to intersect the neighbouring $x = \text{constant}$ lines, FB and GC (Figure 7.3d). This method, while allowing relatively large time increments to be employed, carries the penalty that the solution at A becomes dependent on the concurrent solutions at points F and G and vice versa, i.e. the solution becomes *implicit*. In contrast to the explicit technique in which solutions at

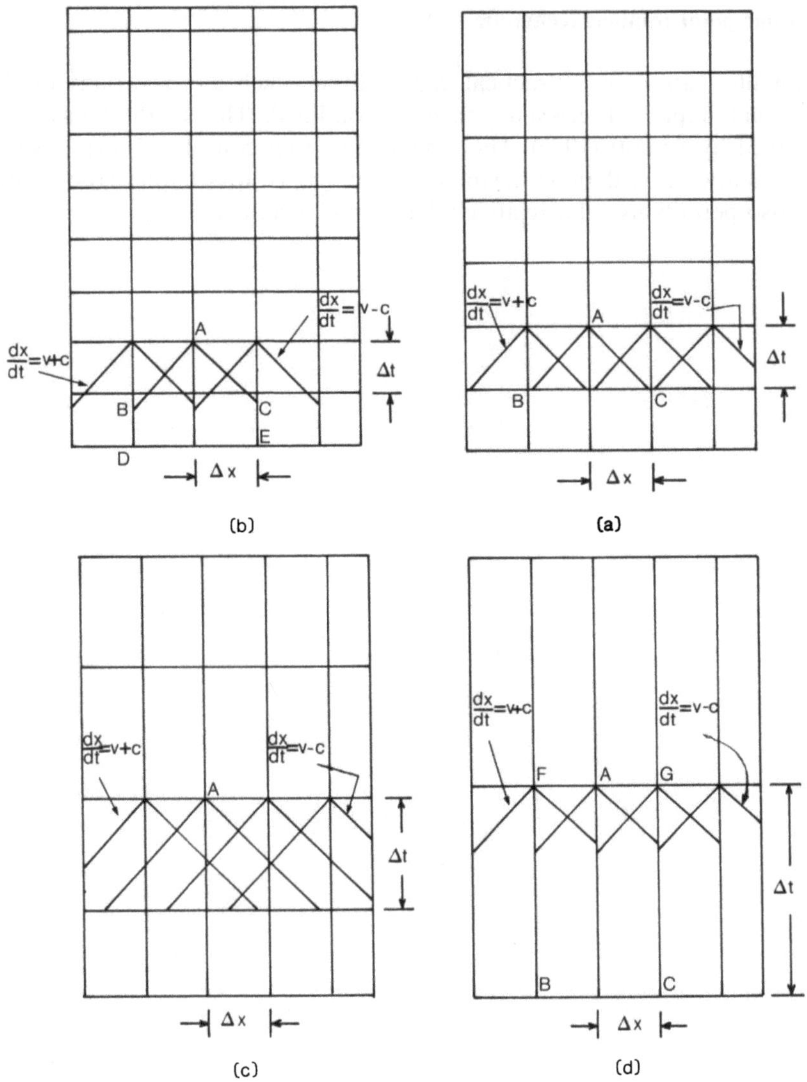

Figure 7.3 Alternative fixed-mesh computational schemes.

each point can be obtained independently, in the implicit techniques solutions are obtained at all computational sections through simultaneous solution of the equations at all points in the network. The advantage of the implicit approach is that relatively large time increments can be used while preserving the freedom to choose the location of cross-sections in the channel. Implicit methods have proved increasingly popular for flood routing applications and are currently in use in many investigations throughout the world.

7.9 Four-point implicit technique

As an illustration of a practical computational scheme a variant of the four-point implicit Preissman scheme is outlined. This method has been described by Abbott (1979). The scheme has been considered attractive in that it allows considerable flexibility in the choice of section arrangement and also permits use of a relatively large time increment.

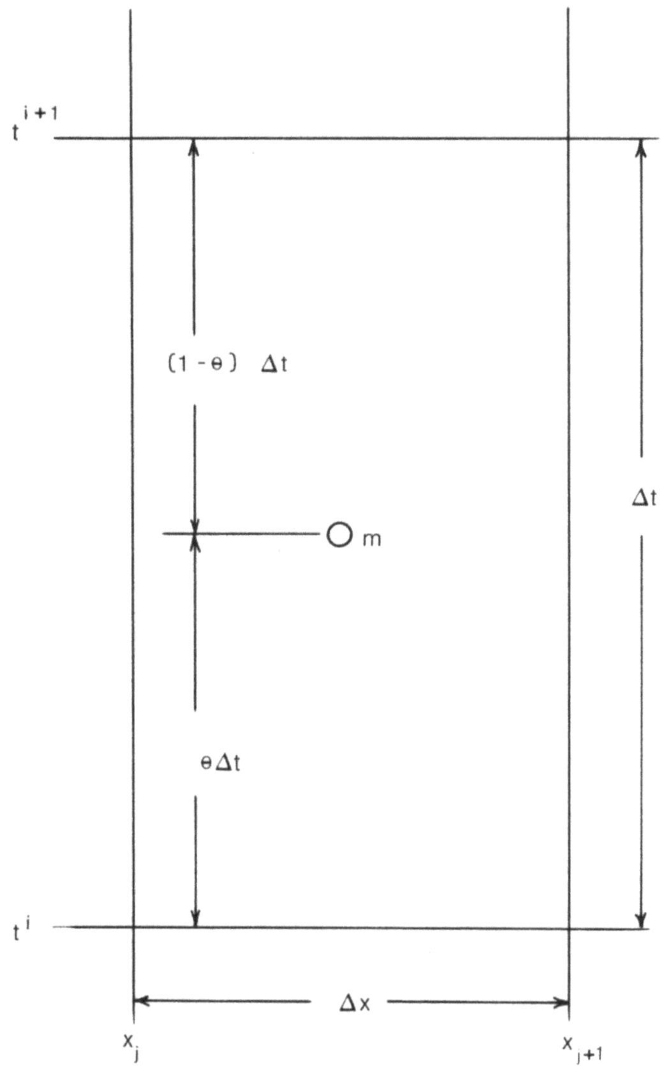

Figure 7.4 Arrangement of four-point implicit scheme.

Solutions are obtained for flow rate and water level at all points of a grid covering the axial distance x, time t, domain (Figure 7.4). For the four-point grid defined by the intersection of the vertical lines x_j and x_{j+1} with the horizontal lines t^i and t^{i+1}, eqns 7.1 and 7.2 are written in finite difference form. At a point m (Figure 7.4) average values and derivatives of any variable j can be written as:

$$f(m) = \frac{(1-\theta)}{2}(f_j^i + f_{j+1}^i) + \frac{\theta}{2}(f_j^{i+1} + f_{j+1}^{i+1}) \tag{7.5}$$

$$\frac{\partial f(m)}{\partial x} = \frac{1}{\Delta x}(1-\theta)(f_{j+1}^i - f_j^i) + \theta(f_{j+1}^{i+1} - f_j^{i+1}) \tag{7.6}$$

and

$$\frac{\partial f(m)}{\partial t} = \frac{1}{2\Delta t}[(f_j^{i+1} + f_{j+1}^{i+1}) - (f_j^i + f_{j+1}^i)] \tag{7.7}$$

where θ is a weighting factor, usually in the range $0.5 < \theta < 1.0$.

Equations 7.1 and 7.2 may now be written in finite difference form. Leaving aside the lateral inflow/outflow term q and the resistance term, eqns 7.1 and 7.2 can be written in the form:

$$\frac{B_j^i}{2\Delta t}(h_j^{i+1} - h_j^i) + \frac{B_{j+1}^i}{2\Delta t}(h_{j+1}^{i+1} - h_{j+1}^i) + \frac{1}{2\Delta x}(Q_{j+1}^{i+1} - Q_j^{i+1}) + \frac{1}{2\Delta x}(Q_{j+1}^i - Q_j^i) = 0 \tag{7.8}$$

and

$$\frac{1}{2g\Delta t}\left(\frac{Q_j^{i+1}}{A_j^i} - \frac{Q_j^i}{A_j^i} + \frac{Q_{j+1}^{i+1}}{A_{j+1}^i} - \frac{Q_{j+1}^i}{A_{j+1}^i}\right) + \frac{\theta}{\Delta x}(h_{j+1}^{i+1} - h_j^{i+1}) + \frac{(1-\theta)}{\Delta x}(h_{j+1}^i - h_j^i) + \frac{\theta}{2g\Delta x}\left[\frac{Q_{j+1}^{i+1}Q_{j+1}^i}{(A_{j+1}^i)^2} - \frac{Q_j^{i+1}Q_j^i}{(A_j^i)^2}\right] + \frac{(1-\theta)}{2g\Delta x}\left[\frac{(Q_{j+1}^i)^2}{(A_{j+1}^i)^2} - \frac{(Q_j^i)^2}{(A_j^i)^2}\right] = 0 \tag{7.9}$$

for the continuity and dynamic equations respectively.

Equations 7.8 and 7.9 form a pair of simultaneous equations for the two unknowns Q and h at the cross-sections bounding the reach of channel. If there are $(n-1)$ reaches, i.e. n sections, in a stretch of channel between upstream and downstream boundaries, then there will be a total of $2n$ unknowns at any time. For each of the $(n-1)$ reaches in the channel stretch there will be two equations of the form of eqns 7.8 and 7.9, giving a total of $2(n-1)$ equations. At each of the boundaries a further relationship will be available. As already mentioned, this may either take the form of an explicit value of one of the dependent variables on the boundary such as flow rate Q at the upstream boundary, or it may take the form of an equation relating the dependent variables on the boundary, such as a rating curve at the downstream boundary. By including these boundary conditions sufficient equations are thus available to allow solution of the $2n$ simultaneous equations. These equations may be solved using a Gaussian elimination technique or a more modern method (Roache, 1972). Having obtained a set of solutions at the latest time t^{i+1}, the solution can then be advanced by a further time increment, and so on until the entire flood event has been computed.

Usually the starting point of a computer run will be a steady-flow profile obtained from backwater analysis calculations using a simpler model. There will arise cases where successive flood events are to be studied, and it is then possible to use the predictions from an earlier computer flood simulation as the initial condition for commencing the latest simulation.

7.10 Representing head losses in open-channel flow

Representing the term for channel resistance to flow in the dynamic eqn 7.2 raises a number of important issues of both a hydraulic and also a numerical nature.

7.10.1 *Assessment of the equivalent roughness height,* k

The equivalent roughness height, k, is required to encompass a wide range of factors influencing head loss in open channels. Its assessment must take into account such varied aspects as: resistance to flow over the channel bed and sides given the non-uniform bed material; the influence of minor irregularities and changes of channel section; obstructions in the section, such as fences, fallen trees, etc., which intrude into the wetted section; plant growth within the cross-section; and also the influence of channel meandering. Chow (1950, pp. 94–123) gives data which allow a preliminary estimate of roughness coefficient to be made and which include the influences mentioned above. It should be remembered that the relative importance of some of these effects is dependent on the stage or water level in the cross-section. At low water levels the influence of minor channel irregularities will be of greater importance than at higher stages. Conversely, as the water level rises the likelihood of trees, fences and other obstructions influencing the flow will tend to increase.

It is important to be able to isolate the different factors influencing channel resistance, particularly if the objective of a study is channel improvement, which may involve straightening, improvement of section shape and so forth. Unless the significance of each alteration to the channel is understood, it becomes more difficult to predict the changes which will occur in the roughness coefficient, which represents the overall resistance to flow, and how this value will vary with stage in the river. Recently the topic of head losses has received considerable attention in an attempt to quantify certain aspects of energy loss more clearly.

7.10.2 *Losses at bends and meanders*

In the case of meanders and channel bends generally, secondary currents or large-scale turbulent eddies occupying most of the cross-section are responsible for energy losses as a result of internal fluid friction and also transverse shear forces (Ervine and Ellis, 1987). Methods of quantifying these effects have been proposed by Kikkawa *et al.* (1976) and in a simplified form by Chang (1983). Interaction between different aspects of head loss can occur. At bends or meanders the appearance of a deep pool on the outside of each bend is commonplace, with deposition of material at other points on the inside of the bend (Morisawa, 1985). Thus there is a connection between the presence of a channel bend and the development of irregularities of cross-sectional shape. Both of these play a part in determining the overall resistance to flow in the channel.

7.10.3 *Resistance with overbank flows*

When water levels exceed the bank-full level in the main river channel section, parts of the flood plain are inundated by the rising waters. Typically these flood plains will have quite different characteristics of roughness and bed form. Also there will be a tendency for some development to have taken place, with walls, fences and other structures occurring, and hedges, orchards and other plantations being present. All of these contribute to resistance to flow across the flood plain. The depth of flow on the flood plain and also the hydraulic radius of this part of the system will be much less than in the river channel, and careful consideration must be given to how best to represent this compound cross-section.

A simple illustration will demonstrate one of the pitfalls which await the inexperienced investigator. Consider the case of a straight river channel with a flat expanse of flood plain (Figure 7.5). For simplicity, assume that the roughness heights of the channel and the flood plain are the same. Up until the bank-full stage, conveyance of the cross-section is computed on the basis of the channel only, giving the portion of conveyance curve AB (Figure 7.5). At a stage marginally above bank-full the wetted perimeter is greatly increased while the flow area is only marginally greater. The result is an abrupt reduction in hydraulic radius and a corresponding apparent reduction in conveyance, point C (Figure 7.5). Computations based upon such a simple approach would not be satisfactory, and, in the course of model calibration

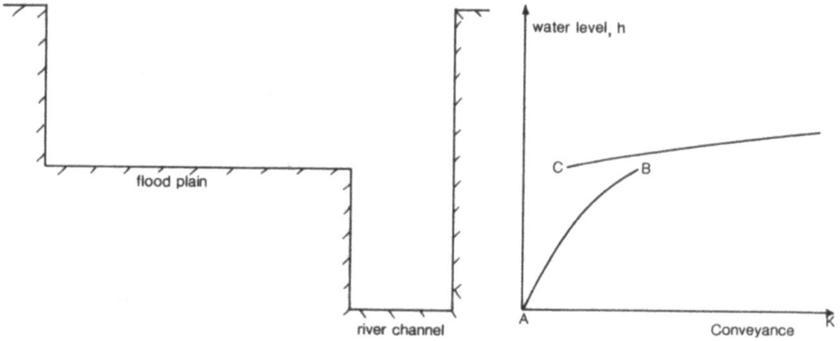

Figure 7.5 Conveyance as a function of water level for a compound channel of idealised shape.

using field observations of water surface profile just above the bank-full stage, the engineer might be tempted to reduce the roughness coefficient unreasonably in order to compensate for the reduced conveyance which would otherwise be computed above the bank-full stage.

An approach such as described above would be unsatisfactory in many cases. Consideration of a system such as distinct co-flowing channels, each with independent roughness conditions and with its own velocity, is more realistic. An interchange of momentum between the separate parts can be included as a result of turbulent shear at the interface between the flows.

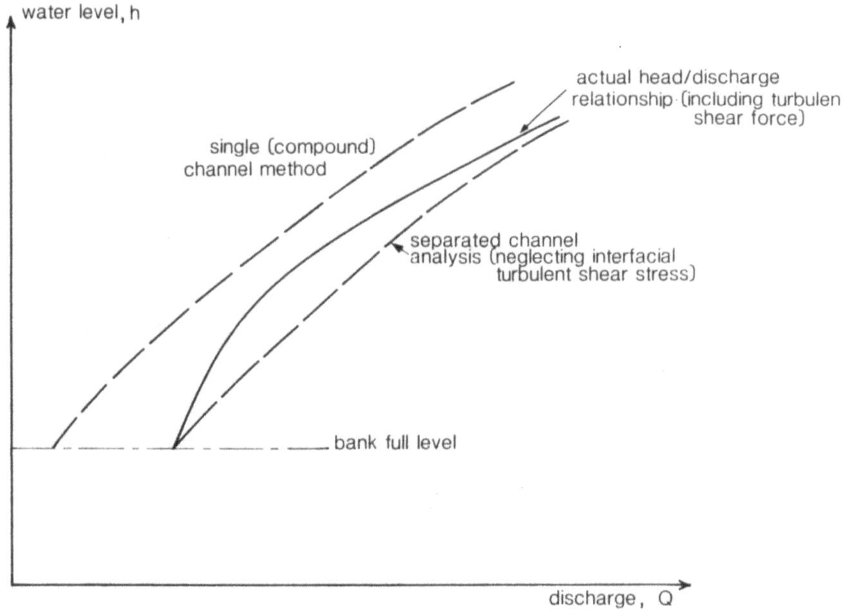

Figure 7.6 Head–discharge relationship for a river channel with flow on adjacent flood plain.

This shear force increases head losses above the bank-full stage. In Figure 7.6 is shown the typical form of stage discharge relationship which can result. This aspect of flow behaviour has received considerable attention, and Ervine and Ellis (1987) contains information on the principal investigators. Fixing the dividing line between main channel and flood plain may be straightforward in some cases, for instance the simple example of Figure 7.5, but other circumstances may be more uncertain, e.g. where the side slopes merge gradually with the flood plain.

7.10.4 *Meandering channels with overbank flow*

When the channel is meandering or has bends, the situation is further complicated under overbank flow conditions by the presence of transverse velocity components passing across the flood plain and encountering the deeper river channel (Figure 7.7). Expansion and contraction effects occur for the flood plain element of flow and should be included in any assessment of resistance for the system. The magnitude of these losses will be a function

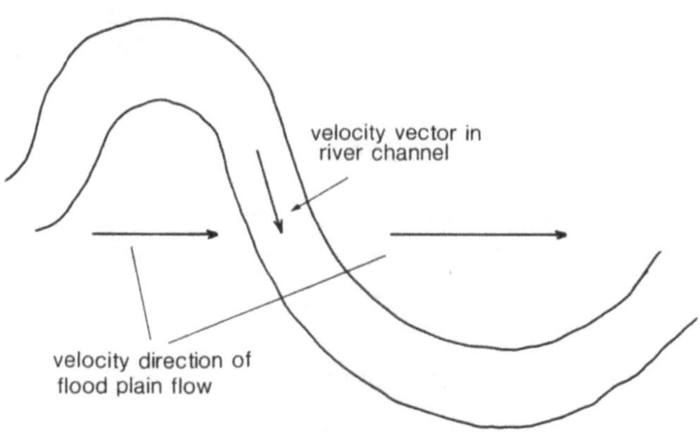

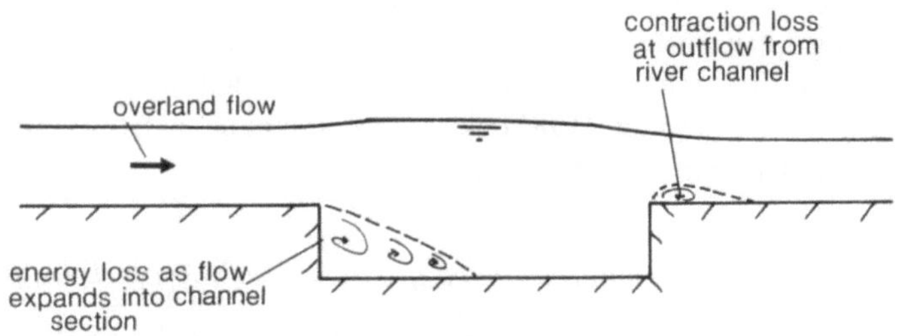

Figure 7.7 Head losses resulting from transverse velocities of overbank flows.

of the geometry of the channel bends or meanders and of the channel shape, including depth of section and side slopes of the channel. Ervine and Ellis (1987) have presented preliminary findings of an analysis of this behaviour, which is presently the subject of research at a number of centres.

The foregoing gives a brief insight into the complexity of determining resistance characteristics of natural river systems as a function of stage. As indicated, some effects will be more important at low stage while other influences will become important at higher stage.

7.10.5 *Numerical aspects of head loss representation*

In addition to the hydraulic aspects of assessing resistance to flow, there are numerical considerations which must be borne in mind. Returning to the computational scheme (Figure 7.4) for simplicity, the rate of head loss resulting from resistance, S, may be written as:

$$S = \frac{Q^2}{K^2} \tag{7.10}$$

where K is the conveyance of the cross-section. Conveyance may be evaluated using any one of a number of resistance laws, such as the Strickler equation:

$$K = \frac{8.41 g^{1/2}}{k^{1/6}} R^{2/3} \tag{7.11}$$

With reference to Figure 7.4, the finite difference expression representing resistance to flow should be representative of 'average' conditions over the reach length, Δx, and timestep, Δt.

7.10.6 *Variation of gradient* S *with time*

The unknown values of friction slope, S_j^{i+1} and S_{j+1}^{i+1}, are functions of Q^2 and K^2 at these points. K in turn is dependent on water level, h. Where it can reasonably be assumed that changes of depth and conveyance are small, it may be possible to adopt values of K at the initial time t^i in any expression for S at time t^{i+1}. However, this can lead to numerical instability in cases where changes are more rapid or where a larger time increment is in use. It is preferable that changes of both Q and K are included in the evaluation of S at time t^{i+1}. Pender (1985) describes a means whereby this can be accommodated within the computational scheme.

7.10.7 *Modelling of average resistance gradient over the reach length*

Some methods of modelling the average slope, S, over the reach length can cause unacceptable errors in certain cases. Suppose a simple arithmetic mean

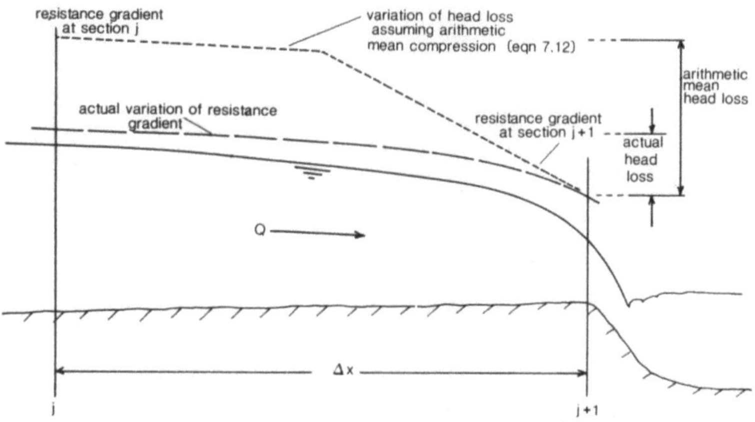

Figure 7.8 Actual and assumed variations of head over a reach length.

of friction slopes is adopted, that is:

$$\bar{S} = (S_j^i + S_{j+1}^i)/2 \tag{7.12}$$

where S is the mean value over the reach length at time t^i. While conditions are varying gradually this approach may be acceptable. If, for example, the gradient steepens towards the downstream end of the reach as the flow approaches a control section, then the curvature of the water surface becomes important, with substantial changes of depth and velocity occurring within a short distance (Figure 7.8). Use of the arithmetic mean (eqn 7.12) in some cases would result in important overestimation of the head loss in the reach. Cunge *et al.* (1980) summarise different methods of averaging resistance slope over a reach length by means of a weighting factor, and Pender (1985) introduced a flexible means of representation which automatically adjusted the weighting between S_j and S_{j+1} to avoid some of the problems outlined above.

7.11 Numerical representation of a river network

As already indicated, the natural river system is to be represented by a set of discrete cross-sections encompassing all important changes of channel geometry and flow characteristics. These sections are usually numbered sequentially from upstream to downstream (Figure 7.9), although in complicated networks, especially under tidal influence, flow may reverse in a channel element and the idea of upstream or downstream may be arbitrary.

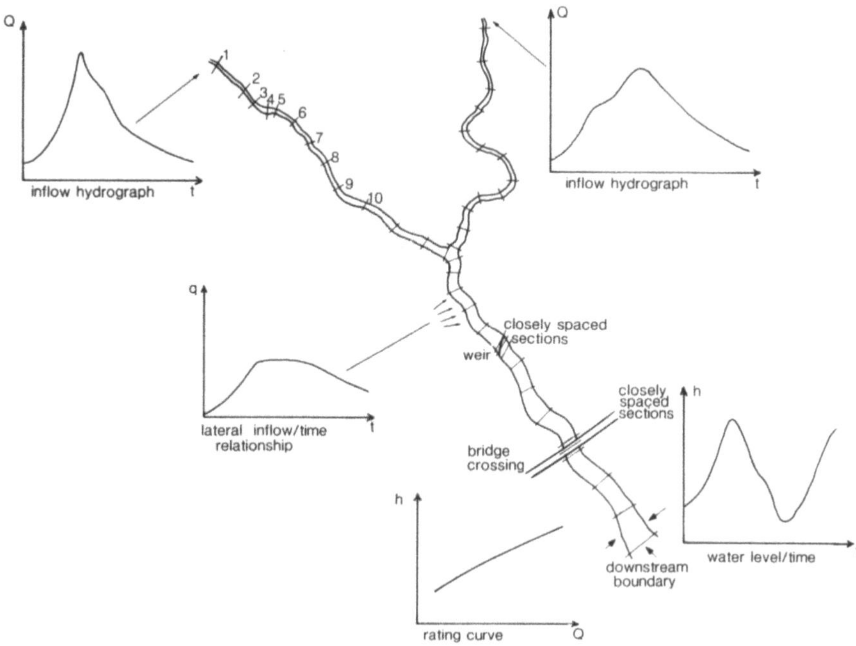

Figure 7.9 Representation of a river system and typical boundary conditions.

7.11.1 *Definition of section shape*

Each cross-section is represented by a set of points joined by straight lines (Figure 7.10). Cross-section properties are determined for any value of water level by summation of the contribution of each triangular or trapezoidal element to the section properties of top width B, wetted perimeter P, cross-section area A, and so forth, thus providing the complete properties of the section. Complicated cross-sections such as bridges can be handled in a similar manner with the numerical device of a small artificial vertical slot in the soffit being used to provide a free surface at all water levels and to connect different parts of the section while not adding to the section properties to any significant extent. At entry and exit from the constrictions created by bridges, etc., local head losses are incurred. Usually the head loss is expressed as a function of the velocity head at the bridge using a loss coefficient. Chow (1950, pp. 476–492) provides a considerable volume of data indicating the effect of constrictions resulting from embankments and bridge piers, although these relate primarily to relatively recent construction. There remain, in developed countries especially, many examples of older arched structures whose influence upon flow profiles may be more difficult to predict. In such cases it may be prudent to construct a 'local' scale model to study the

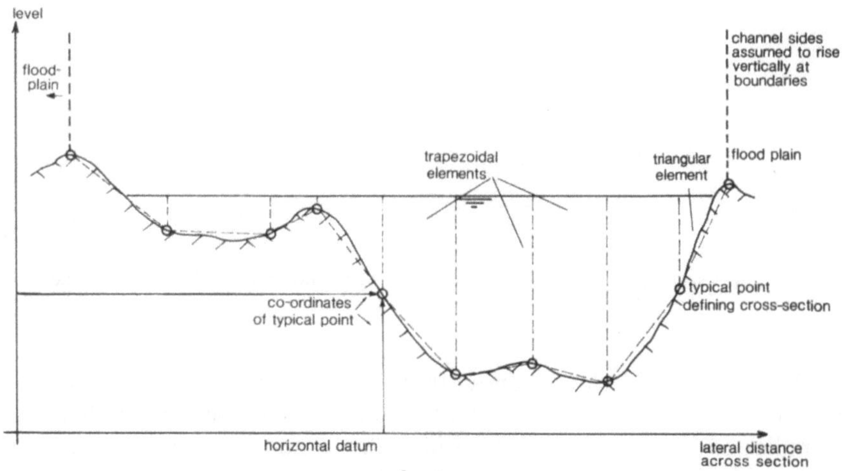

Figure 7.10 Representation of a typical cross-section.

hydraulic behaviour of the structure. It is not uncommon for bridge crossings to be sited close to other channel features such as bends or weirs, and the interaction between these will also make evaluation of head losses more difficult. In such cases the use of scale models offers a means of quantifying the head losses.

7.11.2 *Control sections*

In numerical modelling of constrictions such as bridges and weirs, the possibility of a control section developing under certain conditions must be considered. In the ideal case this will be defined by the equations:

$$\frac{Q^2B}{gA^3} = 1.0 \tag{7.13}$$

and

$$E = h + \frac{A}{2B} \tag{7.14}$$

where E is the energy level. In many cases conditions depart significantly from this ideal condition, and the more general weir flow equation:

$$Q = C_d BH^{3/2} \tag{7.15}$$

where H is the upstream energy level measured from the invert of the control section, allows a relationship to be established between flow rate and water level which includes the variation of discharge coefficient, C_d, as a function of level. Thus a range of non-ideal control section conditions can be accommodated.

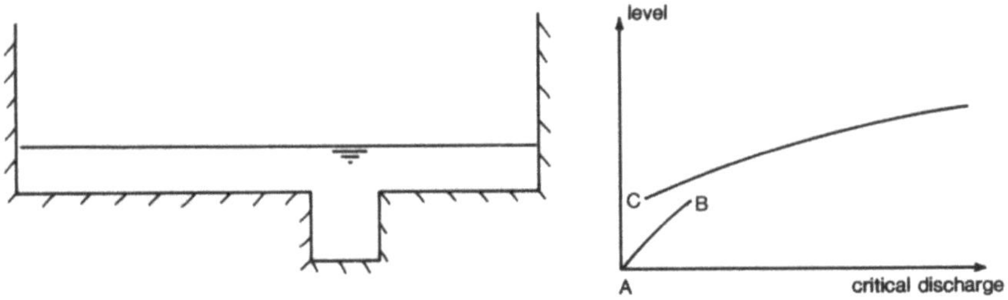

Figure 7.11 Variation of critical flow over a weir with a notch under 'ideal' flow conditions.

The facility to include non-ideal weir flow conditions has long been recognised by river modellers. Care must also be exercised in handling more complicated section shapes. Consider the common case of a structure composed of a weir occupying most of the width of a stream and having a notch cut out part-way along its length (Figure 7.11). Employing the ideal condition equations (7.13 and 7.14), the stage–discharge relationship for this structure can be plotted (Figure 7.11). On part AB the stage is increasing with discharge, but when the notch is just filled and flow extends to a very small depth across the main part of the weir crest the top width is increased dramatically for little increase in the flow area. The discharge, Q, falls sharply to compensate, point C (Figure 7.11). Clearly, as with the case of a compound channel section considered earlier, the different characteristics of the notch and of the main weir have to be taken into account in establishing the true relationship between stage and discharge.

7.12 Overbank storage

The complexity of the subject of overbank flow has already been outlined in relation to the determination of resistance effects. These earlier considerations were largely based upon steady-flow conditions. When flood waves are moving through a river system, transient effects have to be taken into account when studying the interaction of river flow and overbank flow. Figure 7.12 illustrates a typical sequence as river stage rises and falls during a flood event. At the outset of any modelling exercise prevailing conditions are established in the system, that is the initial base flow in the river is used to determine an initial water surface profile. Also, consideration should be given to the possibility of an earlier flood event having left residual water in flood plains, particularly where the river is embanked (Figure 7.12a). As the river level rises and overtops the embankments or bank-full level, flow will proceed onto the flood plain (Figure 7.12b). Even with a relatively modest superelevation over the embankment crest, substantial flows can occur from

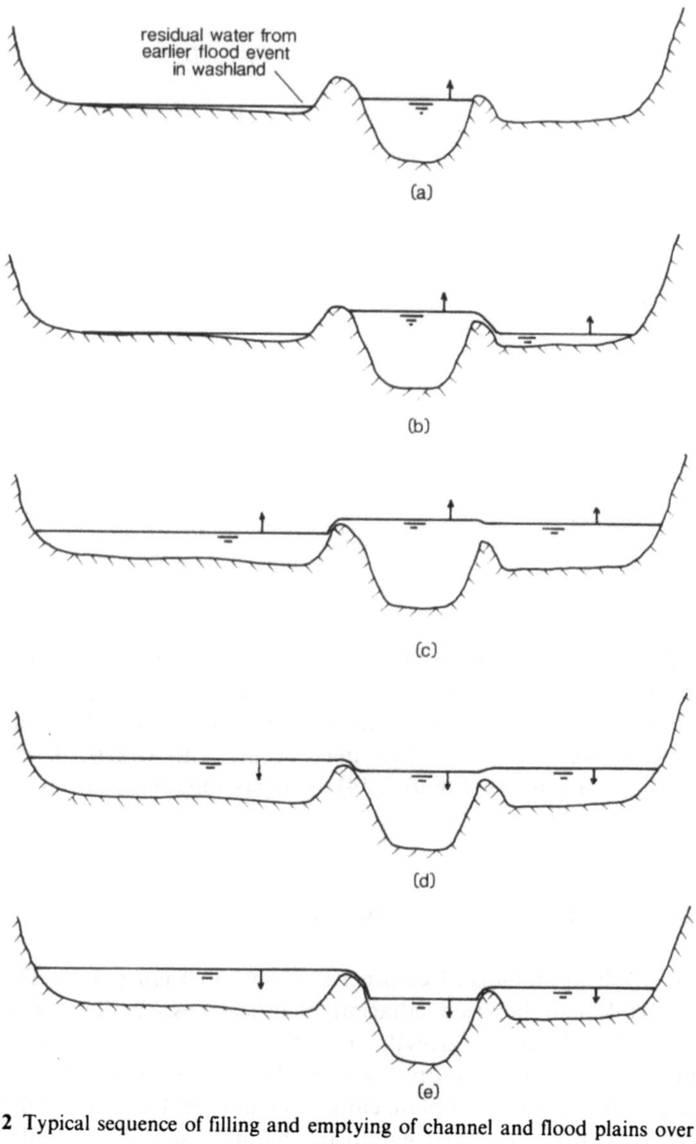

Figure 7.12 Typical sequence of filling and emptying of channel and flood plains over a flood event.

the river to the adjacent flood plain or washland, and a marked alteration in the river stage–discharge relationship can occur (Figure 7.13). When there is little or no water in the flood plain, then flow from the river over the banks will be in the form of a weir flow, albeit with an irregular weir crest. As time passes, levels in the flood plain will increase and the weir flow over the banks will be submerged (Figure 7.12c). Once the flood peak has passed

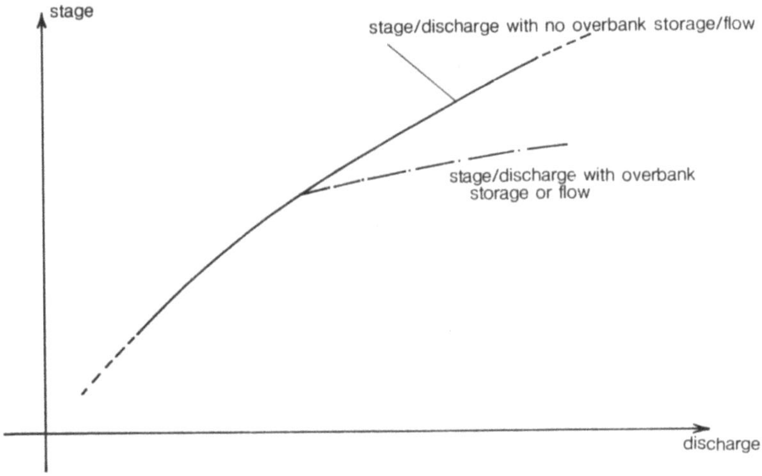

Figure 7.13. Stage–discharge relationships for a channel with and without overbank flow and storage.

and the river starts to subside, flow will occur from the washlands or flood plains back to the river channel (Figure 7.12d and e). Depending on the relative conveyances and gradients in the river channel and flood plains and embankment levels, overland flow may occur, with overbank discharges short-circuiting meanders (Figure 7.14) or bypassing constrictions, weirs and other features in the channel.

7.13 Numerical representation of embankments

A typical reach of embanked channel is shown in Figure 7.15. The profile of the embankment between adjacent channel cross-sections is surveyed, including notes of vegetal growth and other features of the embankment which may have a bearing upon flow over the crest. It should be noted that, where channels are curved in plan, embankment crest lengths will differ from each other and from the axial length of channel itself. The profile of each segment of embankment crest is represented by a set of points in the same way as for channel cross-sections (Figure 7.16). Properties may be computed as a function of water level over the crest to provide tables of discharge values over the crest segment as a function of water level over the crest in the same way as a stage–discharge relationship may be found for a weir. Because of the irregularity of many embankments it is often found that a substantial reduction in the ideal flow–stage relationship, given by eqns 7.13 and 7.14, is necessary to yield the correct flows to match observations. Where

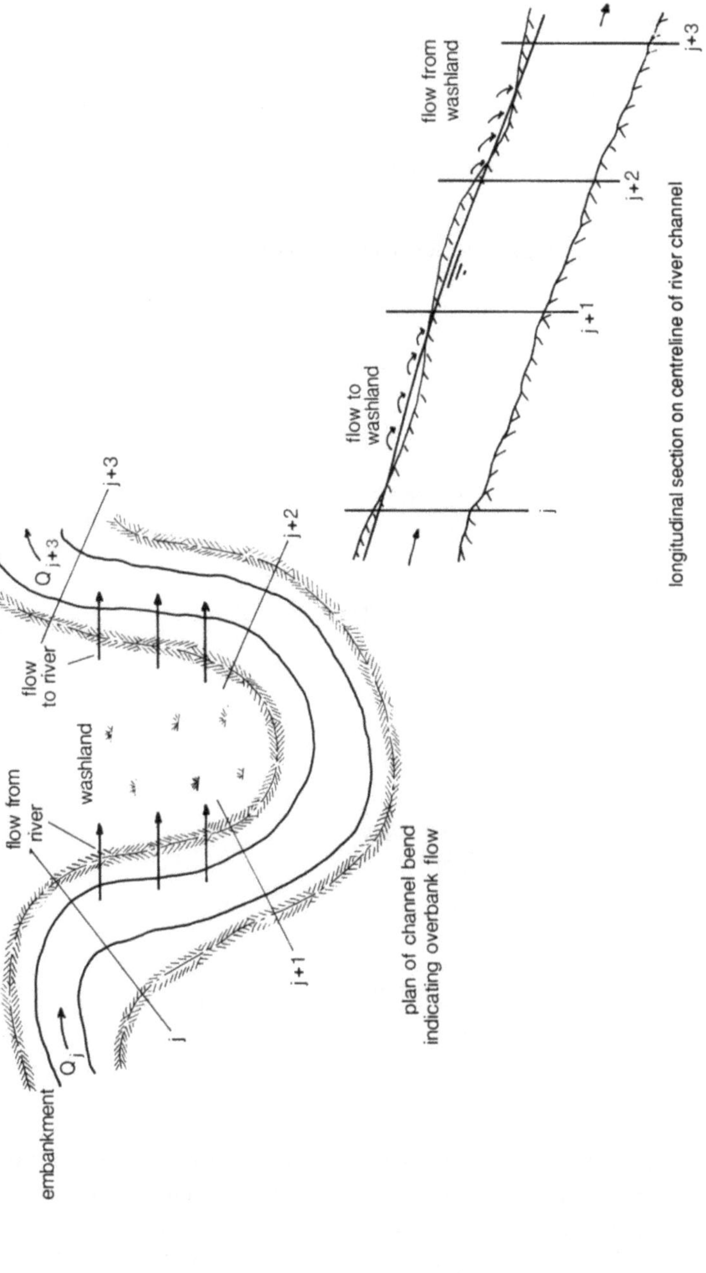

Figure 7.14. Depicting short-circuiting of a channel bend.

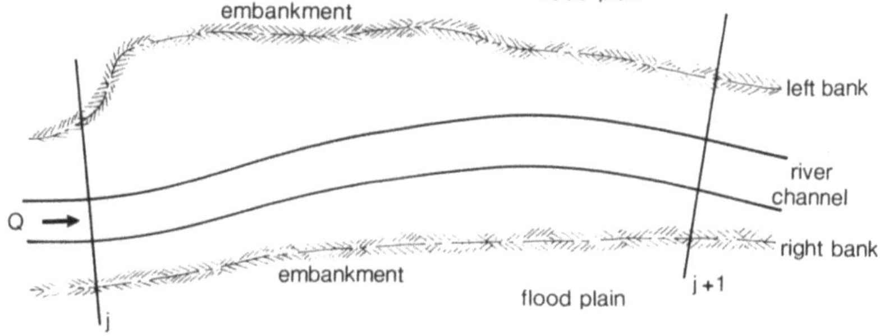

Figure 7.15 Reach of embanked channel.

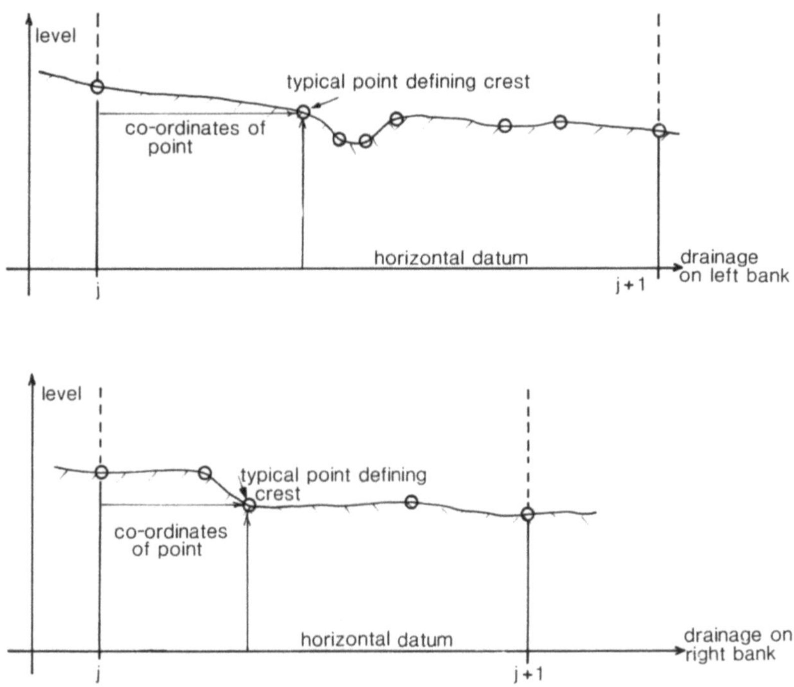

Figure 7.16 Representation of embankment crest in numerical model.

flap valves and other mechanical means such as sluices are incorporated, the stage–discharge relationship for an embankment segment may not be the same for outflow as for inflow to the flood plain, and in any model the facility to incorporate different stage–discharge relationships for inflow and outflow is desirable.

7.14 Flood alleviation

A necessary first step in any study which is intended to develop a plan for flood alleviation or prevention is to define two parts of the system:

'Floodway' means those areas of the system which are responsible for conveying the flood waters.

'Flood fringe' means those other areas of the system which are covered by water but which do not contribute significantly to the actual conveyance or hydraulic properties of the channel system, although they may make an appreciable contribution to water storage.

The extent of the flood fringe is in direct relation to the magnitude of the flood.

A further consideration which should receive early attention is the influence of development or changes in land use upon flood magnitude and behaviour. Particularly important in this respect is urbanisation, which is responsible for a number of major effects on flooding:

Provision of roads, housing, etc., increases the impervious area of catchment, leading to a larger proportion of flow contributing directly to runoff.

Provision of sewerage and culverted streams and improved channels leads to higher flow velocities and thereby shortens the response time of the catchment; thus the inflow hydrographs contributing to the river flows tend to be shorter in duration and with higher peak flows.

Development on and infilling of natural flood storage areas reduces any initial attenuation of the flood wave and contributes to higher flow rates downstream.

Increase of impervious area reduces natural groundwater recharge and in the longer term reduces groundwater levels and lowers dry-weather flows; thus river channels will tend to become smaller and more overgrown, leading to the reduction of carrying capacity of the channel network.

Increased sediment loads are commonly experienced during the several years following the start of development. These loads, being deposited in a largely uncontrolled manner, can have an effect upon flood control methods.

7.15 Flood control schemes

The most obvious means of avoiding flood risk is to situate development and installations outwith the flood fringe. There is considerable pressure to utilise land close to the riversides and within the region of the flood plains. When developments do take place within the flood plains there are some rules which should be adhered to in order to limit the risks. Within that part of the system which has been identified as floodway, in general no development should be permitted which will increase the flood risk. This will inhibit all but very modest structures, such as small pump houses, and even fences should be prohibited as these present a convenient screen on which debris may collect and impose a constricting effect upon the flow. Roads and railways should be designed to provide sufficient freeboard above the afflux level and also to minimise any concentration of the flow. The exception to development within the floodway are those structures which are designed to retard floodwaters upstream by providing temporary storage and thus creating a measure of attenuation of the flood wave and subsidence of the crest.

Within the flood fringe, structures should be provided with adequate freeboard above the design flood afflux level. Embankments and other structures which may divorce part of the flood plain from the river, and thereby reduce the area of storage for flood waters, should be provided with culverts so that storage reduction is minimised. For a more detailed consideration of these topics the reader is referred to the paper by Thompson and Rippin (1985).

In many cases flood control schemes which are of local benefit will have an adverse effect elsewhere, notably further downstream. In order to reduce the risk to the majority of flood plain users it may be necessary to reduce the standard of protection in some places below that which would otherwise be attained. In such circumstances legislation may be necessary relating to compensation and compulsory purchase, although extensive use of such powers should be avoided. Landowners should be convinced that their situation will not be appreciably worsened by any flood protection or prevention scheme, otherwise appeals will be raised and possible delays will result if compensation is not considered adequate. It is preferable that local communities agree to the maximum possible extent if any structural flood alleviation or protection options are to be implemented smoothly.

Flood control schemes fall into two main categories. Firstly structural measures, such as diversion schemes providing improved channel conveyance, off-channel and in-channel water storage or flood retention schemes and other channel improvements, and, secondly, flood warning schemes, together with building control regulations and flood insurance schemes. The normal criterion for evaluating the effectiveness of any proposal is by cost–benefit analysis. The initial cost plus maintenance costs are discounted to a present-day value and compared with the value of anticipated benefits to give a ratio of costs to benefits and thus an index against which alternative proposals may be compared (see also section 9.2 and Penning-Rowsell and Chatterton, 1977).

7.15.1 *Categories of structural scheme*

Structural schemes fall into a number of categories. In general the effects which are of greatest importance are storage, whether overbank or in specially created ponds either off-stream or on-stream using weirs, gates and channel constrictions to control upstream water levels. Also of some importance is attenuation as a result of resistance, i.e. storage in river channels as a consequence of head losses requiring a particular stage to be achieved in order to convey a certain discharge. Starting upstream of the region affected by flooding, there may be opportunities to provide temporary storage. This may take the form of constructing embankments, weirs or gates to provide a temporary reservoir which retains flood waters and provides a measure of attenuation and subsidence of the flood crest. In some cases where several streams converge, the individual flood hydrographs may be in phase, so that their peak discharges coincide, producing relatively short storm duration and high peak discharge. If a retention scheme can be devised which alters the phasing of the hydrographs of one or more of the tributary streams, then the peak flow rate may be significantly reduced.

Several structural forms are possible for each storage area and Hall and Hockin (1980) provide guidance on the dimensioning of storage ponds for modest streams and also present a review of possible structural arrangements.

7.15.2 *Flood walls*

Progressing downstream, the opportunity to provide temporary storage is much more limited, particularly in urban areas. The provision of embankments and flood walls offers a means of preventing flood waters escaping from the river channel system. However, the effect of this is to reduce the attenuation of the flood wave which would otherwise occur as a result of flows passing onto the flood plain. Thus flow rates downstream will be higher, and the risks are increased.

7.15.3 *Channel improvement*

Removal of redundant weirs and regrading of the channel bed to improve the conveyance of the section are further options. These measures alter the stage–discharge relationship of the channel by permitting a larger discharge to pass through that part of the system for a given water level. Measures of this sort can be used to compensate for the tendency to increase water levels which results from providing flood walls. The effect of these improvements is to reduce the attenuation of the flood wave. This will increase the downstream risk, so the measures described cannot be considered in isolation at a particular place, and the entire network liable to be influenced by the changes should be studied.

7.15.4 *Summary*

The increase of upstream storage produces subsidence of the flood crest and attenuation of the wave, whereas in the critical areas prone to flooding improvements to the channel and construction of flood walls reduce the storage in this area as a function of water level and, while protecting the specific area, may cause higher downstream flows. Combinations of these measures should be sought so that protection can be provided without increasing risks elsewhere in the system.

7.15.5 *Non-structural measures*

Use of remote measurement and data transmission systems offers the possibility of providing passive flood warning measures and also, in conjunction with water storage facilities, affords the possibility of optimising use of these facilities. Numerical models may be employed in conjunction with remote measurements where telemetry provides advance prediction of flood hydrographs entering the river system. The numerical model of flood wave propagation can be used to provide predictions of peak water levels and timings of these events at critical areas downstream. Emergency services can be prepared to take measures to alleviate the worst effects of flooding and, also, flood retention structures can be programmed to operate to maximum advantage to provide the optimum storage as a function of time.

7.16 Channel alteration during flood events

In the course of flood wave passage through a network of river channels, and particularly following alteration to the system, there will be a period when erosion and deposition will occur. Finer particles may be removed during a flood event and a natural armouring can be built up from the larger particles remaining. Porosity changes and depth of erosion can change resistance characteristics with time in the channel, as can the accumulation of debris at obstacles within the cross-section. Such effects are difficult to predict but should be considered when any study is undertaken.

8 River engineering

M.J. WAKELIN

8.1 History

Civil engineering is one of the oldest professions in the world, and, within it, river engineering is one of the earliest specialisms to have been established. The parallels between the history of river engineering and the political and economic history of society constitute an absorbing area of study. A large proportion of all the historical engineering works catalogued by engineering institutions around the world concern drainage in one form or another.

The Romans were probably the first to construct large-scale civil engineering works. Many examples exist to this day, some of which still fulfil their original purpose.

In the medieval period, when rural affairs throughout Europe were dominated by the Church, those who ran the monasteries constructed many drainage channels to improve the yield of their lands. Some of these are also still in existence.

The coming of the industrial revolution prompted the next large development of river engineering schemes. This time the aim was not so much drainage as the improvement of the transportation system. However, the underlying motivation was the same, namely the making of profit.

Nowadays, most river engineering is carried out as a public service. Most schemes are commissioned by government agencies of one form or another using national, or in the case of large schemes, international funding, with the actual work being carried out by local, national or international contractors.

Concurrent with the development of river engineering has been the development of river legislation. Much of this is based on custom and established rights, and varies both between and within countries. International treaties govern many of the world's rivers, and in the European Community steps are being taken to harmonise the legislation of member states. The engineer must always take competent legal, and in some cases diplomatic advice at an early stage in any project.

8.2 Types of water course

8.2.1 *Introduction*

There is often a difference between the legal and administrative, and the functional categorisation of water courses. Administrative categories such as main river, highway drain, open or public sewer are frequently used, but it may be difficult to distinguish between some of these categories when they are considered from a hydraulic viewpoint. Thus, for the present purposes it is more helpful to consider a series of functional categories.

(a)

(b)

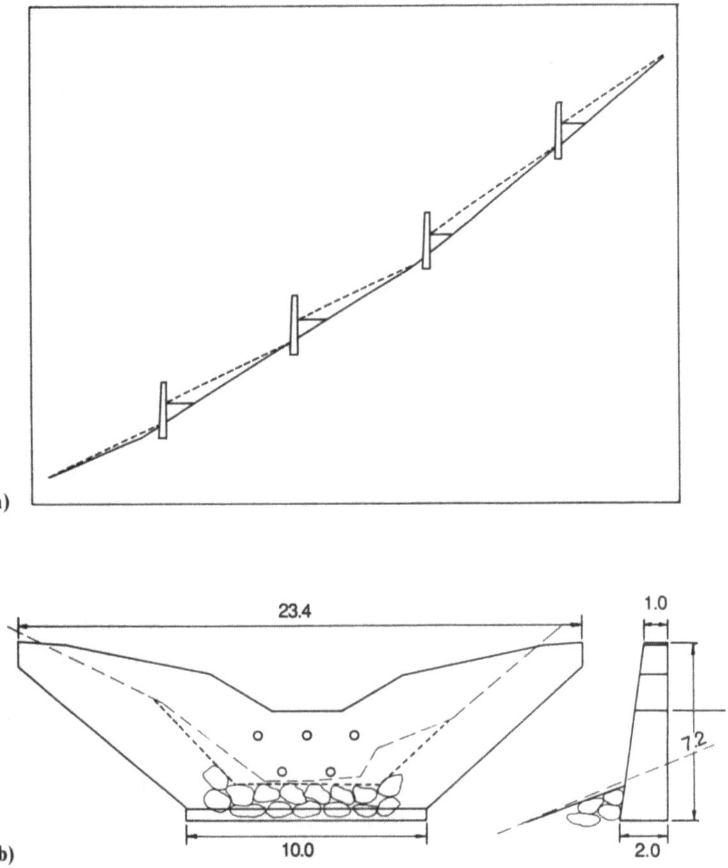

Figure 8.1 (a) Part of a series of check dams to control a mountain torrent, Liesertal and Ossiacher Seebecken, Austria. (b) Details of one of the dams. (Redrawn from material supplied by Wildbach und Lawinenverbauung, Villach.)

8.2.2 *Upland water courses*

In general the problems associated with upland water courses are those of erosion and its control (see Figure 8.1 and Chapter 4). Most drainage work is confined to that necessary for the development of forestry. This, in turn, brings its own set of problems in the adverse effect it has on the amount and quality of the water feeding into the water course. Significant loss of yield has occurred in many upland reservoirs as a result of afforestation.

8.2.3 *Flood plain*

Although not a water course, flood plains call for mention here. In the past, many drainage schemes were carried out to convert riverside meadows into arable land. In the present climate of opinion, any such proposal must be rigorously appraised from the investment planning point of view. Even if economic advantage can be demonstrated, the environmental impact of such a scheme could well be unacceptable. An existing development in a flood plain is different and is regarded, subject to benefit, as deserving flood defence like any other development. An extensive fenland system alongside a river is not, in this context, considered to be a flood plain. For river engineering purposes, an upland channel and its flood plain should both be considered integral parts of the river. Recent developments in the management of rivers and their flood plains, two-stage channels, are considered in more detail in section 8.4.

8.2.4 *Urban channels*

Sometimes the most attractive economic solution to an urban flooding problem is the creation of a lined water course to carry enhanced flows through a town (see Figure 8.2). Such water courses are rarely pretty. Even if they were pretty to begin with, the accumulation of rusty bicycles, lawn clippings and supermarket trolleys which seems to be an inescapable adjunct to town dwelling quickly diminishes the amenity value. For this reason, lined urban channels should be avoided if possible. If this solution to the flooding problem has overwhelming economic advantages, then an on-going maintenance commitment must be accepted and every effort should be made to inhibit would-be vandals by building in attractive environmental features. The channel must be designed for easy access to facilitate maintenance, the removal of debris and the escape of people who fall in.

8.2.5 *Cut-off channels*

From very early times, channels have been constructed around the edges of low-lying areas to intercept runoff from high land and carry it, by gravity, safely around the area. Carr Dyke in England dates from Roman times, and a more

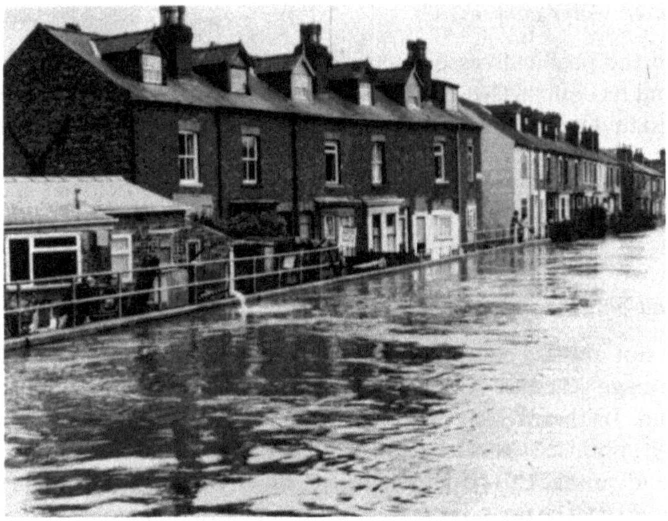

Figure 8.2 Urban channel running brim-full, Sincil Dyke, Lincoln (from Wakelin *et al.*, 1987).

modern example is shown on Figure 8.3 (see Rivet, 1964, for a further discussion of Carr Dyke). Cut-off channels obviate pumping costs, which are a heavy burden on the drainage ratepayer, and future escalations in the cost of fossil fuels may well give added impetus to such energy-conserving schemes. The underlying strata can sometimes cause seepage problems, but this should not deter present-day engineers from designing proper cut-offs (in the geophysical as well as the hydrological sense).

8.2.6 *Raised gravity water courses*

In many low-lying areas, where cut-off channels skirting high land are not practicable, water has been conveyed to the sea across low-lying land by the simple expedient of raising the bank of an existing river. Sometimes channels have been straightened to minimise the costs of bank raising. Older channels of this type, which have existed for centuries, were usually evolved rather than constructed. Often in fenlands as the bordering peatlands shrank, the channel borders rose of their own accord as silt was deposited during periods of inundation. Dredgings may also have been deposited on the banks, and other material may have been imported. The resulting embankments, such as the South Level Barrier in Cambridgeshire and those of the Yellow River in China, have become, almost of their own volition, massive civil engineering structures with a retained flood level six or even more metres above the adjacent land. The analysis of these embankments using soil mechanics principles often yields alarming factors of safety, and the area at risk is often large. Water

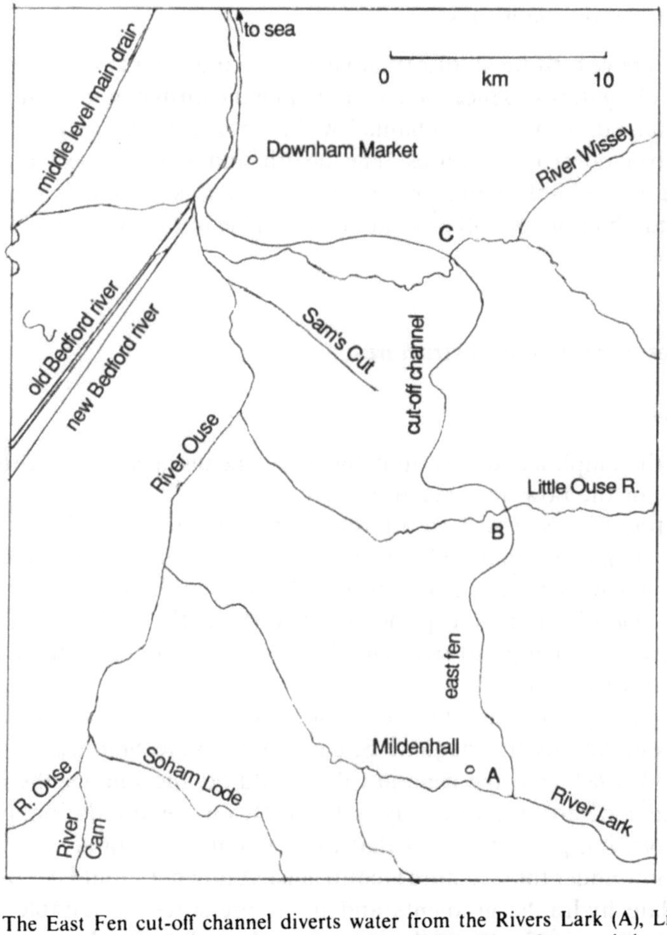

Figure 8.3 The East Fen cut-off channel diverts water from the Rivers Lark (A), Little Ouse (B) and Wissey (C), and then flows northwards to the sea. The River Ouse and the man-made Bedford Rivers carry land water northwards through the middle of the Fens.

courses of this type always carry a heavy maintenance liability and require constant vigilance against damage by cattle, vermin and, not least, farmers anxious to plough to the very last square metre. A programme of inspections, enhanced at the times of high water, is essential for the proper maintenance of the embankments.

8.2.7 *Pumped drains*

Pumped drains, which are often operated by internal drainage boards or their equivalent, are discussed in Chapter 9.

8.2.8 *Navigation waterways*

Many rivers constitute statutory navigations, and the responsible authority then has obligations to meet. These may take the form of a minimum draft to be maintained, a minimum channel width or adequate navigational facilities at river control structures. The health and safety aspect of river engineering is probably more important here, at least as far as the public is concerned, than on any other kind of river. This in turn introduces yet more legislation.

8.3 Types of river control structures

8.3.1 *Weirs*

A weir is the simplest and, no doubt, the oldest means of controlling the level of water, if not the flow, in a reach of a river.

The siting of a weir will, to a large extent, be determined by its intended purpose. It may be required for any of the river uses listed under River management below, except that, ironically, it is unlikely to be for drainage purposes. Despite that, the principles governing the design of a weir are sufficiently fundamental to river engineering to require more than a passing mention in this book.

Having an appropriate site already decided, the designer must be satisfied that the foundations are adequate. Site investigation techniques are described in BS 5930 (1981), but the general rule should be 'the simpler the better'. A reinforced concrete structure may rest directly on the foundation, preferably without bearing piles, provided that the foundation is stable, and provided that the flow under the structure is controlled. A flownet should be constructed to calculate hydraulic gradients and uplift pressures. A suitable cut-off is usually necessary to lengthen the seepage path, and it often happens that two are needed: one at the upstream toe and one at the downstream toe. Cut-offs are usually constructed of steel sheet piling.

Wingwalls are usually necessary to provide a transition between the body of the weir and the riverbank upstream and downstream. They may be of reinforced concrete, masonry or the ubiquitous steel sheet piling. Some flexible (and permeable) revetment helps to form the transition.

It is essential that the energy of the water as it falls over the weir crest is dissipated before it has a chance to erode the banks and bed of the river downstream of the structure (White *et al.*, 1989). A stilling basin of some kind is usually necessary. The greater the flow and the greater the drop across the structure, the more attention needs to be paid to energy dissipation.

The orientation of the structure in the channel is also vital if uneven flow patterns and consequent erosion are to be avoided. If the purpose of the weir is to measure flow (White *et al.*, 1989), it is particularly important to ensure a symmetrical flow pattern. A straight and uniform length of channel is desirable both upstream and downstream of the weir site.

The size of weir contemplated may range from a simple row of timber sheeters driven across a stream to a sophisticated irrigation weir across a major river. Whatever the size, attention should be paid to the principles set out above.

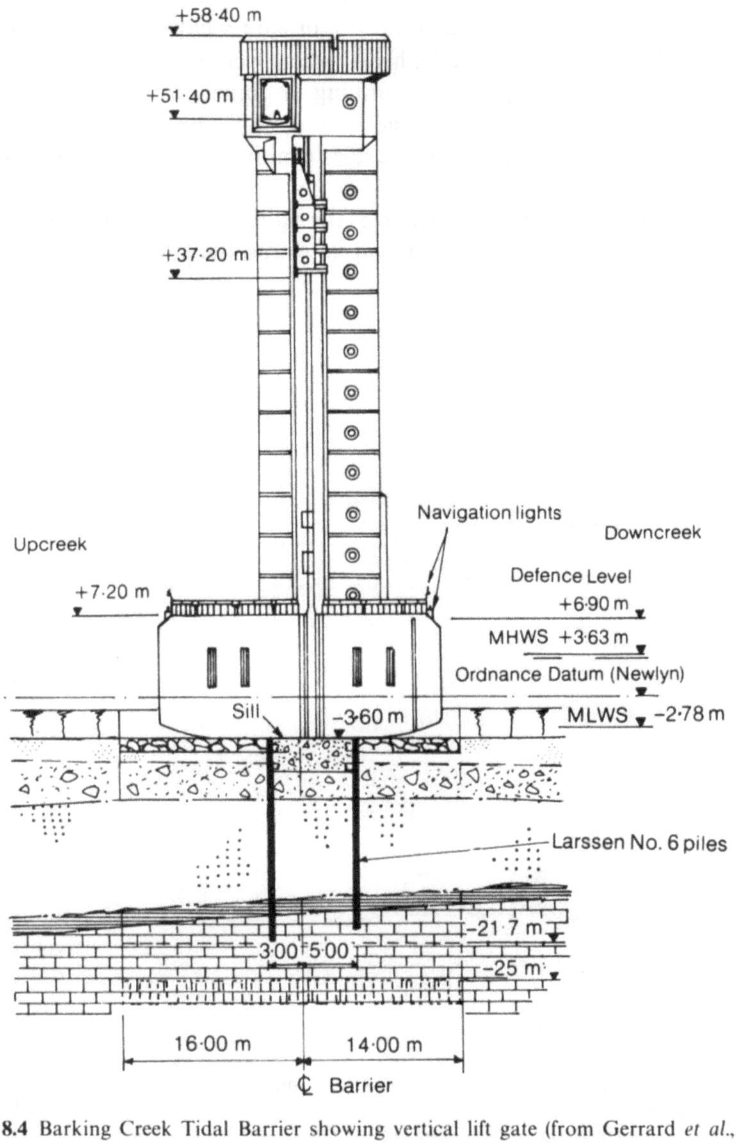

Figure 8.4 Barking Creek Tidal Barrier showing vertical lift gate (from Gerrard *et al.*, 1982).

8.3.2 *Fresh water sluices*

Nearly all the above principles apply as much to sluices as to weirs, and so the two sections should be read together.

The only difference between a sluice and a weir is that the former can pass a varying flow without significant increases in upstream level. The moving parts necessary to achieve this objective involve the skills of mechanical and, probably, electrical engineering. The simplest and commonest form of sluice is the vertical lift gate (Figure 8.4) (White *et al.*, 1989). The gate itself usually takes the form of a steel frame with a steel skinplate welded or riveted on the upstream side. The static hydraulic head is conveyed to a supporting frame by steel wheels mounted on the gate, running in guides, with a suspended rod sealing the vertical edges of the skinplate. The gates are usually counterbalanced and driven by steel cables running over a horizontal shaft at the top of the frame.

Another common form of sluice gate is the radial or Tainter gate (Figure 8.5) (White *et al.*, 1989). It has a curved skinplate, and the static force is taken by

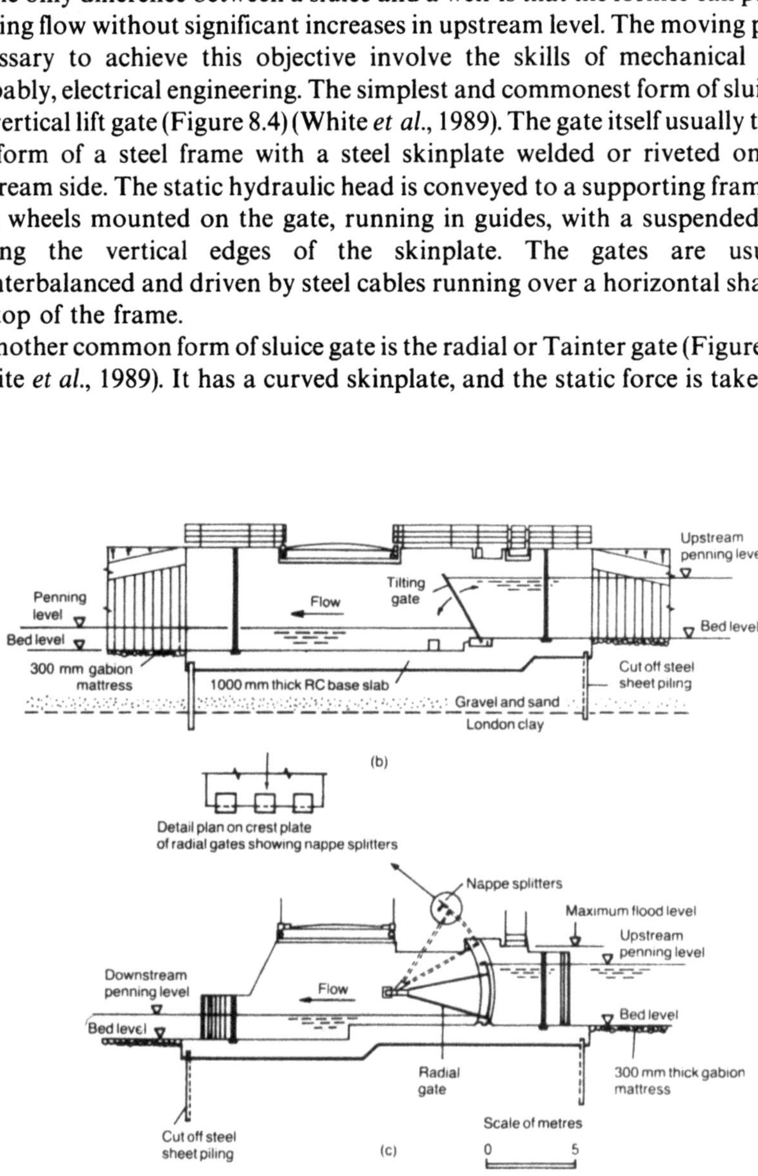

Figure 8.5 Control sluice, River Mole Flood Alleviation Scheme. One tilting gate maintains dry-season water levels and provides some aeration; three radial gates can be raised clear of the water to pass floods (from Foster and Harris, 1988).

radial beams to a trunnion bearing at the centre of curvature. They can be powered by lifting cables, hydraulic rams or, ingeniously, by an arrangement of orifices and tanks which use the upsteam level to govern automatically (without an external power source) the attitude of the gate and, hence, the discharge.

Tilting-bottom, hinged, drop-leaf gates (Figure 8.5) are the least visually intrusive form of sluice, having concealed operating mechanisms. Care must be taken to ensure that the torsional rigidity of the gate is adequate to obviate 'racking' of the gate, particularly if power is applied at one side only. Another pitfall for the unwary is that floating debris, such as large logs, can sometimes not escape from floating behind the nappe. The problem may be avoided by building a physical model to test the hydraulics of the gate before it is built. The nappe should always be ventilated to prevent partial evacuation and adherence of the nappe to the gate itself.

Inflatable rubber dams are a modern alternative to the above types of sluice (NCE, 1990). These consist of a rubber tube anchored to concrete and inflated by either air or water; water may require antifreeze. A single unit 5 m high by 10 m wide was installed across the Ogamigo River, Japan, in 1982, and three units 1.7 m high by 45 m wide were installed across the Iwaki River, Japan, in 1984. These dams are said to be cheap and virtually puncture-proof, and to have a life expectancy of 40 years. An automatic deflation system appears to be fitted as standard but, if this is tripped accidentally, a flood wave may be sent downstream. Inflatable rubber dams are now available from several manufacturers.

8.3.3 *Self-priming syphons*

Self-priming syphons are sometimes used to give a high discharge capacity for small overall size. However, velocities generated are high and can give rise to erosion problems downstream. There is also a very rapid transition from quiescent weiring conditions to turbulent syphonic conditions. This tends to send an unwelcome surge of flow into the downstream reach.

8.3.4 *Tidal sluices*

Control structures at the tidal limit have all the characteristics of freshwater sluices with the added complication of tidal fluctuations on the seaward side (see Chapter 9). The design of the channel upstream of the sluice must take cognisance of any tide-lock period and provide adequate storage for the design fluvial flood. The height of flood defence (which may be the height of the gates themselves or, more likely, the height of the flood wall over the gates) will be determined by design conditions in the estuary. The correlation of fluvial flood return periods with tidal surge return periods represents a challenge to even the most erudite statistician.

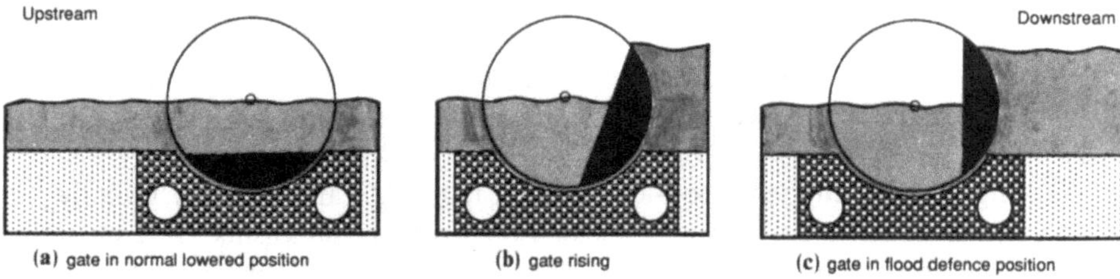

Figure 8.6 Mode of operation of the rising sector getes of the Thames Barrier. (a) Gate in normal lowered position; (b) gate rising; (c) gate in flood defence position holding out a tidal surge. In addition, the gates can be fully inverted for maintenance. (Redrawn from material supplied by the National Rivers Authority.)

Surge-excluding barriers such as the Barking, Hull and Thames Barriers (Figures 8.4 and 8.6), are now seen as a more environmentally acceptable way of protecting an estuary against tidal surges than a full tide-excluding barrage (White *et al.*, 1989). They have the advantage over normal tidal defences that they will be relatively easy to raise in the event of sea levels rising generally as a result of global warming.

8.4 Two-stage channels

Flooding has often been alleviated by straightening, widening, or deepening of a river course, causing removal of trees, natural vegetation, wildlife, and fishlife. A more attractive alternative is the construction of a two-stage channel, where the river is allowed to meander more or less as before, permitting the retention of most of the natural habitat. For example, in Figure 8.7 (a), berms were cut back as far as the limits of the meanders and replanted with grass, forming an upper confined channel or flood plain, which inundates with some regularity during high winter flows. In Figure 8.7 (c), an existing line of trees was retained by forming the upper channel on one side only.

Several questions about the hydraulic design of two-stage channels have arisen:

Can the stage–discharge relationship for a two-stage channel be predicted with accuracy?

What are the most significant channel/floodplain interactions when the main channel meanders across the floodplain, producing bends and cross-over regions in plan form?

What is the effect of floodplain (upper channel) roughness?

What is the effect of the sinuosity of the main (lower) channel?

What is the long-term behaviour of two-stage channels in view of the fact that larger floods, which carry most of the annual sediment transport load, will now carry part of that load onto the side berms? Will these berms silt up again?

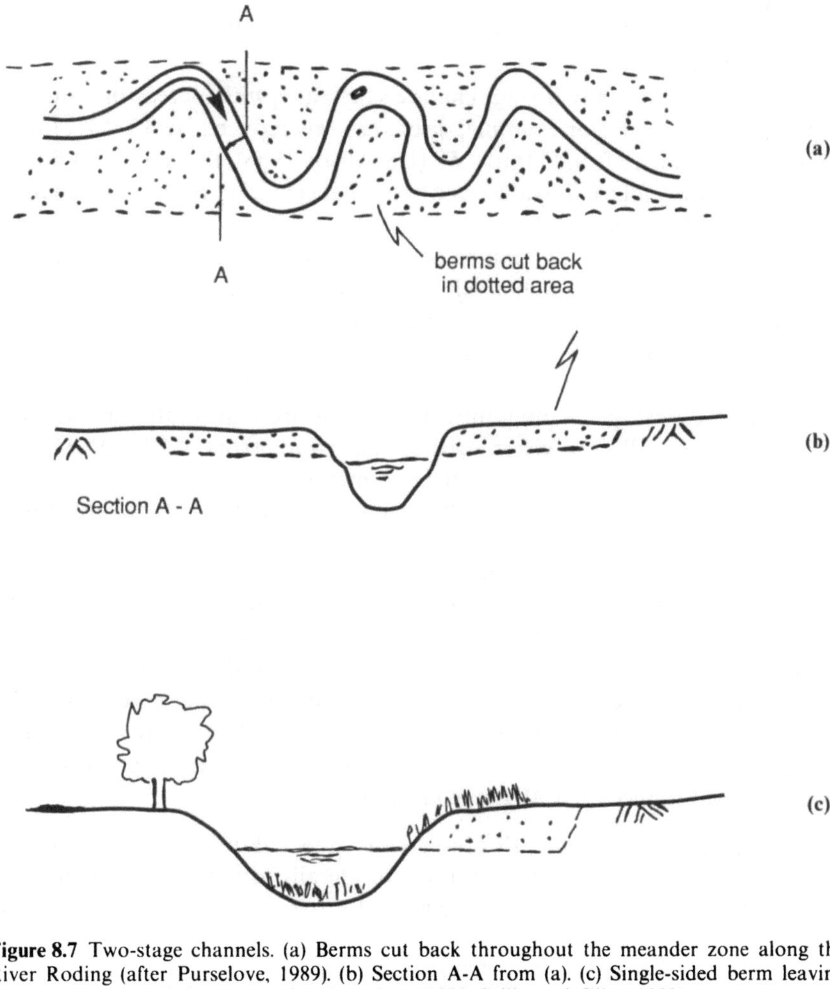

Figure 8.7 Two-stage channels. (a) Berms cut back throughout the meander zone along the River Roding (after Purselove, 1989). (b) Section A-A from (a). (c) Single-sided berm leaving existing trees (after Purselove, 1989; Sellin and Giles, 1988).

These problems are the subject of an on-going, world-wide research effort. Key findings about the behaviour of meandering two-stage channels are:

Flow in meandering compound channels includes a complex mixture of bends and skewed cross-over regions, both with floodplain flow, and is completely dissimilar to the straight parallel case (Ervine and Ellis, 1987).

Large secondary flow structures are set up at compound channel bends, where the secondary cells often rotate in the opposite direction to that at a bend with in-bank flow (Toebes and Sooky, 1967; Stein and Rouve, 1988; Kiely, 1989).

Large secondary flow structures are set up in the cross-over regions driven by floodplain flow passing over the skewed main channel flow below (Ervine and Ellis, 1987; Kiely, 1989; Stein and Rouve, 1989; Elliott and Sellin, 1990; Ervine and Jasem, 1991).

Resistance to flow in two-stage channels increases with increasing sinuosity of the main channel. For example, discharge was reduced by 30–40% for an increase of sinuosity from 1.0 to 1.57 (US Army, 1956). Resistance to flow is also considerably affected by the cross-sectional geometry of the main channel (Willetts and Hardwick, 1990).

Roughness of floodplains or side berms is a significant factor determining flow resistance in two-stage channels; for example, a comparison of compound channels with cut and uncut vegetation showed a 30% reduction in total conveyance (Sellin and Searle, 1987).

Approximate methods of discharge estimation by subdividing a meandering two-stage channel into subsections are inaccurate; for example, using a vertical wall subdivision method has led to errors of 25–50% (Ervine and Jasem, 1991). However, a subdivision method with reasonable accuracy is sketched in Figure 8.8 for the case of a meandering two-stage channel with rough flood plains; this method uses horizontal and vertical subdivisions, with imaginary floodplain roughness extended into the main channel.

Numerical models of skewed and meandering compound flows must be three-dimensional in order to simulate the significant three-dimensional flow structures. However, approximate estimates of stage-discharge are possible using depth-average numerical models, especially if the model includes accurate friction factors for both main channel and floodplain, estimates of lateral turbulent shear stress, and estimates of the secondary circulation term (Knight and Shiono 1990; Wark *et al.*, 1990).

A design manual based on this research is expected in 1991. Samuels (1989) gives a state-of-the art review, and further details are given by Knight and Sellin (1990), Myres and Brennan (1990) and Wormleaton and Merrett (1990).

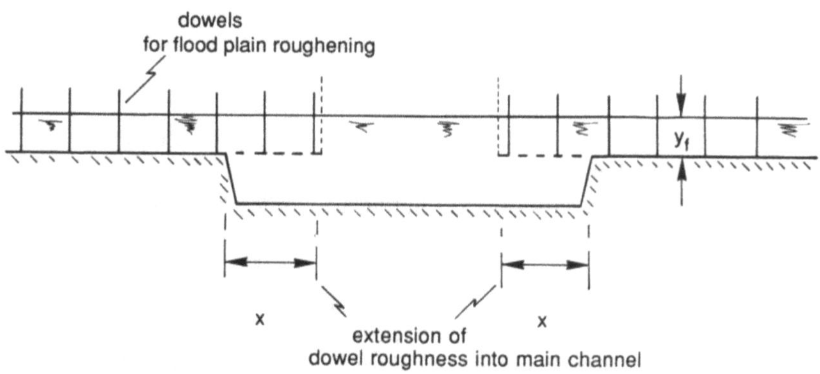

Figure 8.8 Subdivision method for a rough floodplain; dimension $x = 2y_f$ to $3y_f$. (Supplied by D.A. Ervine.)

8.5 Scour

No discussion on river engineering can be considered complete without special mention being made of scour problems. Scour and deposition are natural phenomena occurring throughout a river system. The well-known riffles, pools and bars associated with river meanders provide ample evidence of this. Scour, of course, can and does result from the placing of artificial structures within the river channel. This can lead to spectacular failures, as evidenced by the collapse of the River Ness railway bridge at Inverness in 1989 and the severe damage to the trans-Alpine motorway bridge over the River Inn at Kufstein in Austria in 1990. The river engineer must be careful to distinguish between general and local scour.

8.5.1 *General scour*

General scour produces lowering of the overall river bed, usually along a significant length of river, and results from the river trying to attain its equilibrium or regime depth. General scour can also be induced artificially by restricting the width of a river channel, as would occur when training walls are constructed, say, at approach to a weir or bridge crossing. Farraday and Charlton (1983) have gathered together suitable equations for the prediction of equilibrium flow depth for various types of channel bed material. Comparison of the measured and calculated flow depth allows the scour depth to be predicted. The equations are:

For sand bed channels

$$y = 0.38q^{0.67}D_{50}^{-0.17} \tag{8.1}$$

For gravel bed channels

$$y = 0.47q^{0.8}D_{90}^{-0.12} \tag{8.2}$$

For cohesive bed channels

$$y = 51.4n^{0.86}q^{0.86}\tau_c^{-0.43} \tag{8.3}$$

where y is the mean depth of flow (m), q is the discharge per unit width ($m^3\,s^{-1}\,m^{-1}$), D_{50} is the median size of the bed material (m), D_{90} is the size of bed material (m) such that 90% of the particles by number are smaller, n is the Manning roughness coefficient and τ_c is the critical tractive shear stress ($N\,m^{-2}$).

Multiplying factors are applied to the calculated depth to take account of the channel geometry. These range from 1.25 for straight channel reaches to 2.0 for right-angled bends (Lacey, 1958).

The discharge per unit width, q, is obtained by dividing the channel-forming discharge, Q (often assumed to be the bank-full flow), by the mean channel width, B. For a natural channel, B may be calculated using equations derived from Blench (1969) and Kellerhals (1967) for sand and gravel bed channels respectively, namely:

$$B = 14Q^{0.5}D_{50}^{0.25}F_s^{-0.5} \qquad (8.4)$$

and

$$B = 3.26Q^{0.5} \qquad (8.5)$$

where F_s is the side factor, varying from 0.2 for sandy loam to 0.3 for cohesive bank material.

No similar equation exists for channels with cohesive beds.

For channels artificially confined, say by training walls, *B* is the imposed width.

8.5.2 *Local scour*

Local scour occurs when the channel flow encounters an obstruction. The obstruction may be natural, for example a large boulder or rock bar, or it may be artificial, such as a bridge pier or abutment. In either case a vortex system develops in the flow immediately upstream of the obstruction, producing downward flow which if sufficiently strong will initiate a scour hole. The limiting depth of the scour hole is attained (a) in the case of clear-water scour, when the capacity of the flow to transport material from the hole reduces to zero, and (b) in the case of general bed load movement, when a balance is achieved between the amount of material supplied to the hole and the amount removed from it (Shen *et al.*, 1966).

Depth of scour is influenced mainly by four factors, the magnitude of the mean velocity of the approach flow, the width that the obstruction presents to the flow, the shape of the obstruction and the grain size of the bed material. The form of equation used to predict local scour depth is typified by that given by Shen *et al.* (1969) for clear-water, sand bed scour at a cylindrical bridge pier:

$$d_s = 1.17U_0^{0.62}b^{0.62} \qquad (8.6)$$

where d_s is the local scour depth (m), U_0 is the mean velocity of approach flow ($\mathrm{m\,s^{-1}}$) and *b* is the pier width (m).

Many other equations are given in the literature along with factors to take account of shapes other than cylindrical, angle of attack, etc. The reader is referred to specific texts on the subject such as those by Farraday and Charlton (1983) and Neill (1973).

In the case of local scour at abutments and training works, the general scour depth is calculated by the appropriate equation given in section 8.5.1, and then the maximum local scour depth is obtained by multiplying this by a factor varying from 1.5 for flow parallel to guidebanks to 2.75 for conditions at the ends of groynes or guidebanks (Farraday and Charlton, 1983).

Despite the availability of the equations and tables mentioned above, in many situations it is advisable to commission a physical model study of the

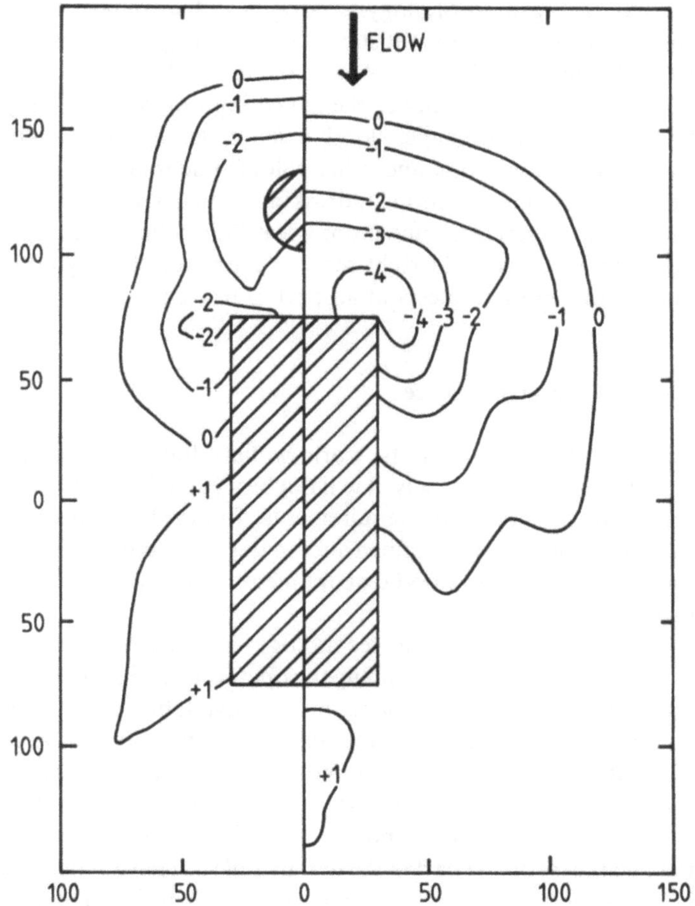

Figure 8.9 A pair of half-plans showing model scour tests: a freestanding pile upstream has reduced the amount of scour. Dimensions are in millimetres; contours are depth of scour (after Ibrahim, 1982.)

particular problem. Figure 8.9 shows the results of a model study. The right half of the figure shows the scour and deposition pattern at a blunt-nosed pier, and the left half the modified pattern produced by placing a cylindrical protective pile upstream of the main pier.

8.6 River management

It will be seen from the foregoing that the river engineer must be competent (or at least capable of taking advice) in the professional disciplines of: civil engineering (soils and structures); economics; electrical engineering; geography; geology; geomorphology; hydraulics; hydrology; hydrogeology; mechanical engineering; and statistics. The river engineer must also have a sensitive understanding of the uses to which rivers and river waters are put and of the likely environmental impact of engineering works on: amenity; angling; commercial fisheries; drainage; flood defence; landscape design; military strategy; nature conservation and other wildlife issues; navigation; pollution; recreation; and water abstraction for drinking, industry, irrigation, and power. Each use has its adherents, some more vocal than others. The secret of river management is to arrive at the right decision every time, having taken account of the often conflicting interests of all parties having legitimate interests.

8.7 Operation and maintenance

The best engineering design in the world will not fulfil its purpose if it is not maintained properly. Conversely, it will not be a good design if it does not take full account of the operators' requirements. Pumped systems in particular must be capable of being maintained and, to this end, access must be available. The same applies to raised flood embankments, which may need to be mown and inspected regularly.

Sophisticated communication technology is available these days and, if properly designed, can greatly simplify the operators' tasks and thereby reduce running costs. Access for maintenance must be available, and the possibility of checking by remote control from the operating centre should be considered.

The layout of ladders, walkways, handrails, etc., for the safe access of staff to work on river control structures is sometimes a bone of contention between operator and designer. It should not be; such problems could be eliminated by a greater awareness on the part of the designer of the relevant health and safety regulations aided by the rigorous application of 'what if' methods.

The capital cost of a project, although large, is a once-only event. Running costs often increase during the lifetime of a structure, and the irritation caused by a badly designed job may lead to a 'don't care' attitude amongst the operators which persists long after the perpetrator has disappeared and which impairs the efficiency of the works.

8.8 Investment appraisal

An essential part, some would say the most important part, of the promotion of a capital project is the appraisal of the client's initial investment proposals. Public money must not only be wisely spent, but it must be seen to be wisely spent.

An appraisal may be carried out in four stages, and at the end of each stage the persons undertaking the appraisal must have the power and the will to take the appropriate decision. This may conflict with the designer's wishes and will, on occasion, result in the abortion of a project.

8.8.1 *Feasibility*

A feasibility study is primarily an exercise in benefit assessment. The problem to be solved must be identified. Possible options must be selected, and the approximate costs of construction estimated. To set against these, the benefits to the community must be quantified, and a comparison made between the costs and the benefits. Proposals which are shown at this stage not to be worthwhile must either be re-examined to find a cheaper solution or abandoned altogether.

8.8.2 *Full appraisal*

The promoter, having satisfied himself that a problem exists and that there is a worthwhile solution to it, must now examine all possible options with a view to selecting the best. Some design work will be needed on all options, and it may appear to the shortsighted that this is wasteful of effort: this is not so. Small amounts of money spent to eliminate unwanted options may save very large amounts later by helping to choose the right path at this critical stage in a project's life.

Included on the 'costs' side of the balance must be: design costs, excluding the cost of appraisal, since that is money which will already have been spent by the time the decision is taken to proceed or not; running costs for the predicted lifetime of the project, discounted back to 'present values'; and construction costs, also discounted (Parker *et al.*, 1988).

The 'benefits' will include: direct benefits, such as flooding damage avoided; and indirect benefits, such as the avoidance of disruption to commerce and communications. Intangible benefits, such as the avoidance of anxiety, are usually omitted from the monetary calculations, but it is legitimate to draw attention to them in the text of the appraisal report (Penning-Rowsell and Chatterton, 1977).

The avoidance of danger to life is also usually excluded, since it is almost impossible to quantify, but, again, if the proposed works would indeed alleviate this danger, then mention should be made of it in the text.

8.8.3 *Preconstruction appraisal*

At the time when the detailed design of the favoured option has been completed, tenders have been received, and a reliable estimate of cost is available, there is an opportunity to pause and consider the implications of proceeding further. It is probably the last chance to avoid major capital expenditure, and the promoter must be sure he is embarking on a wise course of action. If the data used in the earlier appraisal are still valid and the conclusions reached then still hold good, the contract should be let and the works implemented.

8.8.4 *Post-construction appraisal*

Sometimes investments made by a public body are reviewed after completion, either internally or by the national auditor, the EEC, the World Bank, etc. The appraisal may be carried out immediately after completion of the project with a view to assessing the contractor's or the design engineer's performance, and to test the accuracy of the estimating and the quality of workmanship. Alternatively, it may be desired to assess the accrual of benefit over a fairly long period. Benefits of agricultural drainage schemes in particular may not materialise fully for a year or even several years. An appraisal may be carried out after such a time lag to test the overall worth of the investment.

It is too much to expect this to be done even for half of an authority's completed schemes, and it would, in any event, be wasteful of staff resources to do so; but some projects should be reviewed in this way by every well-managed organisation. An appropriate proportion might be one project in 10, but even this is rarely achieved.

8.9 Design

Many aspects of the design of river engineering projects have already been touched upon in the foregoing sections and in the accompanying chapters. Other common techniques with which the designer must be familiar also deserve a mention.

8.9.1 *Return periods*

It could be argued that all engineering design consists of balancing risk against cost, and this is particularly true of river engineering. In flood defence terms, the greater the expenditure the higher the return period which can be safely accommodated, i.e. the lower the risk.

It might be appropriate at this point to give a definition of return period: it is the interval between events of similar severity averaged over a very long time. Clearly it is not practicable to keep records which allow many 1000-year events to be analysed for the same location. Suffice it to say that statistical techniques exist to make meaningful extrapolations of hydrometric records. These are discussed in Chapter 1. Typical design return periods which have been adopted for fluvial flooding are:

Agricultural land	5 years
High-grade agricultural land with scattered housing	50 years
Densely populated areas	100 years

There is a commonsense rule of thumb which says that flooding of populated areas should not be allowed to happen more than once in a lifetime. One has an instinctive feeling that this might be right, but such rough and ready measures will not satisfy the members of an appraisal panel. A proper optimisation exercise should be conducted to select the return period which gives the best value for money.

8.9.2 *Flood storage*

The creation of a 'box' into which to divert flood water until such time as an existing river system can safely accommodate the outflow is often an attractive alternative to major channel-widening schemes. This applies particularly where a town is at risk of flooding and the river flows through developed areas. The storage can be on-line, which is to say impounded in the natural valley, or off-line, that is diverted to a riverside reservoir. Either way, the best value is obtained by exploiting flood forecasting techniques and by remote sensing of hydrometric installations and remote operation of controls or, even better, automatic operation with remote sensing and manual over-ride. A similar concept is discussed with respect to sewer systems in section 5.4.2.

The storage reservoir may contain a permanent shallow depth of water to create wetlands, or it may be dry and put to agricultural or recreational use for most of the time. Such a reservoir must, by definition, contain a large amount of empty space. A flood storage reservoir which is full of water when the flood peak is approaching is of no use to anyone.

Flood storage schemes involve either a large land take or high levels of compensation or both. Methods are available to acquire land and/or the right to flood it (Wakelin *et al.*, 1987).

8.9.3 *Flood embankments*

Many, perhaps most, river engineering projects involve the construction of embankments in one form or another. The established techniques applicable to earth dams should be employed in their design and construction. As in the case of earth dams, it is normally assumed that the embankment will only be over-topped under the most extreme conditions. However, there are situations in which it may be desirable to allow controlled flow over the embankments, either to activate the flood storage mentioned in the previous section, or to direct stored water back into the river system. In these circumstances the relevant sections of the embankments should be designed effectively as large, broad-crested side weirs. In the past, the practice would have been to use rubble or stone embankments at such locations, but nowadays, modern geotextiles allow the use of more environmentally pleasing, reinforced grass embankments. National or local legislation may apply to the safety of embankments, and here again the engineer should seek appropriate advice.

8.9.4 *Steel sheet piling*

Ugly they may be, but steel sheet piles are indispensable to the river designer for temporary and permanent works. It would be difficult to imagine how to tackle many temporary river engineering tasks without them, particularly the construction of cofferdams. For permanent works such as retaining walls, they are not indispensible but will often provide the cheapest way to form a vertical wall. In many instances, such as pumping station foundations, steel sheet piles can be used both for temporary cofferdamming and, later, as part of the permanent structure.

There has never been a wholly satisfactory solution to the problem of corrosion. Special steels and various applied coatings are available. One simple expedient is to overdesign the piles and let them go rusty.

8.9.5 *Erosion control*

The market place contains a bewildering variety of proprietary erosion-control systems. Some are good, some are expensive, some are both. The main types are summarised in Table 8.1. When erosion control is provided in the form of a revetment, this must be flexible so as to accommodate small movements in the foundation. It must be permeable so that pore water pressures cannot build up under 'rapid drawdown', conditions, but it must also prevent the leaching of fine materials. Geotextiles are increasingly used for this purpose (Hemphill and Bramley, 1989).

It is unusual, sea defences apart, to experience heavy wave action in river engineering, although some flood storage reservoirs do have a considerable fetch when full. Whatever the design wave conditions, the revetment should be massive enough to accommodate any predicted wave comfortably. Wave height is a function of wind speed and fetch, and so evaluation or measurement of these parameters along with a chosen factor of safety allows calculation of a design wave height. In Britain such a procedure is given in ICE (1978). It may be necessary further to protect the embankments of storage reservoirs by the use of riprap (Thompson and Shuttler, 1976).

The use of revetment downstream of river control structures has already been mentioned. The turbulent zones here are often inadequately protected against bed and bank scour (see section 8.5).

8.9.6 *Telemetry*

Several references to telemetry have already been made but it is re-emphasised here, since, in operational terms, it is a tool which is very much at the development stage. The intrinsic difficulties of managing a river system are the remoteness of installations and the low density of operational staff on the ground (particularly in rural areas). The next generation of telemetry

Table 8.1 Bed and bank protection

Concrete	Present or future groundwater or river water may required sulphate-resisting concrete (see also below)
Timber	Popular for bank protection despite liability to rotting and to vandals. Softwood needs pressure treatment. Has been used for beds of small streams and inverts of tunnels. When still in place should be treated with care when cleaning or altering the system
Faggot bundles, posts, and logs	Used for minor works and repairs. Willow may sprout into permanent trees
Fascines	Formerly used for banks and sometimes for repairing scour holes in beds: when still in place must be taken into consideration. (Fascines are woven mattresses of osiers or the like; they are either pegged down or weighted with stones; the osiers were often grown specially)
Geotextiles	Useful for banks and possibly for beds; must be pegged down, dug in, or secured to beams. If torn loose, a whole sheet will be lost. Must be protected from traffic and animals. Maintenance requires care. Can be grassed down
Sandbags	Used in emergency to heighten banks and for repairs for breaches and scourholes. Can be filled with concrete to give a permanent repair
Rockfill, gravel, concrete dolines	Used for weighting and protection of geotextiles and fascines and as riprap for protection against waves. Flexible, easy to maintain if layer is thick enough. Rockfill and gravel may weather. Could be introduced to the bed to increase the particle size to provide armouring; maintenance would then require care. Also used as cheap bank protection, often unsatisfactorily. Used in emergencies to fill scour holes. Care is needed lest the rock size be too small
Stone pitching	Used for bed and bank lining. Useful as a permeable filter downstream of solid works. May be partly grouted
Concrete blocks	As stone pitching, but must be laid close together on a relatively impermeable foundation. Gaps may be open, gravel-filled or sealed. Smoother than stone pitching. Loss of one block permits its neighbours to move, but interlocking type is more secure
Cable-tied concrete blocks	More expensive, more secure and less demanding than untied blocks. Can be laid under water
Cellular concrete blocks	Useful for banks and possibly for beds. Often need anchoring by interlocking arrangements or cabling. Grass may be grown in the cells to improve the appearance of the works
Masonry, brickwork	Used for retaining walls and for lining banks and beds. Bricks may need to be sulphate-resisting
Concrete slabs	Used for banks and beds, especially in urban areas, in new cuts and downstream of weirs. Minimise channel width. Require a sound foundation and careful design. Dispersive clay can move up through the joints leading to failure
Asphalt, etc.	An alternative to concrete slabs. More flexible. Minor cracks may be easier to seal. May be made either permeable or impermeable

Table 8.1 Cont'd.

Sheet steel piles and steel sheet trenching	Used for bank protection. Corrosion must be considered, e.g. by increased thickness, galvanising or coating with tar, epoxy paint, etc.
Concrete piles	Used for bank protection
Mass concrete	Used for retaining walls and other structures
Reinforced concrete	Prefabricated units may be suitable for retaining walls, but method of construction must be considered
Rolled concrete	Might be considered for major repairs to banks or beds. Would have to be constructed in the dry
Soil stabilisation	Has been considered for protection of sandy or silty beds in minor schemes. Construction and maintenance would require care
Gabbions	Popular for banks. Used for bed protection both generally and downstream of concrete slabs. Could be used as a subvertical permeable filter downstream of retaining walls. Could be used in emergencies to fill breaches and scour holes, especially when the available rockfill is too small.
Crib walls	Concrete and timber types are used for banks
Puddle clay	Used in the past to line beds and banks. Maintenance requires care. Drying out sometimes leads to cracking. Points where a main river or canal passes over a smaller waterway are particularly vulnerable to breaching
Plants	Subaqueous plants provide little protection but much obstruction; reeds protect the bank from waves, but their roots need protection, and they constrict the channel. Floating vegetation avoids the root problem but may be dangerous. Osiers, willow and alder reinforce the bank but require regular maintenance. Grass protects and reinforces the soil, but must be continuous and tussock-free. All plants take time to establish.

equipment should, if properly applied, be capable of earning major cost savings in both capital and revenue terms.

8.9.7 *Confined spaces*

Many unnecessary deaths result from the neglect of the rules for working in confined spaces. A confined space is defined as a place where there is a possibility of a lack of oxygen or an accumulation of dangerous fumes, probably explosive and possibly poisonous. The two principal routes by which these gases enter confined spaces are from the soil/rock and from the water. Sometimes the rate of entry is minute, and the danger arises because the gases have been allowed to accumulate. Prediction of the risk appears to be virtually impossible and all actions must be based on the assumption that the danger is present.

The principal rules are: the atmosphere of a confined space must be tested by a competent and authorised person before entry; monitoring must be continuous whilst the space is occupied; smoking is forbidden; electrical plant, etc., including camera flashguns, must be flameproof; breathing apparatus, ropes and trained rescuers must all be available before anybody enters such spaces.

In brief, in addition to taking such predictive and preventive measures as are possible, the designer's duties are:

(1) To ensure adequate, permanent and continuous ventilation.
(2) To prevent unauthorised entry.
(3) To provide written instructions for both managers and operators.
(4) If necessary, to provide housing for monitoring instruments, breathing apparatus, safety ropes.
(5) If necessary, to provide telecommunications and escape routes.

8.9.8 *Safety*

The safety of employees, both engineer's and contractor's, and the safety of the public should be matters of direct concern to every designer and every site engineer. In many countries engineers can be held criminally liable if they have failed to make contractors take adequate precautions, or even if they have not prevented contractors following dangerous practices. River engineers must have a working knowledge of the local and national safety legislation.

8.9.9 *Energy dissipation*

Turbulence can be damaging, and the water flowing over a river control structure can acquire large amounts of kinetic energy as it loses potential energy. This unwanted energy must be dissipated before the water is allowed to emerge into an unprotected river. Usually this is achieved by some form of stilling basin within the structure. If the basin within the structure is deep enough, the energy of the falling water will be absorbed in the relatively static water. Baffle blocks in the floor of the basin will allow it to achieve the same effect but at shallower, and hence less costly, depth (Blaisdell, 1948, 1949; Bradley and Peterlea, 1957; White *et al*., 1989).

8.9.10 *Models*

Two type of models are used for studying river engineering problems. Both are very useful in their own way and can often save many times their cost by avoiding abortive work.

The physical model is, as the name suggests, a scale model constructed in an engineering laboratory and used to investigate a variety of problems such as river flooding, potential flood alleviation, scour around bridge piers and river control structures. Although most appropriate for compact projects, very large physical models are sometimes built.

The mathematical or numerical model is a computer model and is used where appropriate instead of a physical model. Studies of all types of problems are carried out, such as river capacity and flood plain flow distribution, sediment transport, pollution and unsteady-state analysis. See Chapters 6 and 7 for further details of mathematical models.

8.9.11 *Environmental assessments*

Virtually every river project has an impact on the environment. Society no longer accepts harsh, environmentally unsympathetic designs. More and more engineers find themselves working as part of a multi-disciplinary team including, for example, botanists and zoologists, at all stages of the design and execution of a project. This trend has to be welcomed, but it is incumbent on educators and professional engineering bodies to ensure that young engineers are sufficiently aware of environmental issues to be able to contribute in other than a purely technical role to projects; in many countries legislation requires the preparation of environmental audits to be undertaken at a very early stage within a project.

Clearly a responsible river engineer should prepare a design which is sympathetic to the environment. Inevitably, however, conflicts of interest will arise. These can sometimes take the form of disagreements between environmental groups. Whenever conflicts arise, every effort should be made by the parties involved to arrive at a mutually acceptable compromise especially as the alternative will almost certainly involve lengthy court cases or government arbitration.

9 Pumped drainage

P. COOK

9.1 Introduction

Pumped drainage will be considered where it is necessary to improve agricultural production limited by high water levels and where floods damage urban areas or prevent the development of such areas. The installation and operation of a pump involves expense comprising initial capital cost and subsequent running costs. If it is possible to obtain satisfactory water levels using natural or gravity flow, then this is likely to be cheaper on both counts.

Water may be maintained at a low level economically where it is possible to isolate the area concerned and pump only that water that falls as rain. The area improved by lower water levels may be called the benefit area, and the area draining to the pump the catchment area. For the greatest economy the two areas should be as nearly coincident as possible. There may be seepage into the pumped area from adjoining land, and occasionally drainage from land outside the catchment has to be accepted into the pumped area. In this case a careful assessment must be made of the flow, which is termed foreign water, and an allowance made when calculating the necessary pump size.

9.2 Benefits

Whether a pumping scheme is to be financed by a private company or a public authority, the persons financing the scheme will need to be satisfied that the anticipated benefits exceed the cost of the work. To obtain a true comparison the total costs must be compared with the total benefits, even in those cases where different persons or bodies pay for various parts of the scheme. The costs include:

Purchase price of pump and motor.
Construction of pumping station.
Construction or modification of approach and discharge channels.
Cost of attendance on pump and weed screen clearing.
Fuel, oils and greases.
Maintenance including overhauls at intervals.

Secondary or pipe drainage.

Purchase price of machinery to farm the improved land or the cost of developing the improved area.

The benefits may be calculated by one of two methods, or in some cases by both. If the pump makes land available for agricultural production or improves production, then the value of the increased crop produced annually must be calculated. In a developed urban area the value of the damage caused by flooding must be assessed and coupled with the frequency of such flooding to produce an average annual cost of flooding. Where the installation of the pump will permit land to be developed, the value of the undeveloped land may be compared with the value of land suitable for development; however, this is frequently difficult to determine and it may be necessary to assess the cost of flood damage assuming the land was fully developed.

Whichever method is appropriate, the value of the anticipated benefits or the value of damage avoided as a result of the installation of a pump must be compared with the total cost of the pumping station. This may be done by using a discount factor to compare the value of money spent now with the value of benefits to be received in future years. The discount factor is

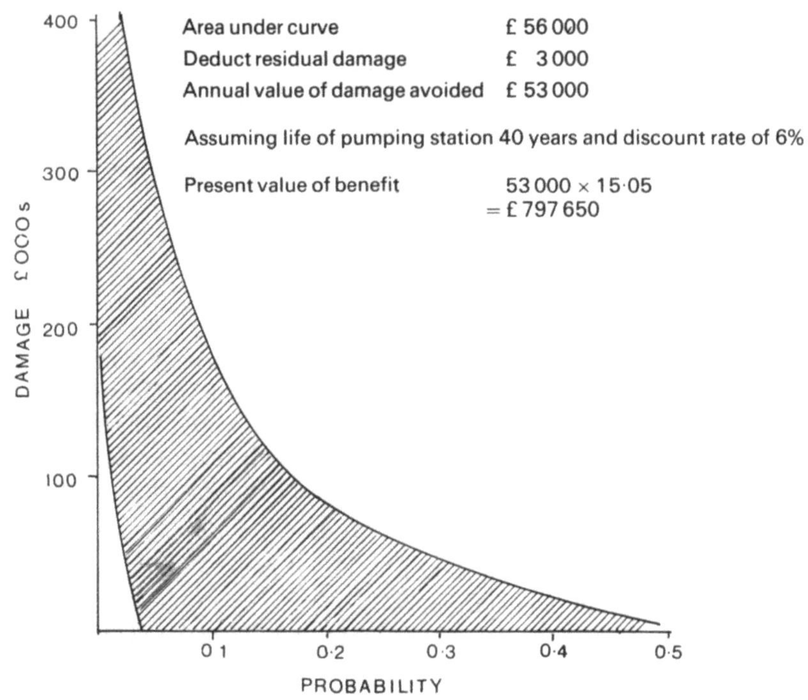

Figure 9.1 The damage probability relationship.

usually related to the general interest rate except where a political decision has been made that it should be otherwise.

It is sometimes necessary at a very early stage to make a rough assessment of the benefit–cost relationship in order to decide whether it is worthwhile to invest money and man–hours on designing a pumping station. A rough estimate of the benefits may be obtained as in the following example. (For further details see section 7.15 and Penning-Rowsell and Chatterton, 1977.)

Example

A group of houses floods on average every third year, and the cost of the damage is £166 200. The average annual value of damage is therefore £166 200/3 = £55 400. In this case the discount factor is 6% and the expected life of the pumping station 30 years. From actuarial tables (valuation tables) is will be found that the present value of an annuity of £1 per annum is £13.765, hence the present value of the benefits is £55 400 × 13.765 = £762 581. If the preliminary rough estimate of the cost of the pumping station is less than this figure then it is likely to be a worthwhile project.

The inaccuracies in this method are obvious, and a more accurate method would involve plotting the flood levels and relating these to a return period, then assessing the value of damage against each return period. It must be remembered that the pumping station will have a maximum capacity which will be exceeded by rare events and the houses will still be flooded on these very rare occasions.

Example (see also Figure 9.1)

A pumping station is to be constructed to deal with floods up to the 60-year frequency. The following table shows the value of damage caused by floods of the corresponding return period:

Return period years	Probability	Damage in pounds
50	0.02	400 000
20	0.05	300 000
10	0.1	170 000
6	0.2	80 000

The value of damage that will occur in the event of a flood exceeding the capacity of the pumping station is calculated and plotted. The area between the two curves represents the value of the annual damage avoided, which will be discounted over the period of the life of the pumping station, as before, to show the present value of damage avoided.

9.3 Design

There is rarely a unique solution to any land drainage problem, but usually one solution will emerge as having advantages over all others. The designer of a scheme for pumped drainage will probably be required to produce a report for those who will finance the scheme. This report must start with a clear statement of the object to be attained, and should be written in terms intelligible to a layman but with sufficient technical evidence to satisfy any engineer to whom it may be referred. The report should be arranged in a logical sequence and the following headings are suggested:

Statement of the problem.
Basic assumptions and data on which the engineer's solution is based.
Details of investigation carried out and design criteria adopted.
Alternative solutions considered with reasons for their rejection.
Description of recommended solution.
Estimates of cost and time for construction.
Conclusions and recommendations.

Catchment areas may be determined from published contour maps. In most schemes for pumped drainage, and invariably in polder situations, a detailed level survey will be needed. For large schemes in inaccessible areas this may be more economically carried out from the air. In good conditions an aerial survey should produce a map with contours at 0.5 m intervals and an accuracy of ± 0.1 m.

The position of dams to isolate the area to be pumped may be determined from the survey. Where water courses which would bring water from adjoining land into the area to be pumped are dammed, alternative channels must be provided to convey this water around the pump area to a satisfactory outfall. Care must be taken when isolating the pumped area not to damage the interests of adjoining landowners or expensive litigation may result.

Where geological maps are published for the area, these should be used to determine the nature of the subsoil. Frequently a site investigation will be required to supplement this information, particularly at the site of the proposed pumping station, where the bearing qualities of the soil must be assessed. The permeability of the soil should be estimated to ensure that the seepage from adjoining areas is not significant. In areas of stable soil and a head difference of 2 m or less, earth dams having 1 m top width and slopes of 1 vertical to $1\frac{1}{2}$ horizontal are sufficient to isolate the area.

In a polder situation it will be necessary to decide at an early stage whether the area should drain to one pumping station or whether the polder may be subdivided into small catchments each with a small pump. The first method has the advantage of low cost but the disadvantage of a higher pumping head because of the backwater effect of a long approach channel. The second method has the advantages that the approach channels may be relatively shallow and pumping heads low; also there is some flexibility to vary the water levels according to cropping or development within the area. The disadvantage is the higher initial cost of constructing several stations.

Local subsidence or earth movement may result in a river flooding large areas. In this case the cost of pumping the full flow of the river must be compared with the cost of embanking the river and pumping drainage water from both sides into the embanked channel. If the former option is adopted then a spillway channel must be provided to carry any flow that exceeds the capacity of the pumping station.

If the pump can be situated at the lowest point of the catchment then a number of difficulties are avoided. In some places, such as deltaic regions and some estuaries, repeated flooding with deposition of silt has caused the banks of the river to be higher than the land more remote. If the pump is situated on the bank of the river, then a long and deep approach channel must be constructed. Alternatively, the pump may be situated some distance from the river at a low place and a discharge channel constructed to carry the water to the river. Deep channels should be avoided, especially where bank stability problems occur. Two-stage pumping may also be considered with the pumps several kilometres apart; then the cost of the additional station must be compared with the cost of additional excavation and possible revetment of the banks.

While the discharge from a pump to a substantial channel will usually only cause a very small increase in water level, this increase should be calculated. Care should be taken that landowners abutting the discharge channel are not disadvantaged by the pumps or compensation may be required.

A gravity discharge by sluice or flap valve should be included, even if this will only permit gravity discharge at a high level, so that the consequences of flooding will be minimised if the pumps fail through mechanical fault, or non-arrival of fuel or of personnel.

9.4 Pumping head

In any catchment there will be one critical point, often but not always the lowest point in the catchment, which will control the highest permissible water level. In any urban catchment, this may be an arbitrary depth below lowest ground level, or a depth which will permit the lowest drainpipe to discharge. In an agricultural catchment, damage to crops must be avoided, in particular damage to the roots of the crop by high water levels. Various crops have various rooting depths, and the most vulnerable period for damage is usually winter and early spring. If the land concerned has been underdrained, either by mole drainage or by pipe drains, then ideally water levels should be arranged so that these discharge freely. In certain stable soils, submergence of underdrains for up to 24 hours will not cause damage.

In reclamation areas where soils are to be underdrained, find the level of the critical point and subtract the minimum depth of cover of the underdrains, then allow a fall along the drain of, say, 0.05–0.1% to obtain the depth of the drain outfall.

Example

Low land level (LLL)		12.1 m above datum
Minimum drain depth	0.70	
250 m from LLL to outfall @ 0.1%	0.25	
	0.95	0.95
Level of drain outfall		11.15 m above datum

From the level of the outfall, a backwater curve may be plotted to the proposed pumping station to determine the highest permissible water level at the pumping station. It may be necessary to repeat this procedure for several places to find the critical point. The designer should bear in mind that there may be small areas of land so low that it is uneconomic to provide the same freeboard as for the majority of the area. If the catchment contains organic soils which may oxidise and shrink, then the drop likely to occur during the life of the pumping station must be estimated and the sill made sufficiently low. In such cases it may be cheapest to dig drains to suit the present land level and to lower them by periodic resectioning as required. In this case, the pumping station sill may include a few courses of brickwork, which are easily knocked out when resectioning.

The total head against which the pump must operate is given by the expression (Figure 9.2):

$$H = H_s + H_d + H_f + \frac{v^2}{2g} \tag{9.1}$$

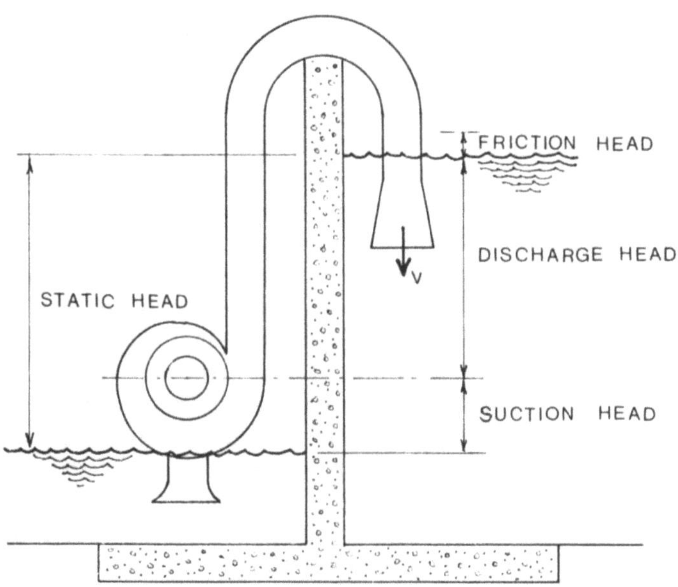

Figure 9.2 Elements of pumping head.

where H is the total head, H_s is the suction head, H_d is the discharge head, H_f is frictional losses and v is the velocity at discharge.

Most rotodynamic pumps are suction-sensitive, and the suction head should be kept to a minimum; frequently the impeller will be below still water level on the suction side. The pressures at all points in the suction and discharge piping should be estimated by Bernoulli's theorem to ensure that at no point, particularly within the pump casing, does the pressure fall close to the vapour pressure of the liquid pumped or cavitation may result. Land drainage water is usually corrosive to some extent, and cavitation will rapidly erode the impeller blades and their shroud.

When the pump is operating, the discharge head is the net distance from the impeller to the discharge water level; but a siphonic discharge (see Figure 9.2), necessitates that, on starting, the pump must lift water to the crest of the siphon and at a sufficient rate to evacuate the air, thus completing the siphon. The pump discharge has a residual velocity head, some of which may be reclaimed by the use of a tapered conical outlet pipe carried beneath the surface of the liquid. A taper of 1 in 10 is frequently adopted.

The pump will cause a drawdown of the water level adjacent to the station. Even where the approach channel is of substantial cross-section, the upstream limit of the drawdown is relatively close; for example, at Newborough Pumping Station there is no discernible fluctuation in the water level 3.7 km upstream of the station to indicate whether the pump is operating or not (Beran, 1982). Storage volume for the pump should therefore be located close to the station, and this is frequently done by widening the approach channel, which has the added benefit of reducing scour. With electrically driven pumps, substantial savings can be achieved by operating only at off-peak periods, hence the storage volume must be sufficient to contain the runoff between these periods. This is best designed by plotting the backwater curves at both switch-off and switch-on levels, and using the cross-sectional areas of the approach channel to determine the volume. When designing the secondary channels feeding the main discharge channel, it is usually sufficiently accurate to assume that the water level is parallel to the bed level, hence the Manning equation can be used in the form:

$$v = \frac{m^{2/3} i^{1/2}}{n} \tag{9.2}$$

where i is the slope of the channel bed (dimensionless), v is velocity ($\mathrm{m\,s^{-1}}$), m is the hydraulic mean depth (m), and n is the roughness coefficient (rugosity factor).

In polder situations where the channels are well maintained, n may be taken as 0.03, and for smaller channels or those less well-maintained as 0.04 (see Table 4.7 for further values). These are only average values, since the actual value of rugosity varies substantially with the amount of weed growth. The roughness coefficient also varies with hydraulic mean depth, hence the

Manning equation gives an approximate value, and it is suggested that the Colebrook White resistance law is used (Brandon, 1987) when greater accuracy is necessary.

9.5 Catchment discharge

In order to obtain a pump of suitable size, it is necessary to determine the discharge from the catchment at a particular return period. Ideally, the discharge from the catchment should be gauged and the results analysed by the methods shown in the Flood Studies Report (NERC, 1975). However, a minimum of 3 years record is required, preferably longer. Occasionally it is possible to obtain data from a similar catchment which can be adjusted to fit the catchment to be pumped. Usually the designer will have no alternative but to estimate the discharge from the catchment characteristics using the procedures given in the Flood Studies Report.

For small (150 hectares) urban catchments, the Wallingford modified rational method (NWC, 1981) may be used to assess peak runoff. However, for small agricultural catchments the original version of the rational formula is perfectly adequate. This in metric form is:

$$Q = \frac{C I A}{360} \tag{9.3}$$

where Q is the discharge ($m^3 s^{-1}$), C is the runoff coefficient, I is the rainfall intensity ($mm\,h^{-1}$) and A is the catchment area (ha). C must be assessed or selected from published tables (see section 1.4.5). I is the intensity of rainfall which will give the greatest runoff, and because the most intense rain occurs in storms of the shortest duration it is therefore necessary to decide on a certain design duration. The time taken for rain falling on the furthest part of the catchment to reach the point of outfall is called the time of concentration (T_c). The maximum runoff is unlikely to be reached until all the catchment contributes, hence T_c will be used as the duration of the storm. There are several formulae for T_c, but that derived by Kirpich (1940) is appropriate to small agricultural catchments:

$$T_c = 0.003245 \frac{L^{1.15}}{H^{0.385}} \tag{9.4}$$

where T_c is the time of concentration (h), L is the length of catchment (m) and H is the height of watershed above outfall.

From published rainfall records (Meteorological Office, 1964; NWC, 1981) in which intensity of rainfall is tabulated against return period and duration of the storm, read off the rainfall intensity, I. The return period appropriate to any particular scheme depends on the type of farming, hence the value of the damage that will be done by a flood.

A pump capable of dealing with the calculated discharge will usually be selected. This method is adequate in small catchments where many of the design parameters are approximate and the pump is a stock machine, not specifically designed for the task. It will be seen that because the design storm is of short period, the discharge calculated is a peak or almost instantaneous quantity, whereas a pump of the same capacity can discharge at this rate virtually indefinitely. However, it is likely that during the life of the pump there will occur precipitation which induces runoff greater than the capacity of the pump, in which case water levels higher than the permitted maximum will occur, and for this reason the motor and circuitry in the pumping station should be situated above flood level.

Because the time of concentration method depends on the slope of the catchment, it is inappropriate to a polder situation. Similarly, the equations in the Flood Studies Report are inappropriate, since among other reasons the stream frequency term is intended for natural catchments, and the man-made polders may yield a misleading figure. The following equation given in the Flood Studies Supplementary Report (NERC, 1978) will provide an approximate figure:

$$\bar{Q} = 0.00066\,\text{AREA}^{0.92}\,\text{SAAR}^{1.22}\,\text{SOIL}^{2.0} \tag{9.5}$$

where $\bar{Q}$ is the mean annual flood ($m^3 s^{-1}$), AREA is the catchment area (km^2), SAAR is the annual average rainfall (mm) and SOIL is an index determined from five standard soil types.

In the Fenlands of eastern England, most land drainage pumps in the 1960s and 1970s were designed to have a capacity of $0.14\,m^3\,s^{-1}\,km^{-2}$. In this area the mean average rainfall is around 600 mm. The high standard of drainage reflects the high value of cash crops which can be grown in the area, provided the water level is maintained at a sufficiently low level. In western England, a capacity of $0.09\,m^3\,s^{-1}\,km^{-2}$ has been used, although the mean annual rainfall is 800 mm. This represents a lower standard of drainage in a predominantly grassland area where some waterlogging will cause little damage.

Larger agricultural areas may be subdivided into smaller catchments and routed to the pumping station using usual flood routing methods. Alternatively, a modified version of the Flood Studies method may be used which employs a trapezoidal hydrograph more appropriate to land drainage than the triangular or peaked hydrograph. The method is set out in Brandon (1987, Chapter 6).

9.6 Selection of pump

Pumps for land drainage purposes must be capable of moving a large volume of water against a comparatively low head. A head of 2–3 m is common, and

5 m is rarely exceeded. Positive displacement pumps, either reciprocating or rotary, do not meet these requirements, and rotodynamic pumps are almost invariably used. Rotodynamic pumps are classified by the direction in which the pumped liquid passes through the impeller into three main types: (1) centrifugal or radial, (2) mixed flow, (3) axial flow.

Centrifugal pumps have a central inlet and a circumferential discharge. Some centrifugal pumps are arranged so that the volute cannot drain out and the pump is therefore self-priming. Larger installations must be primed before starting the pump, and in order to achieve this a sluice valve must be fitted in the discharge piping. With the sluice valve closed, a small auxiliary pump is used to exhaust the air from the pump casing, and the pump is started against a closed valve which is then gradually opened (Figure 9.3).

From the results of a pump test, the pump discharge may be plotted against the corresponding head; usually the power absorbed and the efficiency are plotted on the same graph. The shape of the head–discharge curve is known as the characteristic of the pump, and it is a feature of the centrifugal pump that the power absorbed increases with the discharge. In a land drainage situation, the head against which the pump operates will vary, hence the pump cannot always operate at maximum efficiency. The pump selected should however have an efficiency curve that peaks near the normal pumping range.

The characteristic of the axial-flow pump is entirely different from the centrifugal. The head–discharge curve tends to be steeper but, more importantly, the power absorbed becomes greater as the discharge decreases. For this reason it is unwise to include a sluice valve on the discharge side in case the pump should be inadvertently started when the valve is closed, and discharge should be arranged through a 'flap' valve, by siphonic discharge or through a cascade. The axial-flow pump is suction-sensitive, and the pump should be designed so that the impeller is always below water level if possible. It is unlikely to operate successfully with a suction head exceeding 1 m. The tube-type casing and open impeller enable the pump to pass small objects in suspension which get through the bars of the weed screen. The vertical-spindle, axial-flow pump has the great advantage that the impeller can be located below water level and the electric motor above flood level; furthermore, when the distance between the two is not large, pump and motor can be constructed as one integral unit, thus simplifying work on site.

The mixed-flow pump has an impeller and casing so designed that the flow is partly radial and partly axial. The characteristic of such a pump lies between the centrifugal and the axial type. It can be seen from Figures 9.3 and 9.4 that the head–discharge curve is less steep than that of the axial-flow pump and the power absorbed more constant over a wide range of discharge.

In a polder situation, the archimedean screw-type pump (Figure 9.5) has particular advantages. This pump comprises a metal spiral which revolves in a closely fitting sloping trough, usually of steel or concrete. The lower end

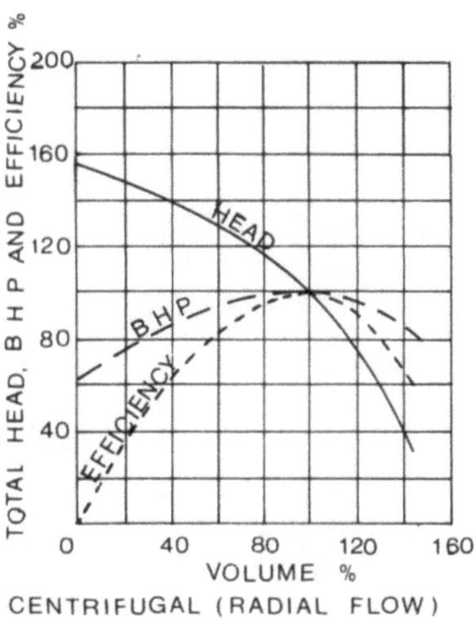

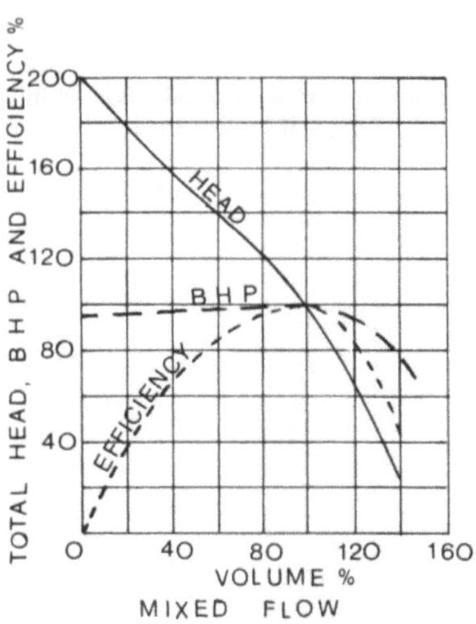

Figure 9.3 Typical pump characteristics (after Terry, NEI Allen Ltd).

of the spiral dips into the water to be pumped, and the spiral is revolved on its axis by a motor at the higher end. Near the top of the trough, a discharge weir is constructed. The advantages of this type of machine are that the motor is situated well above any major flood level and a motor of small power can be used because of the reduction gearing to the slow-moving spiral. It should be noted that, as the pump reduces the water level on the suction side, so the discharge decreases, and this can be very useful in areas where soils are unstable, because scour in the approach channel to the station is limited. The disadvantages are that, within narrow limits, the discharge

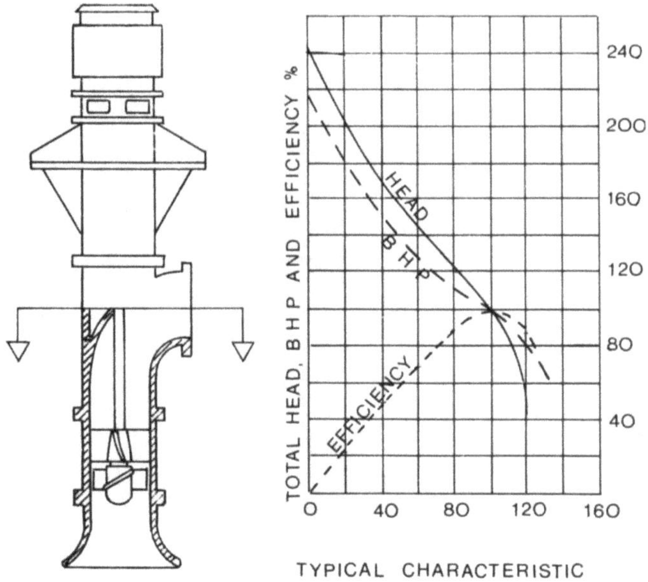

Figure 9.4 Part section through a trunk-suspended axial-flow pump with characteristic (after Terry, NEI Allen Ltd).

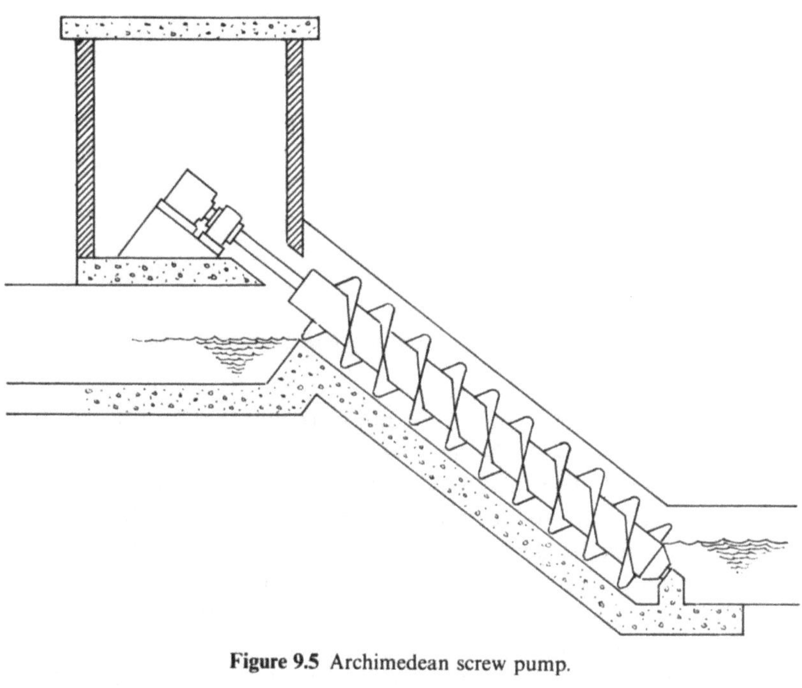

Figure 9.5 Archimedean screw pump.

level is fixed, hence the pump always works against the full head. Secondly, the trough requires very precise construction. Thirdly, the pump occupies a large area compared with other pumps of similar capacity, and the station must be constructed so that differential settlement does not occur.

Only for the very largest pumps is it economical to manufacture a unique machine. Most pump manufacturers produce a range of machines, and by matching stock impellers, motors and casings the whole range of likely requirements can be met. The advantage for the pump user is that spare parts tend to be readily available when required; furthermore, in some cases it is possible to obtain an identical replacement pump while the original is out of service. When the head–discharge range for each pump is plotted as an envelope, then a chart is produced from which the designer may select a machine appropriate to the duty. Because of the economy occasioned by the construction of a large number of pumps, the user may well find that it is cheaper to buy a 'stock' machine which nearly fits his requirements than to have a special machine manufactured to fit exactly.

Land drainage pumping stations with variable-speed motors have been constructed; similarly it is possible to fit variable pitch impellers, but in general such complications are not necessary, and they are accompanied by their own risk of failure. Sufficient flexibility can usually be obtained at any station by installing more than one pump and these of unequal size. Inevitably, two pumps cost more to install and run than one pump of equivalent total capacity. A designer would be well advised to discuss the proposed installation with the pump manufacturers, whose experience and advice may often be incorporated with advantage.

If pump manufacturers are to be invited to tender for the supply of land drainage pumps, then the following information should be provided.

Nature of liquid to be pumped. (Land drainage water may be acidic and usually contains suspended matter, both organic and mineral. This affects the material and blade spacing of the impeller.)

Number of pumps required.

Capacity of each pump.

Prime mover (diesel or electricity).

Whether the equipment will be enclosed or weatherproof.

Suction side—high water level.

Suction side—low water level.

Suction side—flood water level.

Discharge side—high water level.

Discharge side—low water level.

Discharge side—flood water level.

Motor floor level.

Duty working head.

Quantity at duty head.

9.7 Motive power

Before the advent of the steam engine, wind power was used to drive land drainage pumps of the scoop wheel variety, both in The Netherlands and in Great Britain. A large windmill produces only a modest amount of power, hence head or discharge is limited, but, more importantly, winds are fickle, making evacuation of water uncertain. Steam engines, particularly the compound engine, provide a satisfactory power supply, but the inefficiency of a steam plant makes it uncompetitive when compared with diesel or electricity, and even with mechanical stoking full-time attendance is required.

The slow-revving diesel engine with a massive flywheel coupled to a centrifugal or mixed-flow pump is still giving excellent service in many parts of the world. Modern diesel engines take up less space for the same amount of power, are faster revving and, when coupled through a gearbox, can drive any type of pump. With a bevel gearbox, a vertical-spindle pump can be driven. If large fuel storage tanks are provided at the pumping station, then deliveries of fuel may be infrequent. However, unless fuel is to be brought in by boat, an access track must be constructed. Given adequate storage, pumping will not be interrupted by storms which damage electricity supplies, and this can be important where lives are at stake in the benefit area.

Faster revving diesels tend to be noisy, which can make this an unsuitable source of power in an urban area. Air-cooled diesel engines require adequate ventilation, which may render the pumping station vulnerable to intruders. Air for combustion must be brought in and the exhaust taken out of the station. Many diesel-driven pumps start and stop automatically, depending on water levels; however, the system requires electricity, and storage batteries must be provided with means of recharging. An automatic diesel station therefore has a longer train of processes, with more opportunity for mechanical failure.

The diesel engine may be used as a prime mover, usually in the case of a large station, either where the electricity supply company cannot supply the power required or because the company are unwilling to install generating capacity to supply a land drainage pumping station which runs comparatively infrequently and hence yields insufficient revenue to recover the cost.

The electric motor as a prime mover has many advantages, the principal one being that it is compact compared with diesel motors of the same power. Where the motor can be directly coupled to the pump, and where the power supply will permit direct on-line starting, a simple machine results with few opportunities for failure. An electric motor on starting can absorb a large transient current, hence direct on-line starting may be prohibited by the power supply company because of the effect on the other electricity users. In this case, a stage resistance starter or a star-delta resistance must be incorporated. As with all inductive machines, the power factor must be considered, and larger motors will require a capacitor in the circuit. The pumps may be made to start and stop automatically depending on water levels, in smaller stations by means of a float switch and mercury contact or in larger stations by means of metal rods arranged so that the rising water level will complete a circuit and start the motor. A separate rod set at a lower level may be arranged to stop the motor. A recording ammeter is well worth fitting to an automatic station, since this may indicate problems which might otherwise go unnoticed and lead to expensive repairs. The record may show that the pump is switching on and off too frequently, which may indicate some obstruction on the weedscreen, sump or approach channel. Furthermore, an unusually high power consumption may indicate that the pump impeller has become entangled with weed or garbage. An overload preventor should be fitted, so that the motor is disconnected if the load becomes dangerously high. Similarly, a single-phase preventor is required, as is a thermal cut-out, which will again disconnect the motor if temperatures within the machine rise abnormally. The power supply to the pump can be connected to a time clock such that the pump operates only at off-peak, cheap-rate periods. Sufficient storage for water must be provided in this case.

9.8 The pumping station (Figure 9.6)

Once a suitable pump has been selected, the station is designed around the pump. The level of the floor of the sump will be 0.5 times diameter of the pump-suction bell mouth below the lowest water level on the suction side, unless the pump manufacturer recommends otherwise. Pumping stations are

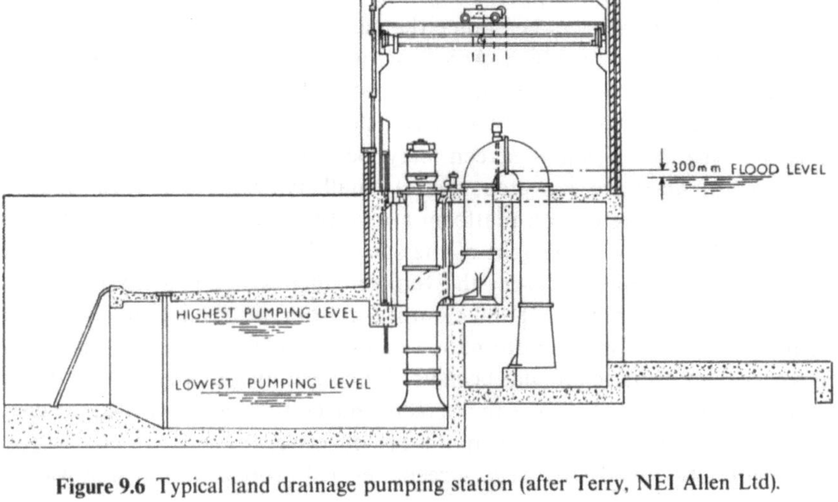

Figure 9.6 Typical land drainage pumping station (after Terry, NEI Allen Ltd).

usually built in saturated soil, and in excavating for the sump difficulties associated with water pressure may be anticipated. For this reason, the use of precast concrete boxes may be considered for small pumping stations, and for larger pumping stations interlocking sheet steel piles braced to form a cofferdam within which a reinforced concrete floor can be cast. The sheet piles must be designed to resist the active earth pressure, and provided they are of sufficient thickness and properly coated to resist corrosion they may be used to form the permanent walls of the sump. On completion of the station the sheet piles forming the wall abutting the approach channel are either withdrawn or burned off at sill level. Alternatively, in order to avoid civil engineering work in difficult ground conditions, the pump may be mounted either on or inside a floating pontoon and a hinged discharge pipe taken ashore and through or over the flood bank. The only difficulties likely to arise with such an arrangement are associated with the hinged or flexible discharge pipe and periodic desilting around and under the pontoon.

Before construction is undertaken, it is advisable to test a physical model of the proposed station with various scale water levels. The formation of vortices can be observed on the model and eliminated by the addition of non-structural concrete shapes into the sump or the erection of flat plates to guide water movement towards the pumps.

The velocity of flow at the entrance to the sump may be sufficient to scour earthbanks and drain bed, particularly when the water level is nearing switch-off point. Bed and bank protection may be required. However, if the approach channel to the pump is enlarged to provide storage, then this has a second benefit of reducing the approach velocity.

The spaces between the impeller blades will pass small-sized solids, but a screen will be required to exclude detritus and protect the machine. The bars should be close enough to exclude sizes that will not pass through the pump, and a spacing of 150 mm is fairly common. The bars should be strong enough to support the difference in head on either side of the screen should it become blocked with weed or rubbish. Any bracing members should be positioned well away from the bars so as not to impede the tines of the rake used to clean the screen. If the bars of the screen slope at approximately 70° it may be easily cleaned. A small screen may be raked by hand. Where large quantities of weed are expected, then a small hydraulic excavator may be converted to operate from a platform above the screen. This platform must be designed to carry the weight of the screen-clearing machine and the wet weed. It may also have to carry the vehicle which will cart away the matter removed from the screen. If the pump is automatic then there is a good argument for providing an automatic weed screen cleaner. A machine having tines on a continuous chain has been used successfully, but a grab-type bucket suspended from a rail above the screen and computer-controlled to clean each section of the screen in turn is more effective.

Immediately outside the weed screen, vertical grooves in the side walls of the sump will enable dam boards or stoplogs to be inserted and facilitate dewatering of the sump for maintenance purposes.

The discharge arrangements must prevent water running backwards through the pump when it is not operating. A simple flap valve over the discharge pipe is relatively cheap. If the valve is of cast iron and the discharge below water level, then care must be taken, because a sudden reversal of head when the pump stops may cause the valve to slam and possibly break. Valves comprising a sheet of rubberised canvas stiffened with metal bars have been used with success in such cases. One alternative to the flap valve is siphonic discharge. This has the advantage that once the siphon has been primed then the pump works only against the static head. Once the pump has stopped, water would siphon back into the pumped area if a siphon breaker valve is not included at the highest point. The siphon breaker valve may require a heater in order to prevent it from freezing. The discharge from the siphon may be conveniently arranged to be vertically downwards onto a flat concrete platform, and at the point of discharge a recovery tube or section of pipe of gradually increasing diameter can further increase the efficiency. Check that on starting the pump can produce a sufficient discharge at the crest of the siphon to evacuate the air and complete the siphon.

Where the discharge pipe leaves the pumping station, provision must be made for differential settlement, and the sections of the pipe should be joined with one of the proprietary joints which permit some movement. Wherever a pipe discharges to a channel there will inevitably be erosion in the vicinity on the opposite bank, which should be protected with riprap.

If the pump discharges by way of a long pipe, it is usually necessary to provide a surge chamber close to the pump, open-topped and sufficiently tall to permit a head of water to develop which will overcome the inertia of the water in a discharge pipe.

Submersible pumps, that is a pump and electric motor designed to operate below water level, may be installed in either a horizontal or a vertical position. Such a pump lying horizontally in a sump, discharging through a concrete flood wall and fitted with a non-return flap valve, permits a pumping station of very simple design. A station constructed with the motor shaft vertical has the advantage that the pump unit may be easily removed (Figure 9.7). The pump may be fitted either inside its own discharge pipe or outside. In the latter case, the pump and motor can be raised and lowered on guide rails, the foot of the discharge pipe being fitted with a lug, which engages in a recess on the pump and motor, to align and clamp them when lowered into position. If the pump is inside its own discharge tube, then a removable pressure-resisting lid must be fitted to allow the pump to be lifted out. Other advantages of submersible pumps are that the whole installation may be either submerged or below ground level with the exception of the electricity control panel, hence the station is unobtrusive; and the submerged motor is very quiet in operation and suitable for urban areas. In addition

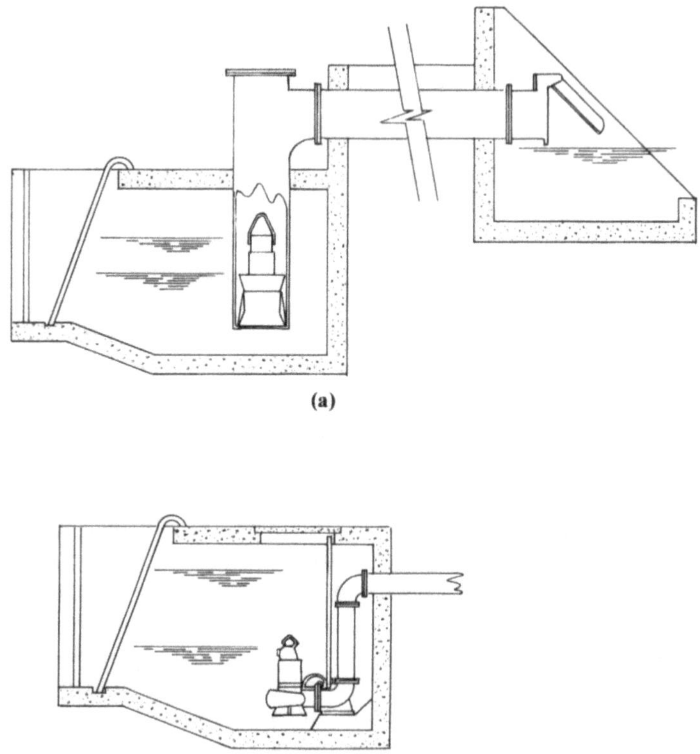

(a)

(b)

Figure 9.7 Pumping station with submersible pump (a) inside discharge tube; (b) outside discharge tube.

to the usual protection for an electric motor, submersible pumps must be fitted with sensors to detect the ingress of water.

A diesel-driven pump will need a pump house to protect it from the elements and to provide shelter for the attendant and equipment. If the pump and motor are enclosed in a pump house, then provision must be made for the removal of the pump and motor periodically for overhaul. A travelling crane of sufficient strength and height to lift the motor and pump and transport them to the door of the pump house will be required. Alternatively, if the roof or part of the roof is removable, then a mobile crane may be brought to site to lift out the pump when required.

The expense of providing a crane and pump house may be avoided if the pumps are driven by weatherproof electric motors. A pumping station without a pump house can make a much smaller impact on the landscape and be more acceptable in environmentally sensitive areas. The control

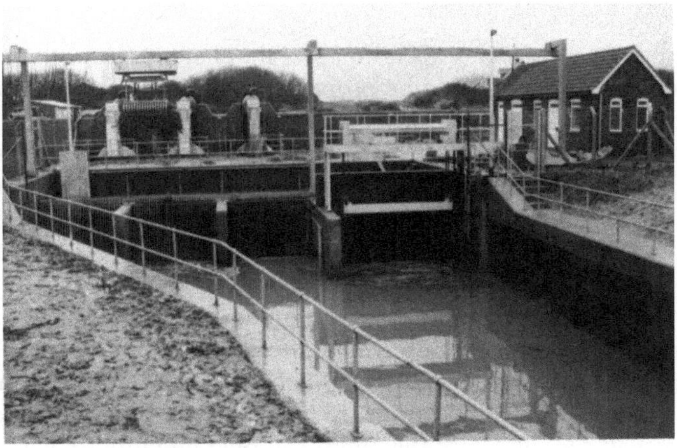

Figure 9.8 Land drainage pumping station with three weatherproof electric pumps, Bosker automated weed screen cleaner and, to the right, an alternative gravity outfall (courtesy of National Rivers Authority).

panel for the pump will require shelter, and a glass fibre or steel cabinet is adequate, although it provides no shelter for an electrician to do any work to the panel or room for the storage of spare parts or pumping record books.

It is possible to purchase a small land drainage pump installed in a polyethylene sump which requires only the construction of the suction and discharge arrangements on site. Medium-sized pumps will have the impeller close-coupled to the electric motor, but for the larger sizes a gearbox is necessary between the motor and the pump in order that the impeller speed should not be so great as to induce cavitation. For the exceptionally large stations, such as the Black Sluice Pumping Station, Boston, England, which has five pumps of over $11\,m^3\,s^{-1}$ capacity each, it was found cheaper to cast the volute of the vertical spindle pumps in concrete rather than produce iron casings. The shuttering for the concrete required very precise setting out and careful supervision of the concrete quality control.

As pumping stations are designed, certain safety precautions should be built in. Sheet-piled channels should have safety chains and a ladder in case personnel fall into the water. Weed screens should have a rail at the top of the screen to prevent persons overbalancing and falling into the water and a safety rail together with a harness to be used by anyone hand raking the screen. Within the station all electrical controls should be contained within an earthed cabinet which will automatically be isolated when the cabinet door is opened. Moving parts on pumps and motors should be enclosed with wire mesh screens to prevent loose clothing from becoming entangled.

9.9 Maintenance

It is essential for satisfactory operation that the channels on both the suction and the discharge sides should be properly maintained. Erosion may occur at the point of discharge and in the approach channel on the suction side, and if soils are very unstable then sheet steel piling may be necessary for some length. The approach channel on the suction side will have been designed using an appropriate roughness coefficient (commonly 0.03–0.04 in polder situations; see Table 4.7 and Chow, 1959), and it is necessary to ensure that the roughness is maintained to this standard. In temperate climates in summertime, transpiration and evaporation are sufficient to take away the average rainfall, but short-duration high-intensity storms will cause the pump to operate. In cooler winter weather, when crop growth is at a minimum, then less of the rainfall will be absorbed by evapotranspiration and a greater percentage will run off, hence the pump will operate more frequently. If the channels on the suction side of the pump have been cut to a satisfactory roughness coefficient, then the variation in roughness will be the result of weed growth on the banks. If the weed growth on the bank is annual, then in the summer it will be fairly soft and floods will temporarily flatten the growth. Annual maintenance will be required to ensure that thick strong plants do not survive from one year to the next, unless the channel has been designed with this in mind.

If, having made the usual assumptions, the equation of continuity is combined with the Manning equation, then the following equation results:

$$Q = A\frac{m^{2/3}i^{1/2}}{n} \qquad (9.6)$$

where Q is the discharge of the channel ($m^3 s^{-1}$), A is the cross-sectional area of the channel (m^2), m is the hydraulic mean depth, i is the slope of the channel (dimensionless) and n is the roughness coefficient (rugosity factor).

Considering for a moment a natural catchment with an inadequate channel which is required to carry a flow of Q_1, and assuming that whatever size the channel will be it is cut to the most economical section (Lewitt, 1958, p. 257), then m is in this sense a constant. In that case, if Q is to be increased then the cross-sectional area or the slope of the channel must be increased or the roughness coefficient must be decreased. It is to increase the slope of the channel, or more precisely the water slope, i, that a pump is introduced into the system. Having once fixed the slope of the channel, then in order to increase Q one may either increase the cross-sectional area or decrease the rugosity. If vegetation is permitted to grow without check, the roughness coefficient may be doubled or tripled (see Table 4.7). If the cross-sectional area were increased to compensate for this, then the area of land required for the channel would probably be excessive, hence there is really no alternative to restricting weed growth on the banks.

Similar remarks may apply to the bed of the channel, and growth in both areas may be controlled by spraying. Unfortunately many of the chemical sprays that control weed growth also damage the environment in other ways, and great care must be taken in the type of spray, the intensity of application and the time of year applied if unacceptable side effects are not to occur. Weed growth may also be controlled by mechanical cutters, and machines capable of running within the banks of a trapezoidal drain, cutting the weed and transporting it to the top of the bank where it may be later collected, operate successfully and very economically. Similarly, boats or pontoons with a scissors-type cutter bar shaped approximately or precisely to the channel can deal with underwater weed. Where channels are both irregular in section and sinuous, both the flail-type mower fitted to an agricultural tractor and the scissors-type cutter bar fitted to the arm of an hydraulic excavator are effective. In order to cause as little environmental impact as possible, the work should be done outside the breeding season for birds and small mammals; hence in temperate climates, autumn is suitable, and usually firm ground will be available for the machine to work on; furthermore, crops on adjoining fields will have been harvested. Weed growth in the channel can be limited naturally by encouraging trees which shade the waterway. Periodically the channel will require desilting, and this work, if done with knowledge and consideration, can enhance the environment. If desilting is carried out either from one side or the other alternately, or if the channel is divided into sections and the sections dealt with in different years in rotation, then small animals can find alternative homes. If channels can be made wider or deeper than required for land drainage purposes, fish breeding can be encouraged and plants necessarily removed in the narrow sections can be replanted in the wider spaces.

9.10 Control

Automatic multi-unit pumping stations are usually arranged so that one pump switches on at a predetermined level and the remaining pumps cut in successively if the level rises. The first pump to cut in is usually referred to as the duty pump, and by altering the electrodes controlling the switch it is possible to rotate the 'duty' around the pumps to equalise wear. It is apparent however that in the case of a summer storm the pumping station can only react as the flood peak arrives. With computer control it is possible to sample water levels in drains remote from the pumping station and evacuate some of the storage capacity before the flood peak arrives. This provides more accurate control of water level, particularly in the vicinity of the station. Such a control system is particularly useful where a number of small pumps discharge into a main drain which is itself pumped to sea. The operation of the smaller pumps can be made to trigger the operation of the main pump.

Various safety precautions must be taken with such a system to ensure that personnel are not in a position of danger when the pump is switched on remotely. The system can be extended such that the computer receives signals from raingauges in the catchment and can operate pumps in a certain sequence.

9.11 Flap-controlled gravity outlets

When the land surface approximates to high tide level or above, it is often possible to obtain a standard of drainage adequate for urban and agricultural areas by gravity alone. The discharge to the sea will be through a sluice comprising either a top-hung flap valve or side-hung pointing doors which open when the water inside is higher than that outside and close automatically as the rising tide reverses the head difference. Design of a tidal outlet will be illustrated by an example.

(1) Decide where the outfall is to be.
(2) At the site of the outfall, measure the height of the tide over a lunar day and plot against time. Repeat for critical conditions such as spring tides at equinoxes and neap tides between equinoxes, e.g. Figure 9.9(b).
(3) Decide the highest permissible water level in the storage area upstream of the sluice, e.g. 2.5 m above datum.
(4) Estimate the average inflow to this storage area, e.g. $13.5 \times 10^3\ m^3\ h^{-1}$.
(5) Calculate the volume of water in the storage area and plot against water level by survey, if storage exists, or from drawings if designing new storage, e.g. Figure 9.9(a)
(6) Plot the highest permissible water level on the falling limb of the tide curve (see Figure 9.9b). This is point A.
(7) Compute the level at which the sluice must close on the rising tide if point A is not to be higher than the permissible level. Procedure: from storage–water level curve determine volume in storage corresponding to highest permissible level. Deduct from this the flow in 1 hour and determine new level. Plot this level on the tide curve (Figure 9.9b) 1 hour to the left of point A. Repeat at hourly intervals until the line of plotted points intersects the rising limb of the tide curve at point B. Here the sluice will close at 0 hours 50 minutes, open at 5 hours 30 minutes and close again at 13 hours 15 minutes (C). Thus the sluice is open 7 hours 45 minutes per half-lunar day (approximately 12.5 hours).
(8) Find the outflow, e.g. $13.5 \times 10^3 \times 12.5/7.75\ m^3$
(9) Decide the level of the sill of the sluice to obtain the advantage of low tide but not so low that siltation problems occur and maintenance becomes difficult.

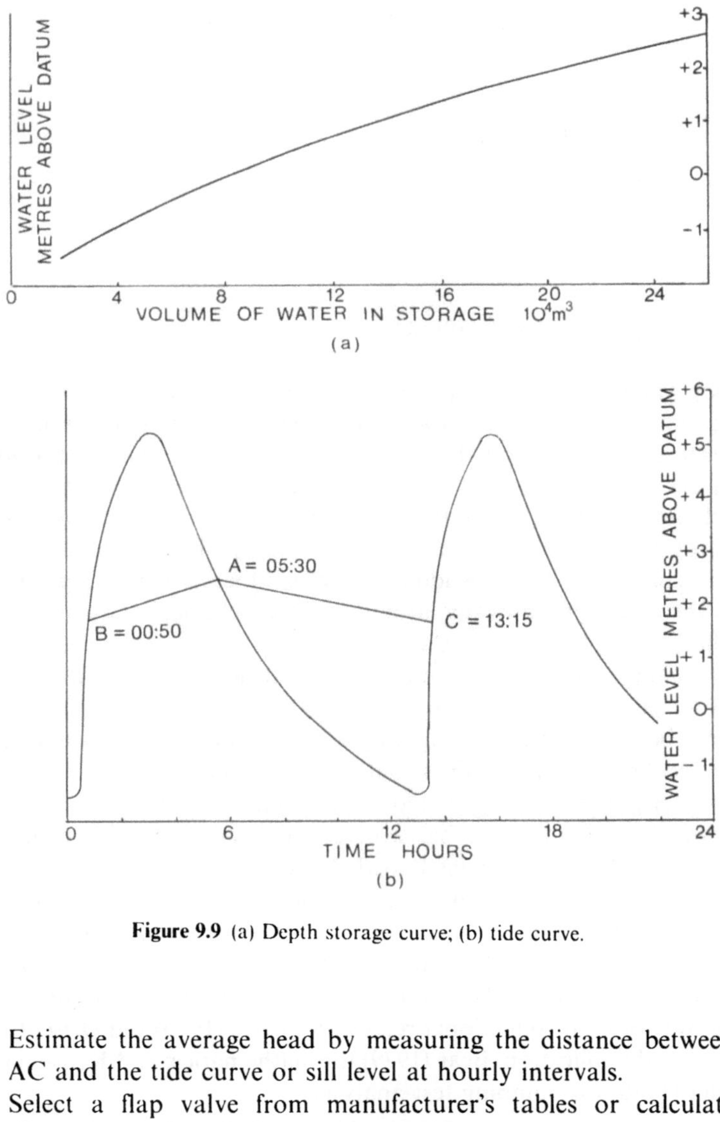

Figure 9.9 (a) Depth storage curve; (b) tide curve.

(10) Estimate the average head by measuring the distance between line AC and the tide curve or sill level at hourly intervals.

(11) Select a flap valve from manufacturer's tables or calculate the dimensions using the formula for discharge over a broad-crested weir or submerged weir (Lewitt, 1958). If it is necessary to adjust for salinity the salt water levels may be increased by a notional 3.5%.

(12) Check by means of an iterative calculation in a similar manner to that described to determine the storage level at each hour using both the spring and neap tide curves.

10 Deep drainage

N.S. ROBINS

10.1 Groundwater, flow and storage

Excluding water trapped in the polar icecaps, groundwater accounts for about 97% of all non-marine water on Earth. It has a far greater significance in terms of drainage and water supply than surface water, but it risks being overlooked even by the engineer because it is easy neither to see nor to quantify. In England and Wales slightly more than one-third of water for public supply derives from groundwater; in Scotland it is only 3%. In arid climates such as large areas of Africa and the Middle East where there are no perennial water courses, the role of groundwater attains a greater significance because it is the only reliable source available to man.

Deep drainage is the process of drawing groundwater from excavations and lifting it to the surface. Drainage may be promoted by pumping from wells, wellpoints, boreholes and trenches or by sump pumping; it may be at relatively shallow depths or in deep mines, but no matter how it is undertaken the mechanics of groundwater flow and storage remain universal.

The study of groundwater has evolved alongside man's ever-increasing demand for water. Our current knowledge of groundwater hydraulics has benefited from contemporary developments in data handling and manipulation, but many drainage problems remain barely soluble. This chapter aims to highlight the main aspects of groundwater circulation and deep drainage. Further explanation of selected topics will be found in: Price (1985) by way of an introduction; Freeze and Cherry (1979) and Driscoll (1986) for theory and application; Bear (1979) for mathematics; and Kruseman and de Ridder (1970) for pumping test analysis.

10.1.1 *Aquifers*

'Aquifer' is a general term for saturated rock which will yield groundwater in economic quantities. In an engineering context all rocks are potential aquifers in that most are able to transmit some groundwater towards, for example, deep drainage schemes.

This chapter is published by permission of the Director, British Geological Survey (NERC).

The water contained within saturated rock beneath the water table is groundwater. It is stored in the intergranular pore spaces of the rock and in any fissures or other openings, at a pressure equal to that of the atmosphere at the water table, and at a pressure which increases with depth beneath it. Groundwater flows from areas of high fluid potential (high head) to areas of low fluid potential, that is it flows from areas where the water table is highest to those where it is lowest along the line of greatest hydraulic gradient.

Although the volume of groundwater stored within saturated rock is equal to the pore volume, the fraction released under free drainage, the specific yield, is less. The retention of porewater is caused by both intergranular surface tension and the sorptive properties of some mineral grains (see also Chapters 2 and 3); the volume retained is specific retention.

Rocks which are less able to transmit groundwater may form a hydraulic barrier, or a confining layer to deeper horizons in which groundwater may move more freely. Such is the case in the London Basin, where London clay confines groundwater in the underlying Tertiary sands and chalk. The sands and the chalk are a confined aquifer beneath parts of London, but are unconfined where they crop out beyond the London clay cover to form the upstanding North and South Downs.

The pore pressure in the tertiary sands at the junction with the confining clay is, for the most part, considerably greater than atmospheric. Indeed, most penetrating boreholes, or piezometers, were once artesian (flowing) because the head, or potentiometric level, was at a greater elevation than that of the ground surface. However, intensive pumping throughout the nineteenth and much of the twentieth centuries has reduced the present head to subartesian (non-flowing but still confined) and even to unconfined water table conditions in the chalk and Lower Tertiary sands beneath the clay in parts of central London.

Groundwater in many aquifers such as the chalk or the Permo-Triassic conglomerates and some sandstones is contained both in intergranular pore spaces and in the many cracks and joints which characterise these rocks. Although intergranular storage is dominant, the transport potential is derived almost entirely from cracks and joints. These aquifers are 'fissured aquifers', and the groundwater within them is subject to fissure flow. Although the aquifer may be homogeneous, it is also anisotropic, and preferential flow directions will arise along major joint and fracture trends.

10.1.2 *Aquifer properties*

The energy required to transmit groundwater through the interconnected pore spaces of an aquifer depends on a function called hydraulic conductivity (k). This has the dimensions L^3 T, L^{-2} and relates rate of groundwater flow, Q^{-1} per unit area of aquifer, A, with prevailing hydraulic gradient, i, according to Darcy's law, whereby Q is given by the product kiA (see section 2.3).

Hydraulic conductivity depends not only on pore size and interconnectivity of the pores but also on the viscosity of the groundwater. With the exception of deeply circulating hot brines, the viscosity of groundwater is normally assumed to be constant. However the properties of the aquifer are sometimes quoted as intrinsic permeability, k', which relates solely to the rock properties and has the dimensions L^2. The relationship between the two parameters is given by $k' = kv/g$, where v is the viscosity of the groundwater and g is the gravitational acceleration.

Transmissivity, T, is the product of hydraulic conductivity and effective aquifer thickness for a single homogeneous formation, or the integral of the product in a layered aquifer. This function enables comparisons to be made between aquifers or saturated horizons and their potential to transmit water. It has the dimensions $L^2 T^{-1}$.

The ratio of the volume of water released under free drainage to the bulk volume of the rock from an unconfined aquifer is the specific yield, S_y. It is unitless (being a ratio) and values are generally less than 10^{-1}. In a confined aquifer, water is released as the result of elastic response, and the ratio of water to rock is called storativity, S. Clearly less water will be released from a confined aquifer per unit decline in head than from an unconfined aquifer, and values of storativity are correspondingly lower, usually less than 10^{-3}.

10.1.3 *Estimates of aquifer properties*

There are a number of 'rules of thumb' in use. Although their mathematical justification may not be exact, they are valid, for the most part, given certain limitations. For example, previous experience with the same rock type enables likely values of aquifer properties to be assigned to particular rock types (Table 10.1). Secondly, it is possible to relate the physical properties of an aquifer to

Table 10.1 Typical Aquifer properties.

Rock type	Hydraulic conductivity ($m\,s^{-1}$)	Porosity	Storativity	Comments
Gravel	10^{-2}–10^{-1}	0.20–0.30	0.10–0.25	
Sand	10^{-4}–10^{-3}	0.25–0.40	0.10–0.25	
Silt	$< 10^{-5}$	0.35–0.45	0.05–0.10	
Consolidated sand/silt	10^{-5}–10^{-4}	0.20–0.40	<0.10	
Sandstone	$< 10^{-4}$	< 0.25	<0.20	Partly fissure flow
Limestone	10^{-5}–10^{-3}	0.05–0.30	< 0.10	Mainly fissure flow
Karst limestone	10^{-2}–10^{-1}	< 0.35	< 0.15	Channel flow
Igneous extrusive	$> 10^{-4}$	< 0.10	0.05–0.10	Fissure flow
Igneous intrusive	$< 10^{-4}$	< 0.02	< 0.01	Fissure flow

probable values of intergranular permeability; soil density obtained from a standard penetration test may be used to obtain estimates of intergranular permeability in terms of granular and cohesive soils and dense, medium-dense and loose soils (Driscoll, 1986). Hydraulic conductivity can also be estimated using the empirical relationship conceived by Hazen (1893) whereby intergranular permeability is related to the square of the effective grain size (d_{10}) provided that the sediment is well sorted and the median grain size (d_{50}) lies within prescribed limits. Otherwise, grain size curves can be matched against families of curves for which the hydraulic conductivity is already known.

10.1.4 *Measurement of aquifer properties*

Reliable measurement of aquifer properties is a taxing exercise. Nevertheless, it is an essential prerequisite to predictive work made at the design stage of any drainage programme. Money spent at this the exploratory stage is usually money saved at the construction phase and, as always, it is better to overcollect data than not to collect enough.

Aquifer properties may be determined from laboratory inspection of borehole core samples and from *in-situ* field tests. For example, porosity can be readily measured in the laboratory, but it can also be indirectly determined with borehole geophysics using, among others, a continuous neutron log. Intergranular permeability is measured in the laboratory on core specimens with a permeameter and either falling or constant head conditions. Hydraulic conductivity, however, can only be measured in the field by first calculating transmissivity from pumping test data. Values of specific yield and storativity can also be obtained from pumping tests.

Pumping tests involve the controlled abstraction of groundwater from a production borehole and the measurement of head changes that occur both in the production borehole and in nearby observation boreholes, or piezometers. The borehole pumping rate should be constant. It is dependent on the pump capacity and the ability to dispose of the discharged water without recycling to the aquifer as well as the capacity of the well and aquifer to produce groundwater. In general, the higher the yield and hence the stress on the aquifer, the more accurate will be the results, provided that there is no deviation from Darcian flow.

Steady-state conditions must prevail before the pumping test commences. The water level in a production borehole will decline during the test at a rate defined by the time since pumping began, t, the physical properties of the aquifer and the borehole efficiency. As the cone of depression deepens and widens, so the water levels in nearby observation boreholes begin to decline; these levels are not affected by the borehole hydraulics, as no flow is taking place across the observation borehole walls, and they reflect the true response of the aquifer to pumping.

The drawdown in the production borehole is the result of both the formation loss and the borehole loss, the latter caused by hydraulic friction in the vicinity of the borehole once the Reynolds number exceeds 2, sometimes described as the skin effect. This effect allows a differential to form between the intersection of the potentiometric level with the borehole and the dynamic water level above the pump in the borehole (Figure 10.1). Determination of borehole loss is essential to any dewatering project.

The borehole loss may be calculated by means of a step discharge test (Bierschenk, 1964). The step discharge test requires a borehole to be pumped at consecutive incremental discharges of about 25, 50, 75 and 100% of the maximum borehole yield. Each step is maintained for the same duration of time (normally 90 or 120 minutes). Measurement of cumulative drawdown, s_w, during each step enables the relationship between yield, Q, and the ratio s_w/Q to be attained. The straight-line best-fit graphical plot of Q versus s_w/Q has a positive intercept, B, and a gradient, C, so that the line has the formula:

$$s_w = BQ + CQ^2 \tag{10.1}$$

where BQ describes the linear relationship between drawdown and yield caused by formation loss and CQ^2 describes the additional component of drawdown caused by borehole loss at any given value of Q. The theory strictly applies to the confined case only but is also applicable in water table conditions provided drawdown is small compared with saturated thickness.

The optimum distance between observation boreholes and production boreholes depends on the nature of the aquifer and its likely hydraulic properties. The cone of depression in a confined aquifer is controlled by pressure change only and will propagate more rapidly than the physically drained cone of depression within an unconfined aquifer. Observation boreholes need to be placed at greater distances from the production borehole in confined aquifers than in unconfined aquifers, but highly permeable aquifers will induce wider responses than weakly permeable aquifers. In general, observation boreholes may be placed at distances of tens of metres in unconfined aquifers and hundreds of metres in confined aquifers, whereas piezometers placed at ones and tens of metres may be more valuable in weakly permeable strata (see BS 6316: 1983).

There are severe constraints which need to be observed with the conventional analysis of pump test data. The boreholes must fully penetrate the aquifer or groundwater unit which is being measured and be in open hydraulic contact with it. The aquifer should effectively be of infinite areal extent, homogeneous, isotropic and of uniform thickness over the area influenced by the pumping test, and there should be no significant vertical flow within the aquifer.

Sympathy with these constraints enables values of k and S or S_y to be obtained for both confined and unconfined conditions. This is accomplished by analysing the water level responses in the production borehole and more

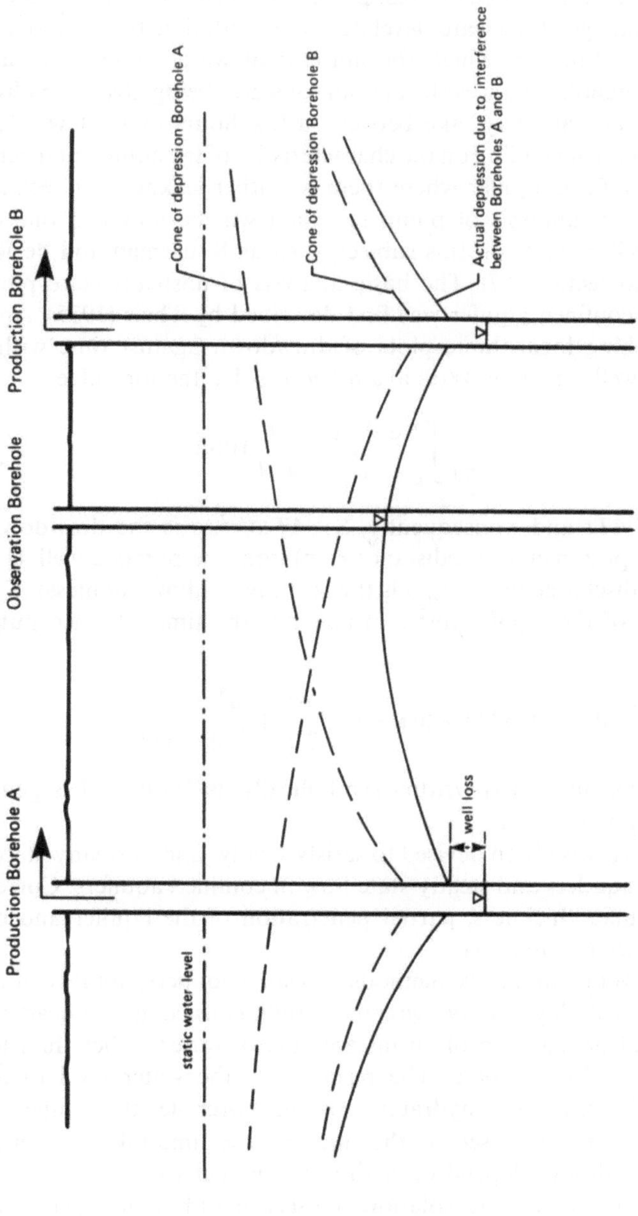

Figure 10.1 Interference between two production boreholes in a uniform homogeneous aquifer.

importantly one or more observation boreholes. The observational time interval increases logarithmically (0.5, 1, 1.5, 2, 3, 4, 6, 8, 10, 15, 20 minutes, etc.) as the rate of change of the water level decreases with time towards an almost steady-state condition in which the amount of water coming in radially towards the borehole balances the amount of water being abstracted from it. This equilibrium state may take between a few hours and a few weeks of pumping to attain depending on the characteristics of the aquifer and can only happen in a confined aquifer where there is neither leakage nor recharge.

Comprehensive analysis of pump test data will be found in one of the numerous excellent texts on this subject, such as Kruseman and de Ridder (1970) (see also section 2.7). The basic analysis of unsteady-state pumping test data in a confined aquifer was first described by Theis (1935). Analysis involves matching logarithmic plots of drawdown against time with type curves of the well functions $W(u)$ against u to solve the formulae:

$$s = \frac{Q}{4\pi T}\int_u^\infty \frac{e^{-y}\,dy}{y} = \frac{Q}{4\pi T} W(u) \tag{10.2}$$

where $u = r^2S/4Tt$ and, consequently, $S = 4Ttu/r^2$, s is the drawdown (m) measured in a piezometer at a distance r (m) from the pumped well, Q is the constant well discharge ($m^3\,s^{-1}$), S is the storativity (dimensionless), T is the transmissivity of the aquifer ($m^2\,s^{-1}$) and t is the time (s) since pumping started.

$$W(u) = -0.5772 - \ln u + u - \frac{u^2}{2.2!} + \frac{u^3}{3.3!} - \frac{u^4}{4.4!} + \cdots \tag{10.3}$$

The exponential integral is written symbolically as $W(u)$, and is generally read as 'well function of u'.

Formulae have also been devised to satisfy steady- and unsteady-state flow in unconfined aquifers and steady-state flow in confined aquifers. Correction factors for aquifer thickness, partial penetration of the aquifer and others can be introduced as required.

There are several alternative methods of testing aquifers, notably slug tests and packer tests. A slug test involves an instantaneous change in head caused by the removal or injection of an instant slug of water rather than longer term abstraction by pumping. The response of the water level to a slug depends on the near-field hydraulics of the borehole; the shape of the time–drawdown curve caused by the slug and the time taken to return to steady-state conditions depend on hydraulic conductivity.

Packer testing involves the isolation of a section of borehole below one or between two temporary plugs or packers. The isolated zone may be subjected to instantaneous pressure changes and the response monitored in order to obtain the value of hydraulic conductivity over that section of the borehole. The Lugeon test is a packer test in which the induced head is raised to 100 m of water pressure. This is a very high pressure, particularly in shallow conditions, and may induce hydrofracturing or surface-water bursts (1 Lugeon is approximately equivalent to $10^{-8}\,m\,s^{-1}$).

Values of storativity derived from time–drawdown data obtained from production boreholes or single-well packer tests are not valid. Values can only be obtained from observation borehole data.

10.1.5 *Field and laboratory determinations*

The adoption of physical property values derived from either field or laboratory tests must be undertaken with caution. Table 10.2 compares laboratory results from tests carried out on core specimens to determine intergranular permeability and porosity with values of hydraulic conductivity and specific yield derived from pumping tests. The data derive from six exploratory boreholes drilled into Permian and Triassic sandstones and conglomerates in south-west Scotland and north-west England. Fissure flow plays a dominant role in these aquifers, and consequently the field hydraulic conductivity (k_t) (a measure of both intergranular and secondary permeability derived from the cracks and joints) is some 10–1000 times greater than the intergranular permeability (k_i). The ratio of laboratory porosity to specific yield ranges from 15 to 260, reflecting both secondary porosity and retention of groundwater under free drainage.

Downhole flowmeter logging can be very instructive. Flowmeter logs may be recorded when the borehole is standing and when it is being pumped. The logs may be run in conjunction with caliper, fluid electrical conductivity and temperature logs, and together they will demonstrate the location and relative inflow or outflow that occurs via each fissure intersecting the borehole. Variations in hydraulic conductivity within the sequence penetrated may allow differential heads to build up at different depths and create the potential for upward or downward flow in certain sections of a borehole. Clearly, it is

Table 10.2 Field and laboratory derived aquifer properties for some Permian and Triassic aquifers.

Place	Map reference	Test yield ($l\,s^{-1}$)	k ($m\,s^{-1}$)	k_i ($m\,s^{-1}$)	k/k_i	S_y	Porosity
Mauchline	NS 488 263	46	10^{-4}	10^{-5}	10	0.01	0.27
Stranraer	NS 037 619	0	0	10^{-9}	low	0	0.08
Dumfries	NX 952 747	53	10^{-5}	10^{-8}	1000	0.01	0.15
Locharbriggs	NX 999 803	8	10^{-4}	10^{-7}	1000	n.d.	0.19
Gretna	NY 311 693	3	10^{-6}	10^{-8}	100	n.d.	0.14
Cliburn	NY 583 260	44	10^{-5}	10^{-6}	10	0.001	0.26

n.d., not done.

essential that such fluxes are recognised at an early stage in any deep drainage proposal.

10.1.6 *Interference modelling*

Time–drawdown prognoses which will assist the design of drainage schemes can be devised. These are based on the measured responses to constant discharge pumping and the derived estimates of k and S. Care must be taken to differentiate between steady-state conditions and dynamic conditions with the application of test pumping results to the design of a pump drainage scheme. Continuous pumping at a low rate will inevitably attain steady-state conditions, while a short duration higher rate of volume, say $8\ \mathrm{h\ d^{-1}}$, will not approach steady state. The appropriate formula must, therefore, be used in any predictive calculation of drawdown with time.

Certain local peculiarities may have come to light during the pump testing programme; these may include knowledge of local barrier boundary or recharge boundary conditions which will have been evaluated using conventional image well theory (Kruseman and de Ridder, 1970). Some idea of the validity of the data so obtained will also be available at this stage. For example, the homogeneity of the aquifer, the degree of partial penetration of the exploratory boreholes, the possibility of fissure flow in selected horizons and the varied thickness of the saturated aquifer horizon may all limit the validity of the interpretive methods that were used to reduce those data to the basic values of k and S.

Given sufficient confidence in the data, predictive analyses can be made at a variety of levels of sophistication. The lower levels of interpretation can be done by hand, but more demanding analyses may require assistance from one of the many commercially available software packages.

Interference modelling is the determination of the potentiometric surface at any given state of pumping at two or more production boreholes. Given steady-state conditions, the effective radius of influence of a pumping well, R_e, is given by the formula:

$$R_e = 1.5\sqrt{\frac{Tt}{S}} \tag{10.4}$$

where t is the time since pumping began.

The important thing here is that the effective radius of influence is independent of the pumping rate, whereas the depth of the cone of depression at any given time, t, is proportional to the pumping rate. Given the potentiometric head in an observation borehole or the corrected value (minus the borehole loss) in a production borehole, the cone of depression can be defined as a straight line, with the distance axis plotted on a log scale, between the observed level in the borehole and the intersection of the cone of depression with the static water table at the radius R_e (Figure 10.1). A second pumping well may be introduced into the system, and the interference between the two is merely the summation of the two cones of depression wherever they intersect.

Three-dimensional modelling requires the use of a digital, or at least an analogue, model. This is particularly the case in an unconfined situation, as the value of T reduces as aquifer thickness declines with drawdown, and a correction for so-called water table conditions needs to be carried out. However, in the confined aquifer, steady-state conditions can never really be achieved in the absence of leakage or recharge, because R_e goes towards infinity as t increases.

The basic dewatering equations under steady-state conditions are as follows:

Unconfined case

$$Q = \frac{k(H^2 - h^2)}{0.733 \log R/r} \tag{10.5}$$

where Q is in $m^3 s^{-1}$, k is in $m s^{-1}$, H is saturated thickness of the aquifer before pumping (m), h is depth of water in the well while pumping (m), R is the radius of the cone of depression (m) and r is the effective radius of the borehole (m).

The depth of the water table, h, at any given distance, r, from the well ($r > 1.5\,H$) is given by:

$$h = \sqrt{H^2 - \frac{0.733Q \log R/r}{k}} \tag{10.6}$$

Confined case

$$Q = \frac{kb(H - h)}{0.366 \log R/r} \tag{10.7}$$

where b is thickness of the aquifer (m), H is the height of the piezometric level from the bottom of the aquifer (m) and the other symbols are as above.

The drawdown, s, at any point within the cone is given by:

$$s = \frac{0.366Q \log R/r}{kb} \tag{10.8}$$

10.2 Groundwater flow regimes

Groundwater flow systems have been classified by Tóth (1963) as local, intermediate or regional in scale. Local flow occurs between adjacent recharge and discharge zones in areas of pronounced relief (e.g. most shallow unconfined flow in the UK). Intermediate systems are more extensive and encompass several local systems (e.g. shallow flow in confined UK aquifers). Regional flow systems, however, extend across whole groundwater basins from the principal watershed to the lowest discharge point. Regional systems cannot develop within the geographical constraints of the UK, but they do occur within continental sedimentary basins.

A typical continental system is the Great Artesian Basin of Australia. This is a confined groundwater basin in which a complex, layered aquifer system is developed within sandstones, siltstones and mudstones of Triassic to Cretaceous age. Precipitation to the Great Dividing Range rapidly drains eastwards to the coast along flowpaths of only 100–200 km or to the west via intermittent surface drainage and the major regional groundwater flow system across the Great Artesian Basin. Discharge from the regional groundwater flow occurs either to the inland drainage of Lake Eyre or to the Darling River (Figure 10.2). The groundwater flowpaths are up to 1000 km long; radiometric dates demonstrate that the age of the water increases down the flowpaths up to a maximum of about 2 million years in the vicinity of Lake Eyre.

By contrast, the maximum age of shallow groundwater in local or intermediate flow systems in the UK ranges from only a few hours to a few tens of years. Exceptionally, water issuing from the thermal springs at Bath (46.5°C) circulates to depths of over 2 km from its recharge area in the Mendip Hills and

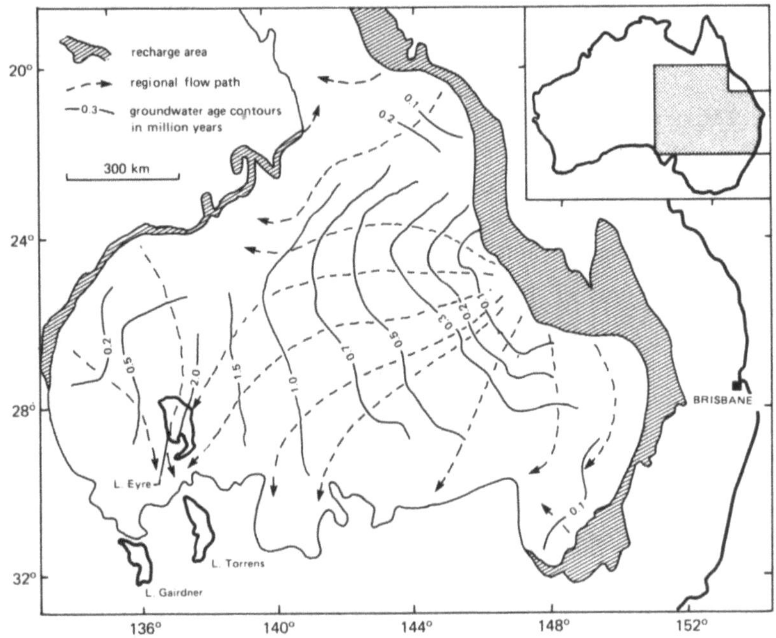

Figure 10.2 Regional groundwater flow in the Great Artesian Basin of Australia.

takes nearly 10 000 years between falling as rainfall on the Mendips to its issue at Bath. The shallower flowpaths in the chalk of the London Basin have yielded radiocarbon dates up to 25 000 years in some areas. Elsewhere groundwater ages are typically measured in tens or at most hundreds of years. However, brines have been found in some strata, for example most probably trapped in the eastern part of the Lincolnshire limestone aquifer when it was first deposited on the floor of the Jurassic sea.

10.2.1 *Groundwater flow analysis*

Groundwater movement is described by Darcy's law, which relates it to the hydraulic conductivity of the rock and the prevailing hydraulic gradient. Analysis of simple two-dimensional flow problems can readily be carried out by conventional flownet analysis in order to obtain a rapid understanding of a particular hydrogeological regime. It should be noted that, since hydraulic conductivity and hydraulic gradient are inversely proportional given a constant throughflow of groundwater, steeper hydraulic gradients often coincide with areas of lower hydraulic conductivity.

A flownet is a two-dimensional map representing the orthogonal grid of mutually intersecting streamlines and their equipotential lines in an isotropic aquifer with specified boundary conditions. Any given stream tube between any pair of streamlines defines a constant discharge which is the product of velocity and the tube cross-sectional area. Given that equipotential lines must intersect impermeable boundaries at right angles, two-dimensional flownets can readily be created and analysed in terms of volume and direction of flow. Real three-dimensional problems are not so easy to evaluate, but useful solutions can be obtained by considering a number of vertical cross-sectional segments. Analysis can also be carried out by electrical analogue simulation (both Darcy's law and Ohm's law are based on linear flow law) or by numerical simulation using the finite difference method or the finite element method (Freeze and Cherry, 1979).

The water table in an area of hilly terrain tends towards a subdued version of the surface relief. This is created by the combined effect of infiltration from rainfall over higher ground and groundwater drainage and discharge to streams at lower elevations. In the confined case the highest elevation obtained by the potentiometric surface cannot exceed the elevation of the recharge area where the aquifer is at outcrop. The lowest point of the potentiometric surface is given by the lowest discharge point from the aquifer.

In general, hydraulic conductivity and storativity are greater, and depths to water table less, beneath valleys than beneath hills. The main reasons for this are:

(1) Valleys tend to be eroded in rock which is more permeable than elsewhere because of the occurrence of joints and other discontinuities produced through chemical dissolution.

(2) The more permeable weathered zone is commonly deepest in the valleys and may only be saturated beneath lower lying elevations.
(3) Stress release as a result of the removal of overburden in the valleys may enhance secondary permeability.
(4) Groundwater flows from highland towards lowland areas, but a groundwater divide need not necessarily coincide with a topographical divide. Lowland areas can thus draw on a greater volume of storage derived from the total catchment area than can sites at higher elevations in the same catchment.

On a site-specific basis, a simple walk-over survey and limited programme of exploratory drilling may often yield sufficient information to be able to ascertain the nature and direction of groundwater flow. Three shallow boreholes, each near the corner of an equilateral triangle, reveal the direction and gradient of the water table, and short-duration pumping tests can provide values for hydraulic conductivity and storativity which in turn enable the approximate rate of flow to be evaluated. However, on a larger scale there are several other important factors. These include the identification of local and intermediate flow patterns, their recharge and discharge zones and the calculation of the total throughput of groundwater. It should be remembered that any spring discharges indicate the elevation of the water table at that particular location, and the occurrence of springlines can provide valuable information as to the whereabouts of the water table along valley sides.

Not all discharge from groundwater is visible as springs at the ground surface. Much groundwater discharge occurs as baseflow to surface rivers and lakes. This may account for up to 90% of the total annual flow of some rivers in the more permeable catchments and 10–20% of the total river flow in the less permeable areas of central Wales and northern Scotland. Discharge in coastal areas may be submarine or obscured by superficial marine deposits.

Recharge to groundwater systems may occur by direct infiltration of rainwater wherever an aquifer crops out. It may be more intense in areas of higher ground where orographic effects concentrate rainfall, and groundwater flow to lower lying areas provides the capacity to receive recharging water. Some groundwater flow paths will become confined by poorly permeable horizons at lower elevations.

10.2.2 *Boundaries, provenance and throughflow*

Water-bearing units have both horizontal and vertical boundaries. These may be low-flow boundaries against relatively impermeable material or recharge boundaries such as a river or lake which maintain a near-constant head. Although complex layered systems occur in which groundwater flow takes place with different velocities in adjacent permeable horizons, consideration of the more common situation of a single unconfined groundwater unit overlying impermeable rock is sufficient to visualise the influence of groundwater flow on the security of a proposed pit or other excavation.

Trial boreholes establish the transmissivity and storativity of the aquifer unit along with the depth of the aquifer and its areal limitations. It is necessary to establish how the proposed pit is likely to interfere with the existing groundwater flow system and whether the interception of groundwater near the pit can be carried out at a rate which exceeds its supply at source (its recharge capacity).

A simple water balance can establish the likely volume of throughflow that will take place within an aquifer. For example, it was established in a small glacial gravel catchment in the Borders of Scotland that rainfall contributed 54 million $m^3 a^{-1}$ above a particular datum in the valley. This input contributed to 15 million $m^3 a^{-1}$ evapotranspiration, 31 million $m^3 a^{-1}$ stream flow and 8 million $m^3 a^{-1}$ aquifer throughflow. The last calculation was verified by establishing the hydraulic gradient along the valley (roughly equal to the topographical gradient of the valley floor), the aquifer cross-section and aquifer hydraulic conductivity near the measuring datum in the valley, in order to verify that throughflow derived from the Darcy equation was of the same order as that derived from the water balance. This done, it was concluded that any excavation at this point in the gravels would have to cope with a potential throughflow of 8 million $m^3 a^{-1}$ within the gravels. In this case exclusion of groundwater was preferable to interception by dewatering boreholes or wellpoints.

Constant-head boundaries must be treated as a special case. No matter how thoroughly a groundwater interception system is designed, water will drain towards it from river, lake or sea at a rate defined by the effective aquifer thickness, the hydraulic conductivity and the induced hydraulic gradient to the pumping water level. Again consideration should be given to groundwater exclusion, particularly if the aquifer is relatively shallow and of moderate to high permeability.

Another difficulty is that the hydraulic properties of a particular aquifer unit, and for that matter an aquitard (a unit of low hydraulic conductivity which is effectively incapable of conducting groundwater), may vary with location as well as depth. A good example of this is the wadi deposits that occur along the Red Sea coast. Measurements of borehole performance as specific capacity (yield divided by drawdown) are plotted along a cross-section from the basement mountain front towards the sea (Figure 10.3). This shows that the hydraulic properties of the coarse-sand and gravel deposits near the mountain front decline towards the finer sediments at the tail of the fan and increase slightly towards the sea where the material has been resorted by wind action. This same situation is quite common in the UK in the fossil wadi deposits of both the Permian and Devonian rocks of England and Scotland. The drainage engineer should, therefore, be aware of the geological history and sedimentology of the material which he proposes to dewater.

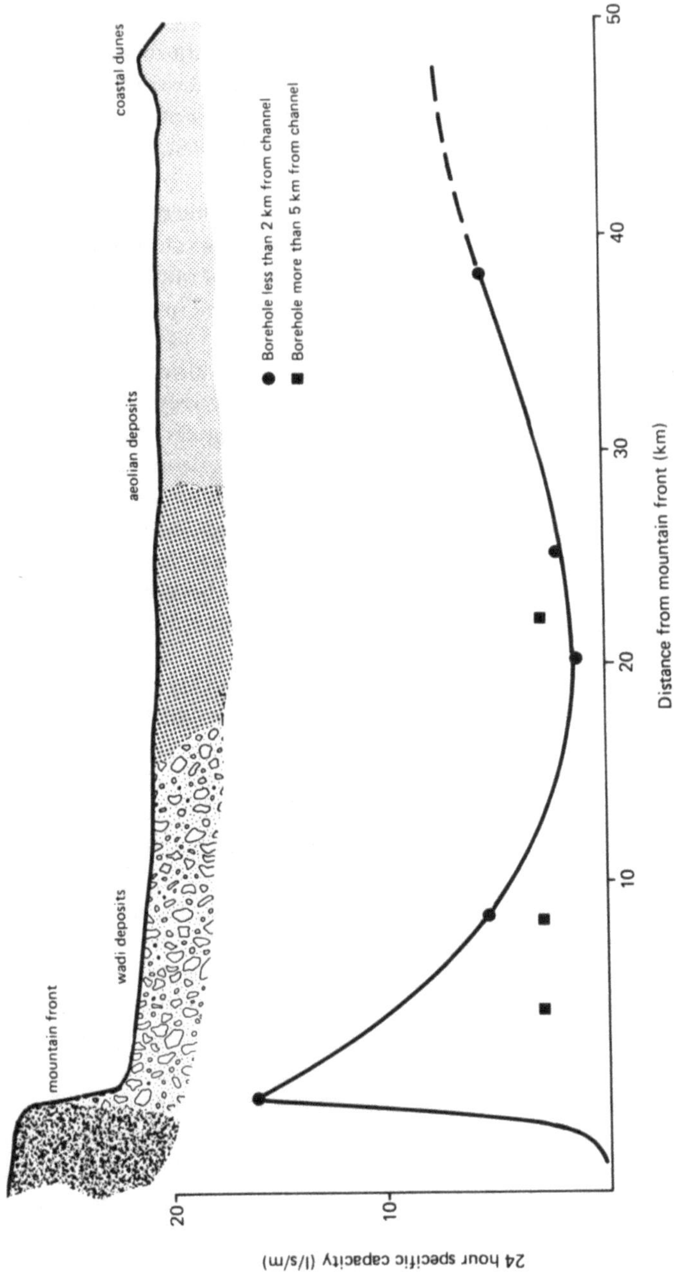

Figure 10.3 Borehole specific capacity (discharge/drawdown) values along a length of Wadi Rima, Yemen Arab Republic.

On a more local scale, the use of dye and other tracers in order to investigate groundwater provenance should be employed with caution. Tracer experiments only tell the investigator where groundwater is flowing when the tracer is positively detected; they do not otherwise tell where groundwater is not flowing. Their use should be restricted to investigations of conduit flow in old mine workings or the evaluation of groundwater flow within karst limestones.

10.3 Induced groundwater flow

Alteration to the natural flow in an aquifer can induce groundwater to move in a new direction. This can be done by pumping a well or borehole or conversely, and sometimes unintentionally, by artificially recharging an area of aquifer by means of recharge lagoons or boreholes. The induced flow patterns are overprinted on the naturally existing flow system and may have the effect of diverting groundwater away from one area towards another. Induced flow systems may be capable of moving large volumes of groundwater, but they are generally only effective over small areas of an aquifer.

The ability of a borehole or well to produce groundwater depends on a number of factors. The main limitations are the formation constants, hydraulic conductivity and storativity, which define the potential of the aquifer to transmit and store groundwater. Another is the hydraulic contact between borehole or well and the aquifer, and it is this which determines the well loss function defined in a step–drawdown test. The last is the capacity of the pump to lift and discharge the water.

The nature of the hydrogeological unit or units which require to be dewatered or regulated dictates the optimum type of installation required to best carry out groundwater interception or groundwater removal. Consideration must also be given to groundwater exclusion. The available options may be summarised as follows.

(1) Removal of groundwater and relief of pressure:
  (a) Sump pumping.
  (b) Groundwater interception by wellpoints or wells.
  (c) Bored wells, relief wells and galleries.
(2) Exclusion of groundwater:
  (a) Sheet piling or diaphragm walls.
  (b) Slurry trench cut-off or thin grout membrane.
  (c) Contiguous bored pile walls.
  (d) Cement, clay, resin or silicate based grouts.
  (e) Ground freezing.
  (f) Compressed air.

The subsequent abandonment of either of the above engineering works will reinstate natural groundwater conditions except where diaphragm walls, grouting or other cut-offs remain. Foundations which are laid in dry conditions thus become saturated and borrow pits flooded.

10.3.1 *Boreholes, wells, wellpoints and piezometers*

Having opted for removal rather than exclusion of groundwater, the most efficient and cost-effective system is designed, installed and tested. A drilled borehole, or dug well, is one of the commonest means of creating a void space in saturated rock into which a pump may be placed. A Hy Mac or similar excavator can attain 5 m depth in soft material. The days of digging a 120-m-deep well by hand into volcanic rock, as they once did for example in parts of the Middle East, are now over.

Shallow unconsolidated drift deposits can be dug to beneath the water table and a shaft of preformed concrete rings let in before backfilling. Stones can be placed in the joints to part adjacent rings and allow water ingress. Coarser backfill should be placed adjacent to the rings; cobbles can be laid on the bottom of the shaft to prevent upwelling of fine material.

Groundwater inflow from the base of the shaft of diameter D m during pumping at $q\,\mathrm{m^3\,d^{-1}}$ (but excluding any inflow from elsewhere in the shaft lining) allows a simple estimate of hydraulic conductivity to be made. According to a formula devised by Hvorslev (1951):

$$q = 2.75\,DkH \tag{10.9}$$

where k is hydraulic conductivity ($\mathrm{m\,d^{-1}}$) and H is drawdown (m).

Harder rock and deeper penetration require the use of drilled boreholes. The completed diameter of the borehole should be adequate to house an electric submersible pump of suitable capacity yet leave sufficient annulus within the borehole not to starve water flowing down to the pump intake. The borehole may be lined with mild steel or, more commonly, plastic or stainless steel liners and screens. The screen is placed adjacent to the producing horizons, and these may need to be identified with the aid of geophysical logs run within the drilled hole prior to casing.

The most common slot width for plastic- and textile-wrapped screens is 2 mm, although others are available, but more careful selection is required for stainless steel wire-wrapped screens. The advantage of the latter is that they offer a greater open area and enable finer grained unconsolidated materials to be exploited. Sieve analyses of unconsolidated sands prescribe the slot width normally selected so that 50–60% of the sample can pass through the screen. Development and washing of the borehole by surge pumping, sometimes using airlift, jetting and swabbing allows fines to pass through the screen and out of the borehole. This produces a graded filter leading from the borehole screen outwards into the aquifer.

A graded filter pack can be employed by placing a rounded filter medium between screen and formation. The practicalities of emplacement require a minimum 50 mm annulus. The pack should be well sorted and of little larger grain size than that of the formation. Packs are particularly useful in fine-grained unconsolidated sands. The median grain size of the pack should be such that it will retain about 60% of the formation, and the screen slot size should be such that it will retain 90% of the pack. A formation stabiliser, however, is a medium- to coarse-grained rounded gravel placed behind the screen and designed to hold the formation from sloughing onto the borehole liner. Its grain size is not critical. It is used in formations such as consolidated but friable sandstones and other strata which would not stand indefinitely as an open hole.

It is good practice to have a sump of plain casing capped at the bottom below the lowest screen section. This allows debris to accumulate clear of the screen. The pump should ideally be placed within a section of plain casing, but this is not always possible. Optimum pump setting depends on design drawdown; a cut-out electrode is useful above the pump intake to protect the pump from drawing air.

Jetting of wells and wellpoints is a simple means of placing a screen into a shallow unconsolidated formation and at the same time creating a graded filter pack around the screen. The action of the jetting removes the fines and some of the coarser material, so making way for the passage of the screen into the formation. This leaves a selectively coarse residue or filter around the screen.

A series of wellpoints sunk into a shallow unconsolidated aquifer can be an effective means of dewatering for trenching, footings or other temporary works. The wellpoints are placed at close intervals (often between 1 and 3 m apart) in order that they interfere one with another to provide a composite 'cone' of depression throughout the area of the wellfield.

Assiduous use of wellhead valves enables several wellpoints to be drawn by a single suction pump via a common main. Suction on each wellpoint can only attain a maximum head of up to 5 m, so second- and even third-stage wellpoints may need to be let into the dewatered and excavated ground as work progresses (Figure 10.4). This and other similar dewatering techniques are discussed further in Chapter 11.

Trenches and infiltration galleries are another means by which shallow groundwater can be intercepted. The infiltration gallery, or horizontal well, is let into a trench below the water table and backfilled using selective coarse material. The trench is designed to drain towards a sump. It may work under steady state or as a transient drain (see section 10.3.3). Conventional field drain or gravel and textile membrane construction may be used. Open trenches can also be utilised as groundwater cut-offs, particularly around the inside perimeter of a gravel pit where a trench can drain to a single sump and relieve seepage through the bund walls of the pit.

Piezometers may be required to monitor changes in groundwater level.

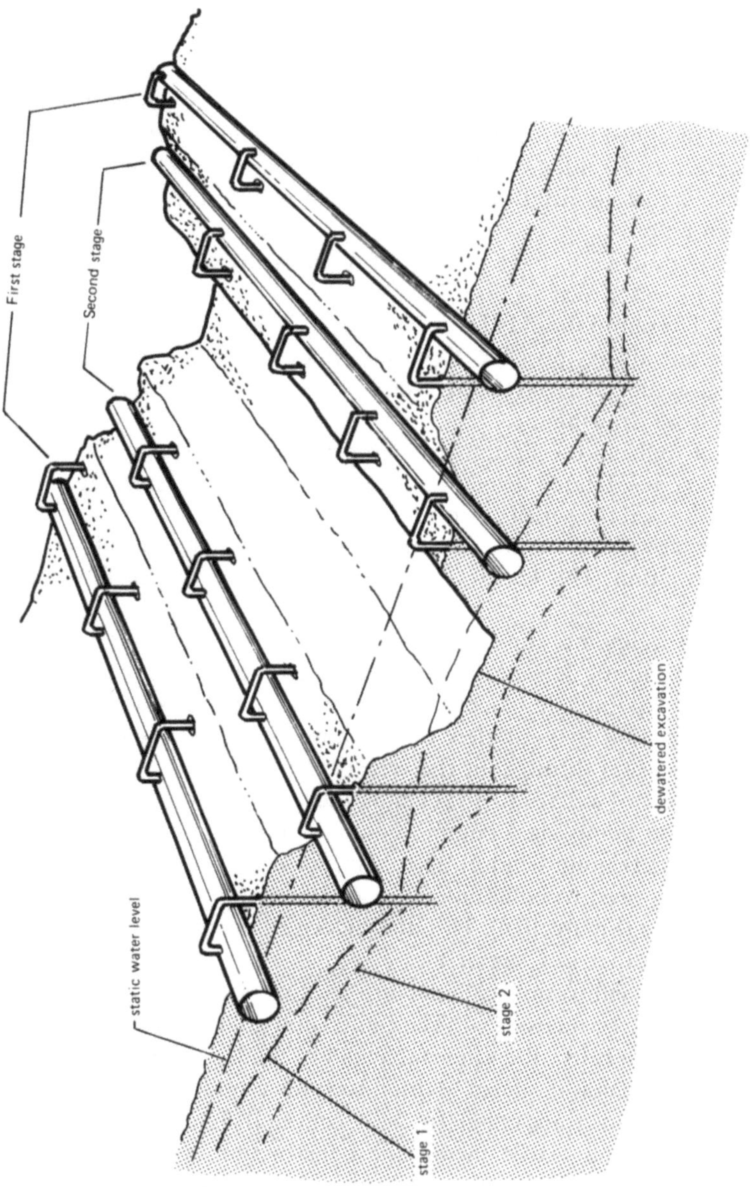

Figure 10.4 Two-stage wellpoint system.

A piezometer is a narrow (50 mm) pipe terminating in a short well screen or ceramic cup so that the head of the groundwater at the screen or cup can be monitored in terms of its effect on water standing in the pipe. The piezometer should be let into a clean-drilled hole of minimum 150 mm diameter in order that the screen or cup can be effectively packed into a permeable filter to ensure adequate hydraulic contact with the horizon being measured. The pack may be sealed on the top with, for example, bentonite pellets, and other piezometers let in at different intervals within the same drilled borehole. Interpretation of water level data obtained from piezometers may require selective judgement regarding the hydraulic efficiency of each piezometer. No significant flow takes place across screen or cup, and clogging can be a problem, causing piezometer levels to be in error.

10.3.2 *Drilling equipment contracts and pitfalls*

There are two basic drilling techniques: percussion and rotary. Traditional percussion or cable tool drilling is the repeated lifting and dropping of a heavy set of drilling tools into the borehole; the bit breaks and crushes the rock into fragments in consolidated ground and loosens the material in unconsolidated formations. Mixed with water, which may be added in dry holes, the resultant slurry is periodically lifted from the hole by a bailer. In very soft ground a sand bailer, or shell, is used. The up and down motion on the bit is imparted by the cable, either by the driller's use of clutch and brake or via a spudding beam.

The efficiency of percussion drilling in consolidated formations depends on the resistance of the rock, the dip of the rock structure, the weight of the drill tools, the length and rate of the stroke and the diameter, sharpness and shape of the bit. Clearance between the tool string and the borehole wall and the density and depth of accumulated slurry at the hole bottom are also important. Efficiency in unconsolidated formations is more dependent on the presence of boulders and cobbles than on the mode of drilling. It is usually necessary to drive casing behind the bit in order to keep the hole open.

Rotary drilling enables faster drilling speeds and greater depths to be attained. The drilling bit is attached to the end of the drill pipe and rotated so that toothed wheels grind the bottom of the hole by a process of cutting and chipping to allow penetration of hard materials. A variety of different bit types is available depending on the nature of the formation to be drilled. Drilling fluid is circulated down the drill pipe and up through the annulus created between drill pipe and hole wall. This serves to cool and lubricate the drilling bit, to remove debris from the hole bottom and to support the hole walls. The rotating action of the bit is generally imparted directly from the drilling rig down the drill pipe. However, the rotary percussion drilling technique uses compressed air to impart a percussive action on the drilling tool and also to rotate it. This method is particularly useful in very hard formations. Downhole motor-driven bits are sometimes used, particularly by the oil industry.

Normal rotary drilling requires the circulation of a drilling fluid; this fluid may be water, compressed air, bentonite-based mud or an organically based fluid designed to reduce to the viscosity of water when treated with acid or other chemicals. The viscosity and density of the circulating fluid are critical for the removal of the drill cuttings.

The selection of an appropriate drilling fluid depends on the nature of the formation to be drilled. Bentonite-based muds cannot readily be removed from fine-grained material adjacent to the borehole even though a filter cake will form on the borehole wall to inhibit their ingress. The mud filter cake should be thinned on completion of drilling by circulating water for several hours before inserting the casing and gravel pack. If this is not done it is generally very difficult to remove residual bentonite from around the borehole during subsequent washing and well development. Water and air are by far the best fluids for circulation, but recourse to more viscous and dense fluids is needed in difficult formations. Thorough programmes of borehole cleaning are always worthwhile and should include airlifting, surging, scouring, jetting, the use of softeners, such as Calgon, and even acid in limestone formations.

It is sometimes necessary to retrieve solid core samples of strata. This can be done using conventional rotary core barrels taking isolated sticks of core or a continuous programme of coring. Care should be taken to select equipment suitable for both rig and ground (Driscoll, 1986). Percussion drilling allows unconsolidated material to be cored using U100 percussion barrels, and techniques are available to obtain least disturbed samples.

The tender document for a drilling contract should, in the UK, follow the procedure set by the Institution of Civil Engineers Standard Contract Form. Otherwise the significant parts of the document are the Specification and the Bill of Quantities. It is good practice to allow potential contractors as much room as is possible and to give them the choice of drilling equipment and a range of sizes, tolerances and materials. Prognosis of the probable ground conditions must be made with caution, and care should be taken not to be too specific if there remains some doubt with regard to geology. Indeed, the contractor would have grounds for a claim if he tooled up the rig for Carboniferous limestone and found he had to drill London clay.

Unlike ordinary construction contracts, the drilling contract should encourage some flexibility because the complete job cannot be surveyed before commencement, and quantities cannot be estimated precisely. A good contract and good supervision of the contractor should allow some element of give and take, and contractual difficulties must *never* be allowed to sour relationships on site. These should be retained for discussion in the office.

10.3.3 *Tunnels, pits and mines*

Analysis of steady-state inflow through a porous medium into a tunnel of infinite length can readily be carried out by two-dimensional flow analysis at right angles to the axis of the tunnel (Figure 10.5). Variations in hydraulic conductivity and in head difference from tunnel to water table can be taken into account along the length of the tunnel. However, where hydraulic conductivity and recharge are insufficient to maintain the flow without a reduction in the piezometric level above the tunnel, and where the tunnel is only partly completed yet already being dewatered, the completed tunnel will act as a transient drain. Prediction of water-filled fissures ahead of the working face can only be made by drilling ahead of the tunnel and remedial action by means of grouting and freezing taken accordingly. Estimation of regional inflow along the tunnel line can, however, be predicted, according to Goodman *et al.* (1965).

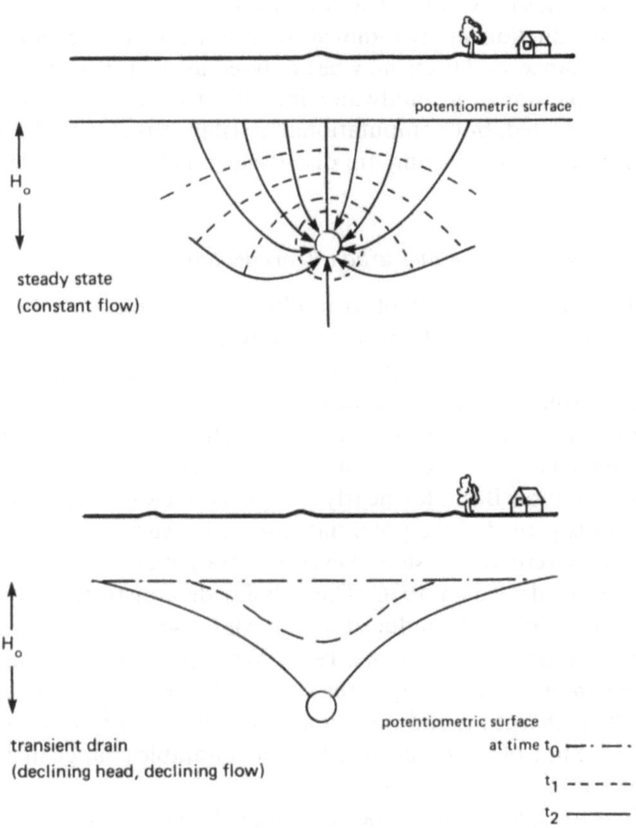

Figure 10.5 Drainage to tunnels.

The steady-state case is given by:

$$Q_0 = \frac{2\pi kH_0}{2.3\log(2H_0/r)} \qquad (10.10)$$

where Q_0 is rate of groundwater inflow per metre length of tunnel ($m^3 s^{-1}$), r is the tunnel radius and k is hydraulic conductivity ($m s^{-1}$).

The transient case is:

$$Q_t = 1.3\sqrt{kH_0^3 S_y t} \qquad (10.11)$$

where Q_t is the rate of groundwater inflow per metre length of tunnel at time t(s) after breakdown of steady-state conditions ($m^3 s^{-1}$) and S_y is specific yield. Equation 10.10 is, however, only valid when the water table has declined to level t_2 in Figure 10.5 and intercepted the tunnel lining.

Prediction of groundwater inflow into pits and excavations is complicated. Analysis depends on both the dewatering technique used (horizontal drains, drainage galleries or wellpoint systems) and the nature of the problem itself. Geometrical reduction into two-dimensional vertical cross-sections is necessary in the first instance, and these may be analysed using normal flownet analysis. The overall picture of groundwater inflow into the pit or excavation can then be constructed, but computational assistance is essential for this work. Further aspects of dewatering are discussed in detail in Chapter 11.

10.3.4 *Artificial recharge and urban hydrogeology*

The artificial replenishment of groundwater resources can be carried out either to improve the quality of the groundwater or, more usually in the UK, to store surplus winter resources for use during the summer as part of a conjunctive ground- and surface-water use scheme. Recharge may be induced via lagoons or irrigation or directly via injection through boreholes.

Artificial recharge through boreholes has been carried out in the Lea Valley area of the London Basin for nearly 100 years. Dewatering of the chalk and Tertiary sands provided the potential storage for surplus surface water from the Lea Valley reservoir system. Seven 0.7-m-diameter recharge/abstraction boreholes were drilled in 1976. These holes demonstrated that 40 million $m^3 a^{-1}$ recharge could be induced in one winter season, of which 75% could later be retrieved (Edworthy *et al.*, 1981). Widespread monitoring of groundwater levels showed the recharge area to be quite large. Following the winter of 1977–78 the recharge mound was some 4 m high and 5 km wide, with a 15-km axis along the line of the River Lea. The most notable change in groundwater quality was that of uptake of sulphate.

Elsewhere in Britain it has been estimated that storage available in the Permo-Triassic aquifers amounts to some 50 times the natural annual infiltration. However, decline in water-intensive industry coupled with induced recharge from cracked sewers and water mains has in any case led to rising groundwater levels in some areas, notably London, Birmingham and Liverpool. For example, in central London up until 1820, groundwater levels were about 5 m above Ordnance Datum and the Tertiary sands beneath the London clay were naturally fully saturated. Groundwater abstraction thereafter induced a steady decline in water levels so that the sand became dewatered some time between 1850 and 1875. More recent years have seen a reversal of this trend, and water levels have begun to recover steadily, so that resaturation of the sands and clays will inevitably occur in due course. This will create some interesting problems with pore pressures in the sands where they are confined by the overlying clays. It will also provide problems of dewatering wherever tunnelling has occurred below the base of the clays and into the Tertiary sands. These sands are pyrite-rich in certain horizons and the resaturation of the oxidised pyrite will allow iron and sulphate to be taken into solution, producing groundwaters rich in sulphuric acid.

In other cities, groundwater levels have been depressed by pumping for so long that it had been assumed that water tables were stable and it was safe to design higher buildings with deeper basements into what was believed to be a permanently unsaturated substratum. The problem is not confined to the UK, and both the New York Transit Authority and the Paris Metro have had problems with recent flooding. Deep groundwater drainage schemes may yet attain a grander scale than anything so far developed.

11 Dewatering

P. CARTER

11.1 Introduction

Groundwater is without doubt the greatest natural cause of problems in civil engineering construction. Dewatering is therefore a very common requirement. It is needed in particular for temporary works, such as excavations below the water table and embankments on waterlogged ground. Dewatering is also needed for some permanent works such as slopes and dams. This chapter gives a review of the subject and further information can be found in Bell (1987), BS 5930 (1981), Cripps *et al.* (1986), Hanrahan *et al.* (1989), ICE (1982, 1987, 1989), Patrick Powers (1981), Somerville (1986) and Weltman and Head (1983).

Groundwater problems sometimes come as a great surprise to the construction engineer, who immediately classifies them as 'unexpected ground conditions'. The cost of dealing with these conditions is then made the basis for a financial claim against the employer. It must be stressed that good ground investigations will do much to take the 'unexpected' out of groundwater problems and will provide the information needed to deal with the situation. A wise employer will therefore appoint a geotechnical consultant who will organise ground investigations and advise on dewatering (McInairnie, 1988; BGS, 1989). In this way, a little more expenditure at the outset of a project can save a great deal more money later on.

11.2 Excavation dewatering—pumping methods

Whenever the construction engineer excavates below ground level there is some danger of penetrating below the water table and encountering groundwater problems. Hazards may include inflow of water, heave of excavation base and collapse of soil material. This is particularly the case in countries which have a generally high water table and extensive areas of recently deposited alluvium or glacial soils. Most of the industrialised countries of the world are affected in this way. Groundwater problems are therefore a worldwide hazard for excavations, and dewatering is used on a worldwide scale.

Dewatering methods for excavations fall into two main groups, pumping

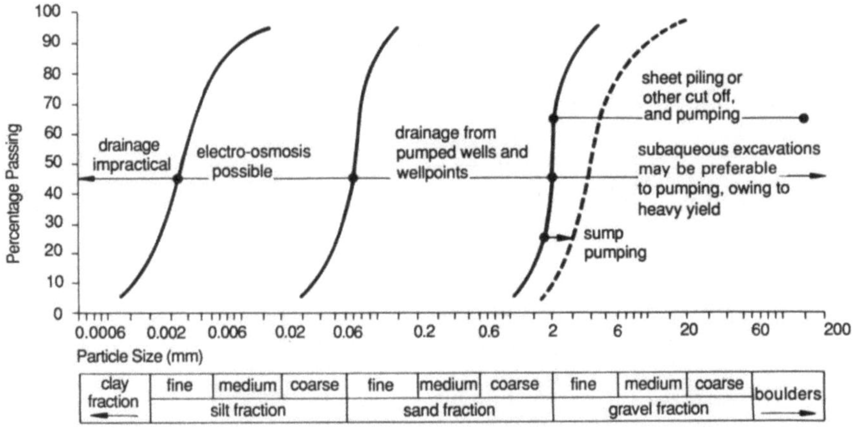

Figure 11.1 Tentative ranges for groundwater-lowering methods (after Somerville, 1986).

methods and exclusion methods. Pumping methods include:

Simple pumping.
Wellpointing.
Specialised wellpointing.
Filter wells.
Electro-osmosis.

The range of applicability of pumping methods is shown on Figure 11.1. These methods are generally best used for sands. Gravels are generally too permeable, and the flows of groundwater too large, for economic pumping. Silts are insufficiently permeable for gravity pumping but electrically induced flow is possible. Drainage of clays for temporary excavations is impractical and not generally required.

11.2.1 *Simple pumping*

Simple drainage and pumping methods are illustrated in Figure 11.2. Surface water inflows are intercepted by surface drainage ditches. Groundwater in shallow sand and gravel deposits can be drawn down by garland drains. These drains surround the excavation and consist of a pipe surrounded by gravel, leading to a pumping point. Sumps are provided for pumping water which collects at the lowest part of the excavation in less permeable soils. The sumps are made large enough to provide some water storage, and drains or ditches are used to lead water to the sumps.

Sump pumping can also be used in permeable soils where it is combined with sheet piling. The piling provides full excavation side support and is also driven down well below the base of the excavation to lengthen the groundwater flow path and prevent heave.

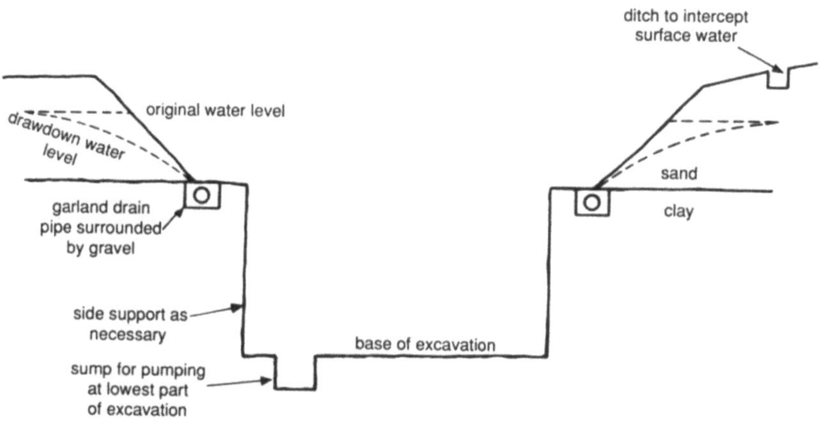

Figure 11.2 Simple drainage from excavation.

It must be noted that ordinary surface-set pumps will operate to a maximum depth of 5–6 m below the pump. Deeper excavations will need stage pumping or submersible pumps.

11.2.2 *Wellpointing*

Pumping from wells sited just outside the excavation is a very common method of dewatering. The principle of well pumping is to produce a lowering of the groundwater table and induce groundwater flow away from the excavation (Figure 11.3).

Wellpoints are very frequently used as method of pumping for excavations, particularly shallow excavations for pipelines. The system is relatively cheap, and much of the equipment can be recovered and re-used. Wellpoint systems consist of a line of wellpoints connected to a common header pipe. Where excavations are deeper than about 5 m, multistage systems will be needed (Figure 10.4).

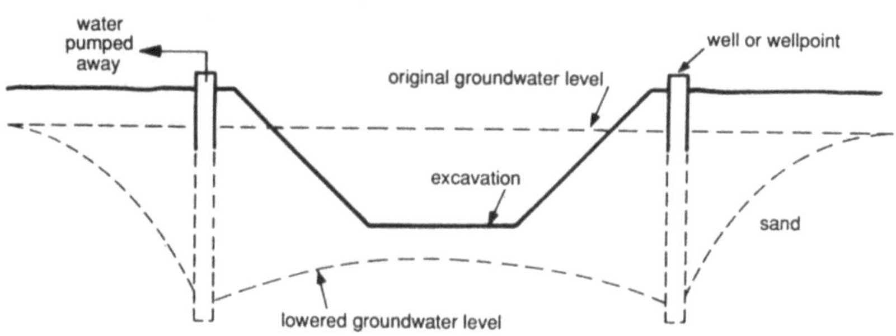

Figure 11.3 Groundwater lowering, flow to wells.

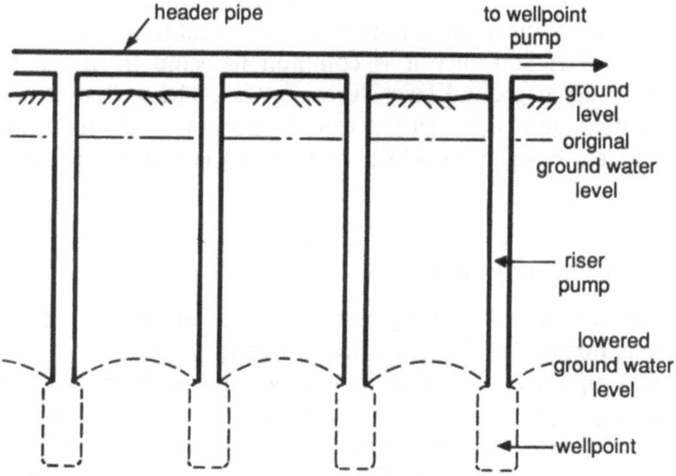

Figure 11.4 Wellpoints.

Wellpoints consist of small well screens about 50 mm in diameter and 1 m long, connected by a riser pipe to the header pipe (Figure 11.4). A centrifugal pump is used to pump water from the header pipe and draw down the groundwater level at the wellpoints. Spacing of the wellpoints will depend on the depth of groundwater lowering required and on the grain size of the sand. For example, for 3- and 6-m drawdowns the following spacings would be required:

Soil	Typical spacing (m) 3-m drawdown	Typical spacing (m) 6-m drawdown
Fine sand	2.4	1.7
Medium sand	1.5	1.0
Coarse sand	1.0	0.7
Sandy gravel	0.7	0.5

Header pipe take-off points for the riser pipes are generally at 1-m intervals, and deep wellpointing in coarse-grained soils becomes impractical as the required wellpoint spacing becomes very close. The time taken to obtain effective drawdown is also very dependent on the nature of the soil. For example, sandy gravels will be dewatered within 1 or 2 days, whereas silty sands may require several weeks.

Wellpoints are normally installed by jetting them into the ground using water under pressure. This is a very rapid process requiring only a few minutes for each wellpoint in loose sands. In coarser, compact materials jetting in may become impractical and a hole puncher is used to assist progress. If the soils are very fine and silty it is common to 'sand in' the wellpoint by introducing sand at ground level during jetting. The wellpoint is extracted when no longer needed by jetting out. Disposable wellpoints are used in particular cases, for example when wellpointing is required for an extended period.

11.2.3 *Specialised wellpointing*

Various specialised wellpointing systems are available, including vacuum wellpointing, horizontal wellpoints and eductor systems.

Vacuum wellpoints are used in fine-grained soils such as silty sands where gravity drainage is very slow. In this case the wellpoints are placed in a sand filter and the hole is sealed at ground level with a bentonite plug to maintain a high vacuum around the filter. The soils are not dewatered but the vacuum provides a pore suction which aids stability. The wellpoints are only effective to a depth of about 4 m and spacing must be very close.

Horizontal wellpoints are used mainly for pipeline work. They consist of perforated pipeline about 100 mm in diameter wrapped in a filter mesh and laid in a narrow trench to a depth of 2–6 m. Trenching, laying and backfilling is completed in a continuous operation using a purpose-built pipe-layer. The perforated pipes are connected by non-perforated suction pipes to pumps at ground level. This system has the advantage of speed and provides a clear working area at ground level. However, drawdown is limited to about 4 m, and the weight of the pipe-laying machine (about 32 tonnes) can cause trench stability problems.

Eductor systems are similar to wellpoints but water-lowering is produced by a vacuum created by a nozzle and Venturi system fed by a high-pressure ring main. They are suitable for low-permeability soils and deeper excavations where the water level requires to be lowered by 10 m or more. The cost of pumping with eductor systems is about four times the cost of pumping from multistage well pointing. However, the amount of land take and excavation required is much reduced.

11.2.4 *Filter wells*

Filter wells are of greater initial cost than wellpoints and the well screens cannot normally be withdrawn for re-use. Their chief adavantage is that groundwater lowering can be taken down to great depths without requiring multistage methods. They are also used in materials that do not allow easy installation of wellpoints.

Filter wells (Figure 11.5) are built in the same manner as water supply

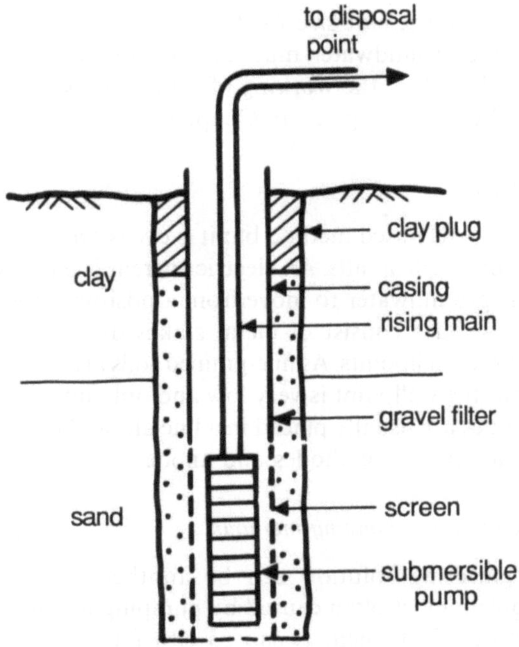

Figure 11.5 Filter well.

wells and include the following:

A screen section, usually 150 or 200 mm in diameter.
Casing from the top of the screen to ground level.
Filter wrapping or a sand filter around the screen.
A submersible electric pump, usually supplied with power by a diesel generator.
A rising main to ground surface and water outlet point.

Boreholes for filter wells are normally bored by cable tool or rotary equipment using temporary casing to support the side of the borehole. The permanent screen and casing is then installed and the filter introduced as the temporary liner is withdrawn. Jetting with compressed air is frequently used to remove any fine material from the screen and to develop the permeability of the ground surrounding the well.

The design of filter wells is dependent on the permeability of the ground and the grain size of the material to be dewatered. Good design of filter wells is of great importance as design failures can lead to ineffective wells. The permeability of the ground will determine the quantity of water to be pumped and hence the size of pump and diameter of screen. The grain size of the material will determine the slot size for the screen and design of the filter. The chemistry of the groundwater must also be known, since clogging or corrosion can greatly reduce the working life of a filter well system. Further details of filter well design are given in Chapter 10.

11.2.5 *Electro-osmosis*

Electro-osmosis is a rarely used method but it is occasionally used to dewater very fine-grained soils such as silts. An electric current is induced through the soil and causes the groundwater to move from a positive anode towards the negative cathode. Anodes consist of metal stakes driven into the ground, and cathodes consist of wellpoints. As fine-grained soils are of low permeability, the rate of flow into the wellpoint is very low and only intermittent pumping is required. Electrodes are usually placed in a line along the excavation about 3–5 m apart with alternating cathodes and anodes.

11.2.6 *Problems caused by pumping methods*

One person's engineering solution can be another person's engineering problem. The problem most often caused by pumping methods is settlement of adjacent structures. Settlement is caused either by loss of fine material into dewatering wells or by inducing consolidation of overlying compressive soils. The latter case can be the more extensive laterally. Dewatering causes a major drop in groundwater pressures, resulting in a commensurate increase in effective earth pressures. Compressible soils such as clay, silt and peat undergo consolidation where this occurs, resulting in settlement and damage at ground surface. This effect can be mitigated by using groundwater recharge to prevent reductions in groundwater level away from the area of the excavation.

11.3 Excavation dewatering—exclusion methods

Exclusion methods operate by excluding groundwater flow and thereby preventing hazards caused by groundwater flow into excavations. Such methods include grouting, freezing, compressed air and cut-offs. The ranges of applicability of these methods are shown in Figure 11.6.

11.3.1 *Grouting*

Grouting involves the infilling of pores or fractures in the ground with a material that replaces the groundwater, seals the water passages and prevents groundwater flow. Grouting methods are continually improving, and grouting is carried out by specialist contractors who have built up considerable experience over the decades.

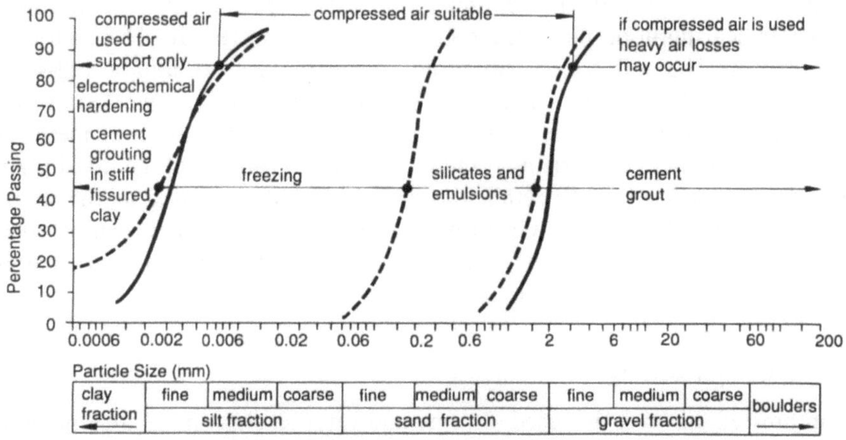

Figure 11.6 Tentative ranges for groundwater exclusion methods (after Somerville, 1986).

Different grouting materials are used depending on the grain size of the material to be grouted. Coarse-grained soils such as gravels can be grouted with particulate grouts such as cement and bentonite, which are often used in combination. Cement–bentonite grouting gives the ground strength as well as impermeability. Medium-grained soils such as sands require solution grouts such as silicates and emulsions. Some of these grouts give additional ground strength but others only give impermeability. Generally the finer grained the soil the more expensive is the grouting. Fine-grained soils such as silt cannot be effectively or economically grouted. Grouts are injected into the ground through boreholes in order to treat the ground to be excavated, or to provide a cut-off around the excavation.

An example of grouting methods is a sewer tunnel constructed beneath a 8-m-high embankment carrying a busy railway line at Dalry in Scotland

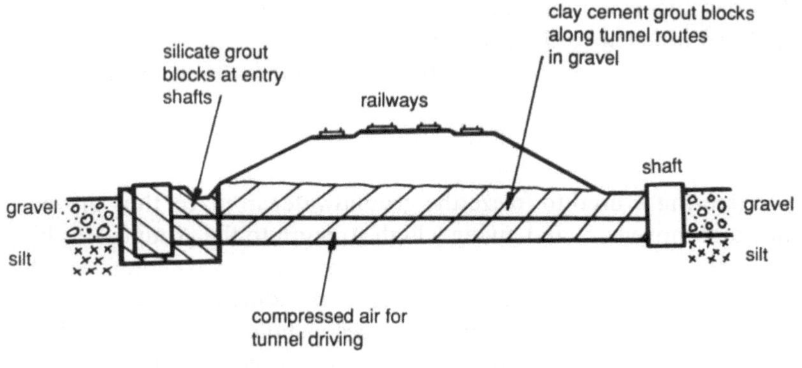

Figure 11.7 Grouting and compressed air for Dalry Tunnel.

(Carter and Forsyth, 1987). The tunnel was excavated in mixed face conditions of water-bearing flood plain gravels overlying soft silt (Figure 11.7), without interrupting the rail traffic. Borehole permeability tests and a full-scale pumping test showed that dewatering by pumping would not work and that compressed air would suffer massive air losses. A combination of methods was therefore used, comprising cement–bentonite grouting of the flood plain gravels, compressed air to retain the silt and silicate grouting at the shafts to permit tunnel breakout. Grouting beneath the embankment was carried out through inclined lances. The cost of the grouting was several times greater than the basic tunnelling cost.

11.3.2 *Compressed air*

Compressed air can be used for groundwater exclusion in an enclosed excavation such as a tunnel. An airlock is fitted to the tunnel entrance and compressed air is fed into the tunnel to maintain an artificially high pressure. The additional air pressure is built up to match the pressure of water to be excluded. For example, with a water table 10 m above tunnel invert level, an additional pressure of 1 atmosphere (1 bar) would be required. In practice it is usual to aim for a balance point about one-third up the tunnel face in order to minimise air loss at the tunnel crown.

Compressed air has a number of disadvantages, including the cost of establishing the airlock and constantly producing compressed air. All manpower, machinery and spoil have to move through the airlock. Losses of air can be high, particularly in coarser grained soils. A rule of thumb for calculating air loss is $7.5\,D^2\,\mathrm{m^3\,min^{-1}}$ where D is the tunnel diameter in metres. The pressures at which men can work safely without health damage are very limited, and this limits the operating depth for use of compressed air. In previous years compressed air was used at high pressure for such estuarial crossings as the Tyne tunnel, but it is now known that high pressures can cause the bends and bone necrosis. Health risks are minimal below 1 bar, but decompression becomes progressively more time-consuming up to 3 bar, above which special air mixtures are also required. Compressed air is now rarely used for tunnels deeper than 10 m below the water table.

11.3.3 *Ground freezing*

Ground freezing is used to freeze the groundwater in place, thus preventing groundwater movement and giving a high strength to the ground. It is highly expensive but is sometimes the only practical way of constructing deep shafts and tunnels, particularly in variable ground, including fine-grained sensitive soils. Freezing is carried out by freezer pipes installed in boreholes through which fluids below 0°C are circulated, such as refrigerated brine and liquid nitrogen. The boreholes may be drilled from the ground surface or from the tunnel or shaft face. The temperature required is dependent on the soil type, typically $-6°C$ in sands but as low as $-30°C$ in soft clay. Circular ice walls have been created using this method for construction of shafts up to 30 m in diameter.

11.3.4 *Cut-offs*

In some cases it may prove more economic or more feasible to provide a positive cut-off to exclude groundwater from the excavation. The cut-off provides an underground barrier penetrating into an impermeable formation below the base of the excavation. Temporary or permanent cut-offs may be provided.

Temporary cut-offs are formed by driving interlocking steel sheet piles. Permanent cut-offs can be formed by a variety of methods including:

Diaphragm walls, which are concrete walls formed in bentonite slurry-supported trenches.
Slurry trenches, which are filled with a slurry consisting of bentonite mixed in with the excavated soil.
Jet grouting, where cement grout is forced under high pressures into the ground, causing hydrofracturing.
Contiguous or secant-bored pile concrete walls.

Where concrete walls are formed they are frequently incorporated into the permanent works.

11.3.5 *Problems caused by exclusion methods*

A variety of problems can be created by groundwater exclusion methods. Barriers to groundwater flow caused by grout curtains or permanent cut-offs can raise the groundwater table and cause flooding of neighbouring underground structures. Some chemical grouts are injurious to health, and this can cause problems for future excavations in the vicinity of grouting operations. Compressed air leakage can result in air escaping into neighbouring properties and causing disruption. An example of this was a tunnel in Grangemouth in Scotland where escaping air caused great blisters to appear overnight in the hallowed turf of a bowling green. When the groundsman stuck a garden fork into one of the blisters it hissed at him! Ground freezing can alter the properties of the soils such that the thawed soil may be weaker than the original unfrozen soil.

11.4 Dewatering for embankments

Embankments constructed across soft fine-grained soils such as silts and soft clays can fail because of the increase in pore water pressure caused by the weight of the embankment.

When a fine-grained waterlogged soil is subject to a vertical load, the water in the pores cannot initially escape because of the low permeability of the soil. As a result the full load is taken by the incompressible water, the pore water pressure increases and the intergranular pressure decreases. Since the soil strength is dependent on the intergranular pressure, the strength consequently also decreases. As a result, and under the shear forces imposed by the embankment, a slip failure may occur.

If failure is prevented by dewatering, the pore water will slowly migrate away from the zone of pressure and the mineral grains will become more tightly packed. The intergranular pressure will increase and the soil strength will also increase and be capable of carrying the increased load caused by the weight of the embankment with safety.

Various dewatering methods are available for constructing embankments across soft cohesive soils including:

Staged construction.
Preconsolidation
Vertical drains.
Horizontal blankets.

11.4.1 *Staged construction*

Staged construction involves building an embankment as a series of layers with set time intervals between the emplacement of each layer. The time interval is set to allow sufficient dewatering of the soil by natural pore water pressure dissipation. For this method to be effective, the permeability and strength of the foundation soil must be known in advance. This requires high-class ground investigation and testing techniques. Stability analyses are carried out for the various stages of embankment construction, and the time interval required between stages is calculated to allow sufficient dissipation and strengthening (Symons, 1976).

An example of staged construction is the construction of a high motorway embankment across the soft alluvial silts and clays of the River Earn in Scotland (Cochrane and Carter, 1990). Investigations and stability analyses led to the creation of a stability chart for controlling embankment construction (Figure 11.8). Piezometers were installed in the soils below the embankment before construction started, and the rate of construction was limited to 0.5 m per month. As shown on the chart, the factor of safety progressivelly fell to about 1.4 by the end of construction. Had the piezometers shown slower rates of pore water dissipation then the rate of embankment construction would have been reduced still further to allow dissipation and to prevent failure.

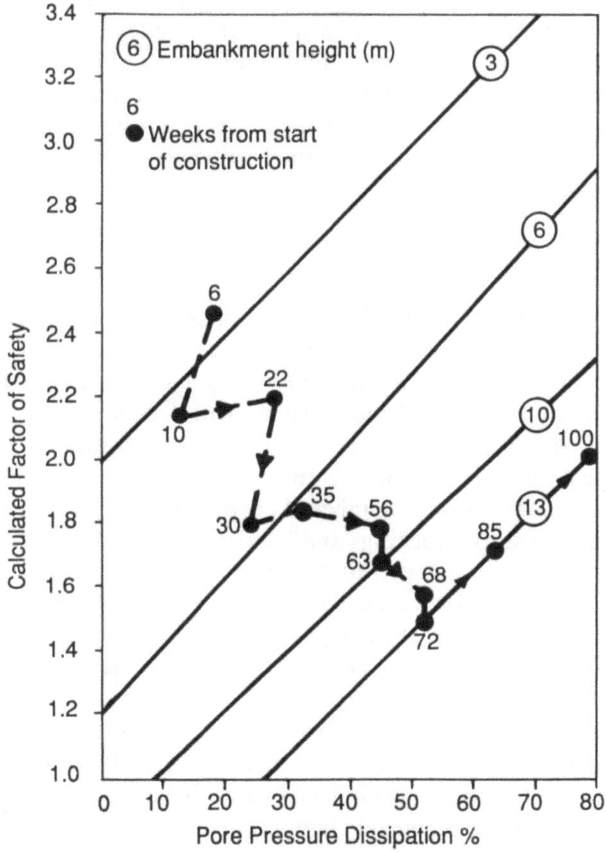

Figure 11.8 Staged construction stability charts for M90 Strathearn embankments.

11.4.2 *Preconsolidation*

Careful staged construction can allow safe construction across soft soils, but this method cannot necessarily prevent excessive post-construction settlement. Construction of a 5-m-high embankment may, for example, ultimately cause 1.0 m of settlement. For stability during construction it may only be necessary to dissipate 50% of the excess pore water pressure. The remaining 50% will cause a settlement of 0.5 m as a result of pore water dissipation after construction has been completed. Such a settlement may cause major road maintenance problems.

One solution is to build the embankment to a greater height than necessary, say 8 m. This will result in increased squeezing out of pore water from beneath the embankment and greater consolidation and settlement during the construction period. The excess 3 m of embankment fill can then be removed and any remaining settlement will be much reduced. This method can only be used if stability can still be maintained during construction. If natural pore water dissipation rates are too slow then artificial aids will be required, such as vertical drains.

11.4.3 *Vertical drains*

Vertical drains can be installed prior to embankment construction to shorten the drainage path for pore water migrating from the stressed areas (Figure 11.9). The vertical drains are generally installed on a diamond pattern at a typical spacing of 2–4 m. Actual spacing will depend on the horizontal coefficient of permeability of the soil and the required rate of construction.

In the past vertical drains were formed by boring holes and filling them with sand. More recently a large number of proprietary drains have come onto the market, such as fabric stockings and band drains. Fabric stockings consist of an outer filter fabric stocking which is filled with sand and placed in a premade hole. Band drains have an outer filter element and an inner core element and are normally driven into the soil.

Vertical drains have been widely used for embankment construction as they represent a seemingly positive engineering solution to an apparent engineering problem. However, both the solution and the problem may be more apparent than real. Some vertical drain systems, particularly those which involve driving the drain into the ground, can cause smearing of the drain sides and disruption of natural permeable laminae. This effect can much reduce if not

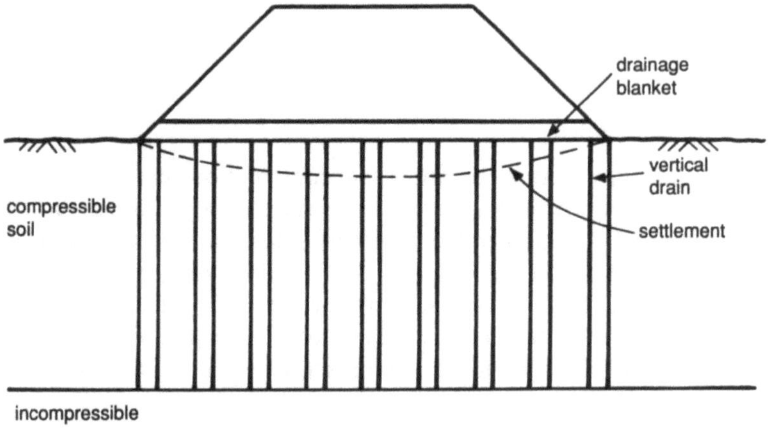

Figure 11.9 Vertical drains beneath embankment.

eliminate the effectiveness of the drains. The problem may also be more apparent than real in that many ground investigation techniques greatly underestimate the natural horizontal permeability of the soil. The soil microfabric may well be able to dissipate the excess pore water pressures without the introduction of artificial drains. Several trials have shown embankments without vertical drains settling at a similar rate to embankments with vertical drains.

11.4.4 *Horizontal blankets*

Embankments constructed over soft soils, with or without vertical drains, frequently require a horizontal blanket at ground level. The purpose of the blanket is to drain away pore water which is squeezed upwards under the weight of the embankment and to provide a blanket of sound material for the commencement of normal earthworks.

Traditionally drainage blankets have been about 1.0 m thick and constructed with coarse granular materials such as river gravel or rockfill. In recent years the use of artificial material has greatly expanded, including geotextiles and geogrids. The purpose of both materials, used in conjunction with a layer of free-draining material, is to provide both permeability and strength (Ingold and Miller, 1988).

11.5 Permanent dewatering

All the dewatering methods discussed so far have related to temporary works. Dewatering measures are also often required as an integral part of permanent works. Generally such measures are designed as gravity systems rather than pumped systems. The most commonly used permanent drainage measures for permanent works are shallow drains, deep drains, relief wells and drainage galleries.

11.5.1 *Shallow drains*

Shallow drains are sometimes used as a cutting slope protection measure. The drains are intended to intercept runoff and to prevent surface precipitation from percolating into the slope. They are also used to intercept groundwater issues or springs and to prevent slope erosion.

Shallow drains are generally filled with drainage aggregate, although open lined drains are also used. The drainage aggregate should be brought right up to ground level and not be covered with soil; the latter practice can often destroy the function of the drain. The drains are generally angled across the slope or arranged in a 'herringbone' pattern to give maximum opportunity for intercepting run-off. If large flows are expected a pipe is provided in the base, typically open-tile pipe, porous concrete or perforated plastic pipe. Geotextiles are often used as a separator between the soil and the drainage aggregate. Some proprietary fin-type drains which are primarily constructed from geofabrics are available.

11.5.2 *Deep drains*

Deep trench drains may be used to stabilise landslides by causing a significant decrease in groundwater pressure. Deep trench drains that intercept the slip plane and provide additional frictional resistance are generally called counterfort drains. Deep drains are infilled with drainage aggregate in the same manner as shallow drains, but the upper part is often replaced with soil as their prime function is deep drainage rather than surface drainage.

Many slip planes are less than 5 m below ground level, and deep drains can readily be excavated to 6 m below ground level using hydraulic backactor machines. The effect of the drains is to promote flow of groundwater out of the soil and into the drains, causing an overall lowering of the groundwater level (Figure 11.10). Groundwater lowering decreases the groundwater pressure on the slip plane, giving an increase in frictional resistance and hence an increase in stability. The spacing of drains for a variety of different conditions can be calculated using graphs presented by Hutchinson (1977), which are summarised by Bromhead (1986).

11.5.3 *Relief wells*

Relief wells are provided in a very wide variety of situations to prevent build-up of excessive water pressures on structures.

Dams are frequently supplied with relief wells on the downstream side of the cut-off in order to control underseepage and prevent build-up of water

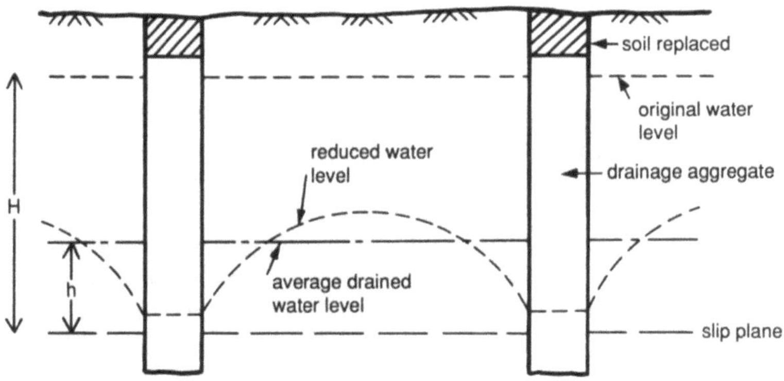

Figure 11.10 Counterfort drains. Water pressure on slip plane reduced from H to h.

pressure beneath the dam foundation. Any such pressure build-up carries the risk of promoting slip failure of the downstream shoulder with consequent massive dam breaching.

Retaining walls act as an impermeable barrier for groundwater flow, and relief holes are provided to allow water flow through the wall. Unacceptable build-up of water pressure behind a retaining wall could lead to overturning or basal sliding.

Tunnels are often driven below groundwater level, and relief wells are sometimes provided to prevent excess build-up of water pressure on the tunnel lining, as for example in the newly renovated Glasgow Subway.

Rising groundwater tables are a new hazard for deep basements in major cities. Groundwater tables have been artificially depressed for decades as a result of pumping for industrial water supply. As the industries have moved out of the cities the wells have fallen into disuse and groundwater tables are re-establishing their former levels. London is a particular case where Simpson *et al.* (1989) have found a large area threatened by a water table which is rebounding at up to 1 m per annum. Studies are also under way for such other cities as Liverpool and Birmingham. Major new structures in London with deep basements such as the new British Library are being fitted with a system of relief wells. Proposals have been made for a London-wide system of relief wells in order to cope with the problem and prevent high costs for individual developers.

11.5.4 *Drainage galleries*

Drainage galleries are tunnels driven into areas requiring very deep dewatering, where the topography allows gravity drainage from the galleries into a surface drainage system. Drainage galleries have been used for landslip stabilisation in particular, for example the tunnels into the Folkestone Warren landslip which are believed to have lowered groundwater levels by up to 20 m. Drainage galleries are however a highly expensive solution, and can be very difficult to construct in failed ground.

References

Abbott, M.B. (1966) *An Introduction to the Method of Characteristics*. London: Thames and Hudson.

Abbott, M.B. (1979) *Elements of the Theory of Free Surface Flow*. London: Pitman.

Abbott, M.B., Bathurst, J.C., Cunge, J.A., O'Connell, P.E. & Rasmussen, J. (1986) An introduction to the European Hydrological System – Système Hydrologique Européen, 'SHE'. 2. Structure of the physically based, distributed modelling system. *Journal of Hydrology* **87**, 61–77.

Abel, P.D. (1989) *Water Pollution Biology*. Chichester: Ellis Horwood.

Ackers, P. & White, W.R. (1973) Sediment transport: New approach and analysis. *Journal of the Hydraulics Division, Proceedings of the American Society of Civil Engineers* **99** (HY 11), 2041–60.

Anderson, K.G. (1987) Legislation—past and present. In T.W. Brandon (Ed.) *River Engineering*. Part 1. *Design Principles*, pp. 1–32. Water Practice Manual Book 7. London: Institution of Water Engineers and Scientists for Institution of Water and Environmental Management.

Ando, Y., Takahasi, Y. & Kuan, M.F. (1984) Relation between land use and final infiltration rate in urban areas. In P. Balmer, P.A. Malmqvist & A. Sjöberg (Eds.) *Proceedings of the Third International Conference on Urban Storm Drainage, Chalmers University of Technology, Gothenburg*.

Aravin, V.I. & Numerov, S.N. (1965) *Theory of Fluid Flow in Undeformable Porous Media* (A. Moscona, Trans.). Jerusalem: Israel Program for Scientific Translations.

Arnell, V. (1982) *Rainfall Data for the Design of Sewer Pipe Systems*. Department of Hydraulics Report Series A:8. Gothenburg: Chalmers University of Technology.

ASAE (1972) Design, layout, construction and maintenance of terrace systems. ASAE Recommendation, p. R268.1. ASAE Yearbook. St Joseph, MI: American Society of Agricultural Engineers.

Bear, J. (1979) *Hydraulics of Groundwater*. New York: McGraw Hill.

Bebelaar, J.P. & Bakker, J.W. (1981) Infiltratie van regenwater door verschillende wegdekken i.v.m. de watervoorziening van straatbomen (Infiltration of rainwater in different pavements in relation to the water supply to trees along roads). Nota 1247. Wageningen: Institute for Land and Water Management.

Bedient, P.B. & Huber, W.C. (1988) *Hydrology and Floodplain Analysis*. Wokingham: Addison Wesley.

Bell, F.G. (Ed). (1987) *Ground Engineers Reference Book*. London: Butterworth.

Beran, M.A. (1982) The drainage of low lying flat lands. *Proceedings of the Conference of River Engineers* (unbound). Wallingford: Institute of Hydrology.

Beven, K. & Germann, P (1982). Macropores and water flow in soils. *Water Resources Research* **18**, 1311–25.

BGS (1989) *The Geotechnical Directory*. British Geotechnical Society.

BHRA (1986) *Proceedings of the Conference on Water Quality Modelling in the Inland Natural Environment, Bournemouth*. British Hydrodynamics Research Association.

BHS (1989) *Weather Radar and the Water Industry*. Occasional paper No. 2. Wallingford: Institute of Hydrology for the British Hydrological Society.

Bierschenk, W.H. (1964) *Determining Well Efficiency by Multiple Step Drawdown Tests*, pp. 493–504. Publication No. 64. Berkeley, CA: International Association of Scientific Hydrology.

Blaisdell, F.W. (1948) Development and hydraulic design, Saint Anthony Falls Stilling Basin. *Transactions of the American Society of Civil Engineers* **113**, 483–520.

Blaisdell, F.W. (1949) The SAF Stilling Basin. SCS-TP-79, US Soil Conservation Service, Washington.

Blench, T. (1969) *Mobile Bed Fluviology*. Edmonton: University of Alberta Press.
Bos, M.G. (1984) Where water leaves the irrigation system, pp. 30–38. IILRI Annual Report. Wageningen: International Institute for Land Reclamation and Improvement.
Bradley, J.M. & Peterka, A.J. (1957) The hydraulic design of stilling basins. *Journal of the Hydraulics Division, Proceedings of the American Society of Civil Engineering*, **83** (HY5).
Brady, N.C. (1990) *The Nature and Properties of Soils*. New York: Macmillan.
Brandon, T.W. (Ed.) (1987) *River Engineering*. Part 1. *Design Principles*. Water Practice Manual Book 7. London: Institution of Water Engineers and Scientists for Institution of Water and Environmental Management.
Brandon, T.W. (Ed.) (1989) *River Engineering*. Part 2. *Structures and Coastal Defence Works*. Water Practice Manual Book 8. London: Institution of Water and Environmental Management.
British Steel (1988) *Piling Handbook*, 6th edn. Scunthorpe: British Steel Plc.
Bromhead, E.N. (1986) *The Stability of Slopes*. Glasgow: Blackie.
Browning, K.A. & Collier, C.G. (1989) Nowcasting of precipitation systems. *Reviews of Geophysics* **27**(3), 345–70: American Geophysical Union.
Bryson Jr, A.E. & Yu-Chi Ho (1975) *Applied Optimal Control*. New York: Wiley.
BS 5930 (1981) *Code of Practice for Site Investigations*. London: British Standards Institution.
BS 6316 (1983) *Code of Practice for Test Pumping of Water Wells*. London: British Standards Institution.
Carter, P.G. & Forsyth, F.M. (1987) Groundwater investigations and control for the Dalry Tunnels. In E.T. Hanrahan *et al.* (Eds.) *Proceedings of the Ninth European Conference on Soil Mechanics and Foundation Engineering*. Rotterdam: Balkema.
Castle, D., McCunnall, J. & Tring, I. (1984) *Field Drainage Principles and Practice*. London: Batsford.
Cavelaars, J.C. (1973). Subsurface field drainage systems. In *Drainage Principles and Practice*. IILRI Publication No. 16, Vol. 4. Wageningen: International Institute for Land Reclamation and Improvement.
Chang, H.H. (1983) Energy expenditure in curved open channels. *Journal of Hydraulic Engineering, Proceedings of the American Society of Civil Engineers* **109**, 1012–22.
Charnley, P.R., Beran, M.A., Samuels, P.G., Terry, J.B., Hann, M.J. & Dennis, C.W. (1987) Lowland drainage. In T.W. Brandon (Ed.) *River Engineering*. Part 1. *Design Principles*, pp. 173–224. Water Practice Manual Book 7. London: Institution of Water Engineers and Scientists for Institution of Water and Environmental Management.
Childs, E.C. (1945) The water table, equipotentials and streamlines in drained land. III. *Soil Science* **59**, 405–15.
Childs, E.C. (1968) The achievements of drainage theory in relation to practical needs: Taking stock. *Transactions of the IXth International Congress of Soil Science* **1**, 349–56.
Childs, E.C. (1969) *An Introduction to the Physical Basis of Soil Water Phenomena*. London: Wiley.
Childs, E.C. (1970) Land drainage: An exercise in physics. *Outlook on Agriculture* **6**, 158–65.
Chisci, G. (1976) Influence of tillage and drainage systems on physical conditions for clay soil cultivation. *Annali Instituto Sperimentale Studio Difesa Suolo, Firenze* **7**, 55–66.
Chisci, G. & Lodi, G. (1974) Ricerche parcellari sulla argillosi. VIII. Influenza delle caratteristiche del suolo e del drennaggio sula produzione e sulla composizione botanica di un prato polifito asciutto. *Annali Instituto Sperimentale Studio Difesa Suolo, Firenze* **5**, 85–102.
Chisci, G. & Zanchi, C. (1981) The influence of different tillage systems and different crops on soil losses on hilly silty-clayey soil. In R.P.C. Morgan (Ed.) *Soil Conservation: Problems and Prospects*, pp. 211–17. Chichester: Wiley.
Chisci, G., Zanchi, C. & D'Edigio, G. (1981) Erosion investigation plots. In *Erosion and Sediment Transport Measurement. Field Excursion Guide*, pp. 40–45. Oxford: Blackwell Scientific Publications for International Association of Scientific Hydrology.
Chow, V.T. (1950, 1959) *Open Channel Hydraulics*. New York: McGraw Hill.
Chow, V.T. (1964) *Handbook of Applied Hydrology*. New York: McGraw Hill.
Chow, V.T., Maidment, D.R. & Mays, L.W. (1988) *Applied Hydrology*. New York: McGraw Hill.
Cochrane, G.A. & Carter, P.G. (1990). Highway embankment construction across the Strathearn Buried Valley. In *Proceedings of the Conference on Engineering Geology, Edinburgh, 1989*.

Coppin, N.J. & Richards, I.G. (1990) *The Use of Vegetation in Civil Engineering*. London: Butterworths for Construction Industry Research and Information Association.

Crank, J. (1956) *The Mathematics of Diffusion*. Oxford University Press.

Crawford, N.H. & Linsley, R.K. (1966) *Digital Simulations in Hydrology. Stanford Watershed Model IV. T.R. 39*. Stanford University Department of Civil Engineering.

Cripps, J.C. *et al.* (Eds.) (1986) *Groundwater in Engineering Geology*. London: Geological Society of London.

Cunge, J.A., Holly, F.M. & Verway, A. (1980) *Practical Aspects of Computational River Hydraulics*. London: Pitman.

De Crecy, J. (1982). Structural behaviour of heavy soils and drainage systems. In M.J. Gardiner (Ed.) *Land Drainage*, pp. 73–84. Rotterdam: Balkema.

van Deemter, J.J. (1950) Bijdragen tot de kennis van enige natuurkundige grootheden van de grond. 11. Theoretische en numerieke behandeling van ontwaterings- en infiltratie-stromingsproblemen. *Verslagen van Landbouwkundige Onderzoekingen* **56.7**, 1–67.

De Vleeschauer, D., Lal, R. & De Boodt, M. (1979) Influence of soil conditioners on water movement through some tropical soils, In R. Lal & D.J. Greenland (Eds.) *Soil Physical Properties and Crop Production in the Tropics*, pp. 149–58. Chichester: Wiley.

Derby, H.C. (1956) *The Draining of the Fens*. Cambridge University Press.

Dieleman, P.J. & Trafford, B.D. (1976) *Drainage Testing*. Irrigation and Drainage Paper No. 28. Rome: Food and Agriculture Organisation.

Doorenbos, J. & Pruitt, W.O. (1977) *Crop Water Requirements*. Irrigation and Drainage Paper No. 24. Rome: Food and Agriculture Organisation.

Driscoll, F.G. (1986). *Groundwater and Wells*. St Paul, MN: Johnson Division.

Dumm, L.D. (1954) Drain spacing formula. *Agricultural Engineering* **35**, 726–30.

Dumm, L.E. & Winger, R.J. (1964) Subsurface drainage for irrigated areas using transient flow concepts. *Transactions of the American Society of Agricultural Engineers* **7**, 2.

Edworthy, K.J., Headworth, H.G. & Hawnt, R.J.E. (1981) Application of artificial recharge techniques in the UK. In *A Survey of British Hydrogeology 1980*, pp. 141–52. London: Royal Society.

EEC (1975) *Directive of 16 June 1975 Concerning the Quality Required of Surface Water Intended for the Abstraction of Drinking Water in the Member States*. 74/440/EEC; oj 1 194. Brussels: Commission of the European Communities.

EEC (1976) *Directive of 8 December 1975 Concerning the Quality of Bathing Water*. 76/160/EEC; oj 1 194. Brussels: Commission of the European Communities.

Elliott, S.C. & Sellin, R.H.J. (1990) SERC Flood Channel Facility, skewed flow experiments. *Journal of Hydraulic Research (International Association for Hydraulic Research)* **28**, 197–214.

Engelund, F. (1951) Mathematical discussion of drainage problems. *Transactions of the Danish Academy of Technical Sciences* **3**, 1–64.

EPA (1972) *A Flushing System for Combined Sewer Cleansing*. Report 11020 DNO. US Environmental Protection Agency.

Eriksson, J. (1979) Soil functions and drainage. In J. Wesseling (Ed.) *Proceedings of the International Drainage Workshop*, pp. 180–212. Wageningen: International Land Research Institute Publication No. 25.

Ervine, D.A. & Ellis, J. (1987) Experimental and computational aspects of overbank flood plain flow. *Transactions of the Royal Society of Edinburgh, Earth Sciences* **78**, 315–25.

Ervine, D.A. & Jasem, H.K. (1991) Two-stage channels with the main channel skewed relative to the floodplain direction. Paper submitted to *Journal of Hydraulics Division, Proceedings of the American Society of Civil Engineers*.

Falk, J. & Niemczynowicz, J. (1979) *Modelling of Runoff from Impermeable Surfaces*. Reports of the Department of Water Resource Engineering 3024. Lund: Lund Institute of Technology, University of Lund.

Farquharson, F.A.K., Green, C.S., Meigh, J.R. & Sutcliffe, J.V. (1987) Comparison of flood frequency curves for many different regions of the world. In V.P. Singh (Ed.) *Regional Flood Frequency Analysis*, pp. 223–56. Dordrecht: Reidel.

Farr, E. & Henderson, W.C. (1986) *Land Drainage*. Harlow: Longman.

Farraday, R.V. & Charlton, F.G. (1983) *Hydraulic Factors in Bridge Design*. Wallingford: Hydraulics Research Ltd.

Fausey, N.D. & Schwab, G.O. (1969) Soil moisture content, tilth and soybean response with surface and subsurface drainage. *Agronomy Journal* **61**, 554–57.

FitzPatrick, E.A. (1986) *An Introduction to Soil Science.* Harlow: Longman.

Fleming, G. (1975) *Computer Simulation Techniques in Hydrology.* New York: Elsevier.

Forstner, U. & Wittman, G.T.W. (1981) *Metal Pollution in the Aquatic Environment.* Berlin: Springer.

Foster, W.E. & Harris, W.B. (1988) Flood alleviation scheme for Lower River Mole. *Proceedings of the Institution of Civil Engineers Part 1* **84**, 235–263.

Freeze, R.A. & Cherry, J.A. (1979) *Groundwater.* New Jersey: Prentice-Hall.

Gardner, W.R. (1958) Some steady state solutions of the unsaturated moisture flow equation with application to evaporation from a water table. *Soil Science* **85**, 244–49.

Geiger, W.E. *et al.* (1987) Quantity of stormwater. In *Manual on Design of Drainage Systems in Urbanized Areas.* Paris: UNESCO.

Gerrard, R.T., Long, J.J. & Shah, H.R. (1982) Barking Creek Tidal Barrier. *Proceedings of the Institution of Civil Engineers Part 1* **72**, 533–562.

Goodman, R.E., Moye, D.G., van Schalkwyk, A. & Javendal, I. (1965) Ground water inflows during tunnel driving. *Engineering Geology* **2**, 39–56.

Gray, D.H. & Leiser, A.T. (1982) *Biotechnical Slope Protection and Erosion Control.* New York: Van Nostrand.

Gray, D.M. (1970) *Handbook on the Principles of Hydrology.* Ottawa: National Research Council of Canada.

Green, W.H. & Ampt, G.A. (1911) Studies in soil physics. I. The flow of air and water through soils. *Journal of Agricultural Science* **4**, 1–24.

Grimmond, C.S.B. & Oke, T.R. (1986). Urban water balance 2; results from a suburb of Vancouver, British Columbia. *Water Resource Research* **22**, 1404–12.

Hall, M.J. & Ellis, J.B. (1985) Water quality problems of urban areas. *GeoJournal* **11**, 265–75.

Hall, M.J. & Hockin, D.L. (1980) *Guide to the Design of Storage Ponds for Flood Control in Partly Urbanised Catchments.* Technical Note No. 100. London: Construction Industry Research and Information Association.

Hanks, R.J. & Ashcroft, G.L. (1980) *Applied Soil Physics.* Berlin: Springer.

Hanrahan, E.T. *et al.* (1989) Groundwater effects on geotechnical engineering. In *Proceedings of the Ninth European Conference on Soil Mechanics and Foundation Engineering.* Rotterdam: Balkema.

Harbeck, G.E. (1962) *A Practical Field Technique for Measuring Reservoir Evaporation Utilising Mass Transfer Theory.* Professional Paper No. 272-E. US Geological Survey.

Harr, M.E. (1962) *Groundwater and Seepage.* New York: McGraw Hill.

Hazen, A. (1893) Some physical properties of sands and gravels. *24th Annual Report.* Massachusetts State Board of Health.

Helliwell, P. (Ed.) (1978) *Urban Storm Drainage.* Pentech Press.

Hemphill, R.W. & Bramley, M.E. (1989) *Protection of River and Canal Banks—a Guide to Selection and Design.* London: Butterworths for Construction Industry Research and Information Association.

Henderson, F.M. (1966) *Open Channel Flow.* New York: MacMillan.

Herschy, R.W. (Ed.) (1978) *Hydrometry, Principles and Practices.* Chichester: Wiley.

Hewlett, H.W.M., Boorman, L.A. & Bramley, M.E. (1987) *Design of Reinforced Grass Waterways.* Report 116. London: Construction Industry Research and Information Association.

Hillel, D. (1980a) *Fundamentals of Soil Physics.* New York: Academic Press.

Hillel, D. (1980b) *Applications of Soil Physics.* New York: Academic Press.

Hillel, D. (1982) *Introduction to Soil Physics.* New York: Academic Press.

HMSO (1974) *The Health and Safety at Work Act.* London: Her Majesty's Stationery Office.

Hogland, W. & Niemczynowicz, J. (1980) Kvantitativ och kvalitativ vatten omsättningsbudget för Lunds centralort; kompletterande mätningar och metodik. Reports of the Department of Water Resource Engineering 3038. Lund: Lund Institute of Technology, University of Lund.

Hooghoudt, S.B. (1940) Bijdragen tot de kennis van enige natuurkundige grootheden van de grond. 7. Algemeene beschouwing van het probleem van de detail ontwatering en de infiltratie door middel van parallel loopende drains, greppels, slooten en kanalen. *Verslagen van Landbouwkundige Onderzoekingen* **46**, 515–707.

Hove, D. ten & Wensveen, L.D.M. (1986) *Rendement Randvoorzieningen Bergbezinkbassin* (Efficiency of Stormwater Sedimentation Tanks). NWRW Investigation Theme 8.
Huber, W.C. & Dickinson, R.E. (1988) *Storm Water Management Model User's Manual Version 4*. EPA/600/3-88/0001a (PB88-236641/AS). Athens, GA: Environmental Protection Agency.
Hudson, N.W. (1981) *Soil Conservation*. London: Batsford.
Hudson, N.W. (1987) *Soil and Water Conservation in Semi-arid Areas*. Soils Bulletin No. 57. Rome: Food and Agriculture Organisation.
Hundal, S.S., Schwab, G.O. & Taylor, G.S. (1976) Drainage system effects on physical properties of a lakebed clay soil. *Soil Science Society of America Journal* **40**, 300–05.
Hutchinson, J.N. (1977) Assessment of the effectiveness of corrective measures in relation to geological conditions and types of slope movement. *Bulletin of the International Association of Engineering Geologists* **16**, 131–55.
Hvorslev, M.J. (1951) *Time Lag and Soil Permeability in Groundwater Observations*. Bulletin 36. Vicksburg, MS: Waterways Experimental Station, US Army Corps of Engineers.
Hynes, H.B.N. (1971) *The Biology of Polluted Water*. Liverpool University Press.
Ibrahim, A.A. (1982) *Analytical and Laboratory Study of Local Scour Round Bridge Piers*. Glasgow University MSc Thesis.
ICE (1978) *Floods and Reservoirs Safety: an Engineering Guide* (prepared by Institution of Civil Engineers). London: Institution of Civil Engineers.
ICE (1981) Vertical drains: Symposium in print. *Géotechnique* **31**, 1–90.
ICE (1987) *Specification for Ground Treatment and Notes for Guidance* (prepared by Institution of Civil Engineers). Thomas Telford Ltd.
ICE (1989) *Specification for Ground Investigation*. Thomas Telford Ltd.
Ingold, T.S. & Miller, K.S. (1988) *Geotextiles Handbook*. Thomas Telford Ltd.
James, A. (Ed.) (1984) *An Introduction to Water Quality Modelling*. Chichester: Wiley.
Jensen, S.J., Stårup, J., Sørensen, B.E. & Jakobsen, C. (1985) Regnafstrømningsprojekt i Mølleåsystemet; Supplerende målinger 1981–1983. Lyngby: Department of Environmental Engineering, Technical University of Denmark.
Karplus, W.J. (1958) *Analog Simulation*. New York: McGraw Hill.
Kellerhals, R. (1967) Stable channels with gravel-paved beds. *Journal of the Waterways and Harbours Division, Proceedings of the American Society of Civil Engineers* **93** (WW1), 62–84.
Kiely, G.K. (1989) *An Experimental Study of Overbank Flow in Straight and Meandering Compound Channels*. Ph.D. thesis. Department of Civil Engineering, University College Cork, Ireland.
Kidd, C.H.R. (Ed.) (1978) *Rainfall-Runoff Processes over Urban Surfaces: Proceedings of an International Workshop*. Report 53. Wallingford: Institute of Hydrology.
Kikkawa, H., Ikeda, S. & Kitagawa, A. (1976) Flow and bed topography in curved open channels. *Journal of Hydraulics, Proceedings of the American Society of Civil Engineers* **102**, 1327–42.
Kirk, D.E. (1970) *Optimal Control Theory*. Englewood Cliffs, NJ: Prentice-Hall.
Kirkham, D. (1949) Flow of ponded water into drain tubes in soil overlying an impervious layer. *Transactions of the American Geophysical Union* **30**, 369–85.
Kirkham, D. & Powers, W.L. (1972) *Advanced Soil Physics*. New York: Wiley.
Kirkus, A.M. (1959) *The Records of the Commissioners of Sewers in the Parts of Holland, 1547–1603*, Vol. 1. Lincoln: Lincoln Record Society.
Kirpich, Z.P. (1940) Time of concentration of small agricultural watersheds. *Civil Engineer* **10**, 362.
Klein, L. (1962) *River Pollution. 2: Causes and Effects*. London: Butterworths.
Klute, A. (Ed.) (1986) *Methods of Soil Analysis*. Part 1. *Physical and Mineralogical Methods*. Madison, WI: American Society of Agronomy.
Knight, D.W. & Sellin R.H.J. (1990) The SERC flood channel facility. *Journal of the Institution of Water and Environment Management* **1**, 192–204.
Knight, D.W. & Shiono, K. (1990) Turbulence measure measurements in a shear layer region of a compound channel. *Journal of Hydraulic Research* (*International Association for Hydraulic Research*) **28**, 175–196.
Krantz, B.A. (1981) Water conservation, management and utilisation in semi-arid lands. In *Advances in Food Producing Systems for Arid and Semi-arid Lands*, pp. 339–78. Davis, CA: University of California.

Kruseman, G.P. & de Ridder, N.A. (1970) *Analysis and Evaluation of Pumping Test Data.* Bulletin 11. Wageningen: International Institute for Land Reclamation and Improvement.
Lal, H. (1985) Animal drawn wheeled tool carrier: An appropriate mechanization for improved farming systems. *Agricultural Mechanization in Asia, Africa and Latin America* **16**, 38–44.
Lacey, G. (1958) Flow in alluvial channels with sandy mobile beds. *Proceedings of the Institution of Civil Engineers* **9**, 145–64, **11**, 219–51.
Lasdon, L.S. (1970) *Optimization Theory for Large Systems.* London: Macmillan.
Laurenson, E.M. (1964) A catchment storage model for runoff routing. *Journal of Hydrology* **2**, 141–63.
Lewitt, E.H. (1958) *Hydraulics and Fluid Mechanics.* London: Pitman.
Leyton, L. & Yadav, J.S.P. (1960) Effect of drainage on certain physical properties of a heavy clay soil. *Journal of Soil Science* **11**, 305–12.
LGORU (1973) *The Economics of Flood Alleviation.* Report C155. Reading: Local Government Operational Research Unit.
Linsley, R.K., Kohler, M.A. & Paulhus, J.L.H. (1988) *Hydrology for Engineers, SI Metric Edition.* New York: McGraw Hill.
Lovell, C.J. & Youngs, E.G. (1984) A comparison of steady-state land-drainage equations. *Agricultural Water Management* **9**, 1–21.
Luthin, J.N. (Ed.) (1957) *Drainage of Agricultural Lands.* Monograph No. 7. Madison, WI: American Society of Agronomy.
McIlveen, J.R.F. (1986) *Basic Meteorology, a Physical Outline.* Wokingham: Van Nostrand Reinhold.
McInairnie, E. (1988) *The Geologists' Directory.* Institution of Geologists.
Maddaus, W.O. & Eagleson, P.S. (1969) *A Distributed Linear Representation of Surface Runoff.* Hydromechanics Laboratory Report No. 115. Cambridge, MA: MIT Department of Civil Engineering.
MAFF (1974) *Arterial Drainage and Agriculture.* Drainage Leaflet No. 16. London: Ministry of Agriculture, Fisheries and Food.
MAFF (1983) *The Design of Field Drainage Pipe Systems.* Ministry of Agriculture, Fisheries and Food Reference Book No. 345. London: HMSO.
Mann, W.R. & Green, J.A. (1978) *The Economics of Pumped Drainage.* Report No C271. Reading: Local Government Operational Research Unit.
Marshall, T.J. & Holmes, J.W. (1979) *Soil Physics.* Cambridge University Press.
Mason, C.F. (1981) *Biology of Freshwater Pollution.* London: Longman.
Matkin, E.A. & Smart, P. (1987) A comparison of tests of soil structural stability. *Journal of Soil Science* **38**, 123–35.
Meteorological Office (1964) *Hydrological Memorandum No. 33.*
Meteorological Office (1969) *Observers' Handbook*, 3rd Edn. London: HMSO.
Meyer, L.D. & Wischmeier, W.H. (1969) Mathematical simulation of the process of soil erosion by water. *Transactions of the American Society of Agricultural Engineers* **12**, 754–58, 762.
Ministry of Housing (1970) *Report of Technical Committee on Storm Overflows and the Treatment of Storm Sewage. Ministry of Housing and Local Government.* London: HMSO.
Morgan, R.P.C. (1986) *Soil Erosion and Conservation.* London: Longman.
Morgan, R.P.C. (1989) Design of in-field shelter systems for wind erosion control. In U. Schwertmann, R.J. Rickson & K. Auerswald (Eds.) *Soil Erosion Protection Measures in Europe*, pp. 15–23. Soil Technology Series 1. Brussels: Commission of the European Communities.
Morisawa, M. (1985) *Rivers—Form and Process.* London: Longman.
MOUSE (1989) *MOUSE User's Guide and Documentation.* Gentofte, Denmark: Mouse Service Centre.
Muskat, M. (1937) *The Flow of Homogeneous Fluids Through Porous Media.* New York: McGraw Hill.
Mutchler, C.K. & Young, R.A. (1975) Soil detachment by raindrops. In *Present and Prospective Technology for Predicting Sediment Yields and Sources*, pp. 113–17. Agricultural Research Service Publication ARS-S-40. Washington, DC: United States Department of Agriculture.
Myres, W.R.C. & Brennan, E. (1990) Flow resistance in compound channels. *Journal of Hydraulic Research (International Association for Hydraulic Research)* **28**, 141–156.
Nash, J.E. (1960) A unit hydrograph study with particular reference to British catchments. *Proceedings of the Institution of Civil Engineers* **17**, 249–82.

NCE (1990) Inflated ideas. *New Civil Engineer* **913**, 34–38.
Neill, C.R. (1973) *Guide to Bridge Hydraulics*. University of Toronto Press for Road and Transport Association of Canada.
NERC (1975) *Flood Studies Report*, five volumes. London: Natural Environment Research Council.
NERC (1978) *Flood Studies Supplementary Report No. 6*. London: Natural Environment Research Council.
Newbold, C., Purseglove, J. & Holmes, N. (1983). *Nature Conservation and River Engineering*. Nature Conservancy Council.
Nicholson, H.H. (1942) *The Principles of Field Drainage*. Cambridge University Press.
NWC (1981) *Design and Analysis of Urban Storm Drainage. The Wallingford Procedure*, five volumes. London: Department of the Environment and National Water Council.
Oldenkamp, A. (1988) *De maandelijkse waterbalans van een woonwijk en een parkeerterrein in Lelystad (1968–1984)*. Lelystad: IJsselmeerpolders Development Authority.
Palmer, R.S. (1964) *The Influence of a Thin Water Layer on Waterdrop Impact Forces*, pp. 141–48. International Association of Scientific Hydrology, Publication No. 65.
Parker, D.J., Green, C.H. & Thomson, P.M. (1988) *Urban Flood Relief Benefits*. Enfield: Flood Hazard Research Centre, Middlesex Polytechnic.
Pathak, P., Miranda, S.M. & El-Swaify, S.A. (1985) Improved rainfed farming for semi-arid tropics—implications for soil and water conservation. In S.A. El-Swaify, W.C. Moldenhauer & A. Lo (Eds.) *Soil Erosion and Conservation*, pp. 338–54. Ankeny, IA: Soil Conservation Society of America.
Patrick Powers, J. (1981) *Construction Dewatering, a Guide to Theory and Practice*. Chichester: Wiley.
Pender, G. (1985) *The Numerical Modelling of Tide and Flood Movement in Two-dimensional Space using Implicit Finite-difference Methods*. Strathclyde University, PhD Thesis.
Penning-Rowsell, E.C. & Chatterton, J.B. (1977) *The Benefits of Flood Alleviation: A Manual of Assessment Techniques*. Farnborough: Saxon House.
Philip, J.R. (1957) The theory of infiltration: 4. Sorptivity and algebraic infiltration equations. *Soil Science* **84**, 257–64.
Pidgeon, J.D. & Soane, B.D. (1978) Soil structure and strength relations following tillage, zero tillage and wheel traffic in Scotland. In W.W. Emerson, R.D. Bond & A.R. Dexter (Eds.) *Modification of Soil Structure*, pp. 371–78. Chichester: Wiley.
Pilgrim, D.H. (Ed.) (1987) *Australian Rainfall and Runoff, a Guide to Flood Estimation*. Barton, ACT: The Institution of Engineers of Australia.
Pitt, R. (1985) *Characterizing and Controlling Urban Runoff Through Street and Sewage Cleaning*. Report 600/2-85/038. US Environmental Protection Agency.
Polubarinova-Kochina, P.Ya. (1962) *Theory of Groundwater Movement* (J.M. Roger de Weist, Trans.). Princeton University Press.
Price, M. (1985) *Introducing Groundwater*. London: Allen & Unwin.
Price, R.K. (1978) *FLOUT—a River Catchment Flood Model*. Report No. IT 168, 2nd impression. Wallingford: Hydraulics Research Station.
Price, R.K. (1980) *FLOUT—a River Catchment Flood Model*. Report No. IT 168 revised. Wallingford: Hydraulics Research Ltd.
Price, R.K. & Slade, J.E. (1982) *A Model for the Design Analysis and Operation of Pumped Drainage*. Wallingford: Hydraulics Research Ltd.
Purseglove, J. (1989) *Taming the Flood: A History and Natural History of Rivers and Wetlands*. Oxford University Press with Channel 4 Television Company.
Ree, W.O. (1949) Hydraulic characteristics of vegetation for vegetated waterways. *Agricultural Engineering* **30**, 184–87, 189.
Richards, L.A. (1931) Capillary conduction of liquids through porous mediums. *Physics* **1**, 318–33.
Rickson, R.J. (1990) The role of simulated vegetation in soil erosion control. In J. Thornes (Ed.) *Vegetation and Geomorphology*, pp. 99–112. Chichester: Wiley.
Rickson, R.J. & Morgan, R.P.C. (1988) Approaches to modelling the effects of vegetation on soil erosion by water. In R.P.C. Morgan & R.J. Rickson (Eds.) *Erosion Assessment and Modelling*, pp. 237–54. Soil Technology Series 1. Brussels: Commission of the European Communities.

Rivet, A.L.F. (1964) *Town and Country in Roman Britain.* London: Hutchinson.
Roache, P.J. (1972) *Computational Fluid Dynamics.* Albuquerque, NM: Hermosa.
Rodier, J.A. & Roche, M. (1984) *World Catalogue of Maximum Observed Floods.* Publication No. 143. Wallingford: International Association of Scientific Hydrology.
Roesner, L.A., Aldrich, J.A. & Dickinson, R.E. (1988). *Storm Water Management Model User's Manual, Version 4: Addendum I, EXTRAN.* EPA/600/3-84/001b (NTIS PB88-236658/AS). Athens, GA: Environmental Protection Agency.
Royal Commission (1865–68) *Royal Commission on River Pollution. 1st Commission, 1865–68.*
Royster, D.L. (1979) Some observations on the use of horizontal drains in the correction and prevention of landslides. *Bulletin of the Association of Engineering Geologists* **16**, 301–52.
Russam, K. (1969) *The Hydraulic Efficiency and Spacing of Road Gullies.* Laboratory Report No. 277. Crowthorne, Berkshire: Transport and Road Research Laboratory.
Rycroft, D.W. & Thorburn, A.A. (1974) Water stability tests on clay soils in relation to mole drainage. *Soil Science* **107**, 306–10.
Samuels, P.G. (1989) The hydraulics of two-stage channels; review of current knowledge. *Institution of Water and Environmental Management, Conference on River Engineering.* Loughborough University of Technology.
dos Santos Jùnior, A.G. & Youngs, E.G. (1969) A study of the specific yield in land-drainage situations. *Journal of Hydrology* **8**, 59–81.
van Schilfgaarde, J. (Ed.) (1974) *Drainage for Agriculture.* Monograph No. 17. Madison, WI: American Society of Agronomy.
Schilling, W. *et al.* (1987) *Real Time Control of Urban Drainage Systems: the State-of-the Art.* Report of the IAWPRC/IAHR Taskgroup on RTCUDS.
Schwab, G.O., Frevert, R.K., Edminster, T.W. & Barnes, K.K. (1981) *Soil and Water Conservation Engineering.* New York: Wiley.
Sellars, W.D. (1965) *Physical Climatology.* University of Chicago Press.
Sellin, R.H.J. & Giles, A. (1988) *Two Stage Channel Flow.* University of Bristol, Department of Civil Engineering.
Sellin R.H.J. & Searle, D.J. (1987) Modelling channel roughness caused by flood plain vegetation. *Proceedings of the XXII Congress of the International Association for Hydraulic Research, Lausanne.*
Severn–Trent Water (1988) *Water Quality 1987/88.* Birmingham: Severn–Trent Water Authority.
Sevruk, B. & Geiger, H. (1981) *Selection of Distribution Types for Extremes of Precipitation.* Operational Hydrology Report No. 15, WMO-no. 560. Geneve.
Sharpe, D.E. & Kirkbride, T.W. (1959) Storm water overflows, the operation and design of a stilling pond. *Proceedings of the Institution of Civil Engineers* **13**, 445–66.
Shaw, E.M. (1988) *Hydrology in Practice*, 2nd Edn. London: Van Nostrand Reinhold.
Shen, H.W., Schneider, V.R. & Karaki, S.S. (1966) *Mechanics of Local Scour.* Report No. CER66HWS22. Colorado State University.
Shen, H.W., Schneider, V.R. & Karaki, S. (1969) Local scour around bridge piers. *Journal of the Hydraulics Division, Proceedings of the American Society of Civil Engineers* **95** (HY6), 1919–1940.
Shuttleworth, W.J. (1979) *Evaporation.* Report No. 56. Wallingford: Institute of Hydrology, Natural Environment Research Council.
Simpson, B., Blower, T., Craig, R.N. & Wilkinson, W.B. (1989) *The Engineering Implications of Rising Groundwater Levels in the Deep Aquifer Beneath London.* Special Publication No. 69. London: Construction Industry Research and Information Association.
Simpson, R.W. & Thorpe, G.R. (1982) Use of a generalised computer program for resource systems optimisation in developing countries. In *Exeter Symposium*, pp. 285–98. Publication No. 135. Wallingford: International Association of Scientific Hydrology.
Singleton, J.A. & Guppy, A.W. (1972) *Starting a Pump.* Bedford: NEI Allen Ltd.
Slade, J.E. (1985) *Simulation of the Operation of Pumped Drainage Systems in Low Lying Catchments.* Wallingford: Hydraulics Research Ltd.
Smedema, L.K. & Rycroft, D.W. (1983) *Land Drainage: Planning and Design of Agricultural Drainage Systems.* London: Batsford.
Smith, K.A. & Mullins, C.E. (Eds.) (1991) *Soil Analysis: Physical Methods.* New York: Marcel Dekker.

Snyder, F.F. (1938) Synthetic unitgraphs. *Transactions of the American Geophysical Union* **19**(1), 447–54.

Somerville, S.H. (1986) *Control of Ground Water for Temporary Works.* Report No. 113. London: Construction Industry Research and Information Association.

Sprague, M.A. & Triplett, G.B. (1986) *No Tillage and Surface Tillage Agriculture.* New York: Wiley.

Stein, C.J. & Rouve, G. (1988) 2D-LDV-Technique for measuring flow in a meandering channel with wetted flood plains, a new application and first results. *Proceedings of the International Conference on Fluvial Hydraulics, Budapest.*

Stein, C.J. & Rouve, G. (1989) 2D Depth averaged numerical predictions of the flow in a meandering channel with compound cross section. *Hydrosoft Journal* **2**.

Sumner, G.N. (1988) *Precipitation, Process and Analysis.* Chichester: Wiley.

Sutcliffe, J.V. (1978) *Methods of Flood Estimation, a Guide to the Flood Studies Report.* Report No. 49. Wallingford: Institute of Hydrology.

Symons, I.F. (1976) *Assessment and Control of Stability for Road Embankments Constructed on Soft Subsoils.* Laboratory Report No. 711. Crowthorne, Berkshire: Transport and Road Research Laboratory.

Tatham, E. (1989) *The Causes and Control of Tramline Erosion.* Cranfield Institute of Technology (Silsoe College) MSc Thesis.

Tebbutt, T.H.Y. (1971, 1987) *Principles of Water Quality Control.* Oxford: Pergamon.

Terry, J.B. (undated) *Pumps for Land Drainage and Irrigation.* Bedford: NEI Allen Ltd.

Theis, C.V. (1935) The lowering of the piezometric surface and the rate and discharge of a well using ground-water storage. *Transactions of the American Geophysical Union* **16**, 519–24.

Thompson, D.M. & Shuttler, R.M. (1976) *Design of Riprap Slope Protection against Wind Waves.* Report No. 61. London: Construction Industry Research and Information Association.

Thompson, G. & Rippin, K.G. (1985) Rural flood plain management. In *Proceedings of the Second International Conference on Floods and Flood Control.* British Hydrodynamics Research Association.

Toebes, G.H. & Sooky, A.A. (1967) Hydraulics of meandering rivers with flood plains. *Publications of the American Society of Civil Engineers, Journal of Waterways and Harbours Division* **93**, 213–226.

Torri, D. & Sfalanga M. (1984) Some problems of soil erosion modelling. In A. Giorgini & F. Zingales (Eds.) *Agricultural Non-point Source Pollution: Model Selection and Application,* pp. 161–72. Amsterdam: Elsevier.

Tóth, J. (1963) A theoretical analysis of groundwater flow in small drainage basins. *Journal of Geophysical Research* **68**, 4795–812.

Towner, G.D. (1989) The application of classical physics transport theory to water movement in soil: Development and deficiencies. *Journal of Soil Science* **40**, 251–60.

Triplett Jr, G.B. & Van Doren, D.M. (1977) Agriculture without tillage. *Scientific American* **236**(1), 28–33.

US Army Corps of Engineers (1956) *Hydraulic Capacity of Meandering Channels in Straight Floodways.* Waterways Experiment Station, Vicksburg, MS. Technical memo (2-429).

Van Dam, C.H. & Schotkamp, J. (1983). *Infiltratie in Bestrating* (Infiltration in Pavement). RIJP-report 1983-38 Abw. Lelystad: IJsselmeerpolders Development Authority.

Van de Ven, F.H.M. (1985) From rainfall to sewer inflow: a process with consequences. In J.C. Hooghart (Ed.) *Water in Urban Areas: Proceedings of Technical Meeting 42.* Proceedings and Information/TNO Committee on Hydrological Research No. 33. The Hague.

Van de Ven, F.M.H. (1988) Urban hydrological cycle. In *Hydrological Processes and Water Management in Urban Areas: Urban Water 88: Invited Lectures.* Koblenz: IHP/OHP Sekretariat, Bundesanstalt für Gewasserkunde.

Van de Ven, F.H.M. (1989*a*) *Van Neerslag tot Rioolinloop in Vlak Gebied* (From Rainfall to Sewer Inflow in Flatlands). Van Zee tot Land 57. Lelystad: Rijkswaterstaat, Directie Flevoland.

Van de Ven, F.H.M. (1989*b*). *Van Neerslag tot Rioolinloop in Vlak Gebied* (From Rainfall to Sewer Inflow in Flat Areas). Delft University of Technology PhD Thesis.

Van den Berg, J.A. (1978) *Quick and Slow Response to Rainfall by an Urban Area.* RIJP-report 1978-1. Lelystad: IJsselmeerpolder Development Authority.

Vardy, A.E. (1976) On the use of the method of characteristics for the solution of unsteady flow in networks. In *Proceedings of the Second International Conference on Pressure Surges.* Cranfield: British Hydrodynamics Research Association.

Varnes, D.J. (1958) Landslide types and processes. In E.B. Eckel (Ed.) *Landslides and Engineering Practice*. Special Publication No. 29; NAS-NRC Publication No. 544. Washington, DC: Highway Research Board.

Verruijt, A. (1970) *Theory of Groundwater Flow*. London: Macmillan.

Wakelin, M.J., Walker, T.G. & Wilson, D. (1987) Lincoln flood alleviation scheme. *Proceedings of the Institution of Civil Engineers, Part 1 Design and Construction* **82**, 755–76.

Wark, J.B., Samuels, P.G. & Ervine, D.A. (1990) A practical method of estimating velocity and discharge in compound channels. *Proceedings of the International Conference on River Flood Hydraulics, Wallingford, UK*, pp. 163–172.

Watkins, L.H. (1962) *The Design of Urban Sewer Systems. Research into the Relation Between the Rate of Rainfall and the Rate of Flow in Sewers*. Road Research Technical Paper No. 55. HMSO.

Weltman, A.J. & Head, J.M. (1983) *Site Investigation Manual*. Special Publication No. 25. London: Construction Industry Research and Information Association.

Whiffin, A.C. & Young, C.P. (1973) *Drainage of Level or Nearly Level Roads*. Laboratory Report No. 602. Crowthorne, Berkshire: Transport and Road Research Laboratory.

White, J.B. (1987) *Wastewater Engineering*. London: Edward Arnold.

White, R.E. (1987) *Introduction to the Principles and Practice of Soil Science*. Oxford: Blackwell Scientific Publications.

White, W.R. *et al.* (1989) River structures. In T.W. Brandon (Ed.) *River Engineering*. Part 2. *Structures and Coastal Defence Works*, pp. 87–156. Water Practice Manual Book 8. London: Institution of Water and Environmental Management.

Wild, A. (Ed.) (1988) *Russell's Soil Conditions and Plant Growth*, 11th Edn. Harlow: Longman.

Willetts, P.J. & Hardwick, R. (1990) *Proceedings of the International Conference on River Flood Hydraulics, Wallingford, UK*, pp. 197–205.

Wilson, E.M. (1983) *Engineering Hydrology*. London: Macmillan.

Wischmeier, W.H. & Smith, D.D. (1978) *Predicting Rainfall Erosion Losses*. Agricultural Research Service Handbook No. 537. Washington, DC: United States Department of Agriculture.

Wormleaton, P.R. & Merrett, D. (1990) Discharge calculation methods in compound channels. *Journal of Hydraulic Research (International Association for Hydraulic Research)* **28**, 157–174.

Wylie, E.B. (1980) Inaccuracies in the characteristics method. In *Computer and Physical Modelling in Hydraulic Engineering*, pp. 165–76. New York: American Society of Civil Engineers.

Yevjevich, V. (1984) Extremes in hydrology. In T. de Oliveira (Ed.) *Statistical Extremes and Applications*. Dordrecht: Reidel.

Youngs, E.G. (1965) Horizontal seepage through unconfined aquifers with hydraulic conductivity varying with depth. *Journal of Hydrology* **3**, 283–96.

Youngs, E.G. (1980) The analysis of groundwater seepage in heterogeneous aquifers. *Hydrological Sciences Bulletin* **25**, 155–65.

Youngs, E.G. (1982) Calculation of ponded water drainage for flow regions of various geometries to demonstrate effect of disturbed soil-zone shape on drain performance. *Journal of Agricultural Engineering Research* **27**, 441–54.

Youngs, E.G. (1983) The contribution of physics to land drainage. *Journal of Soil Science* **34**, 1–21.

Youngs, E.G. (1984) Developments in the physics of land drainage. *Journal of Agricultural Engineering Research* **29**, 167–75.

Youngs, E.G. (1985) A simple drainage equation for predicting water-table drawdowns. *Journal of Agricultural Engineering Research* **31**, 321–28.

Youngs, E.G. (1986a) Water-table heights and discharge rates with artesian flow to interceptor drains. *Journal of Hydrology* **86**, 255–66.

Youngs, E.G. (1986b) Water-table heights in drained anisotropic soils. *Agricultural Water Management* **11**, 1–11.

Youngs, E.G. (1988) Soil physics and hydrology. *Journal of Hydrology* **100**, 411–31.

Youngs, E.G. (1990) An examination of computed steady-state water-table heights in unconfined aquifers: Dupuit–Forchheimer estimates and exact analytical results. *Journal of Hydrology*, **119**, 201–214.

Youngs, E.G. & Leeds-Harrison, P.B. (1990) Aspects of transport processes in aggregated soils. *Journal of Soil Science* **41**, 665–675.

Youngs, E.G., Leeds-Harrison, P.B. & Chapman, J.M. (1989) Modelling water-table movement in flat low-lying lands. *Hydrological Processes* **3**, 301–15.

Zanchi, C. (1989) Drainage as a soil conservation and soil stabilizing practice on hilly slopes.

In U. Schwertmann, R.J. Rickson, & K. Auerswald (Eds.) *Soil Erosion Protection Measures in Europe*, pp. 73–82. Soil Technology Series 1. Brussels: Commission of the European Communities.

Zaruba, Q. & Mencl. V. (1969) *Landslides and their Control*. New York: Elsevier.

Zienkiewicz, O.C. (1971) *The Finite Element Method in Engineering Science*. London: McGraw Hill.

Index

MIX
Papier aus verantwortungsvollen Quellen
Paper from responsible sources
FSC® C105338

If you have any concerns about our products,
you can contact us on
ProductSafety@springernature.com

In case Publisher is established outside the EU,
the EU authorized representative is:
Springer Nature Customer Service Center GmbH
Europaplatz 3, 69115 Heidelberg, Germany

Printed by Libri Plureos GmbH
in Hamburg, Germany